# THE
# BREATHING
# CURE

# THE
# BREATHING
# CURE

## DEVELOP NEW HABITS FOR
## A HEALTHIER, HAPPIER, AND LONGER LIFE

## PATRICK McKEOWN

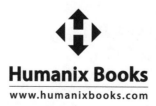

**Humanix Books**
www.humanixbooks.com

Humanix Books

The Breathing Cure
Copyright © 2021 by Patrick McKeown
All rights reserved

Humanix Books, P.O. Box 20989, West Palm Beach, FL 33416, USA
www.humanixbooks.com | info@humanixbooks.com

**Disclaimer:** The information presented in this book is not specific medical advice for any individual and should not substitute medical advice from a health professional. If you have (or think you may have) a medical problem, speak to your doctor or a health professional immediately about your risk and possible treatments. Do not engage in any care or treatment without consulting a medical professional.

Humanix Books is a division of Humanix Publishing, LLC. Its trademark, consisting of the words "Humanix Books," is registered in the Patent and Trademark Office and in other countries.

ISBN  9-781-63006-197-5  (Hardcover)
ISBN  9-781-63006-198-2  (E-book)

Illustrations by Bex Burgess

Printed in the United States of America
10 9 8 7 6 5 4 3 2 1

"A new scientific truth does not triumph by convincing its opponents and making them see the light, but rather because its opponents eventually die and a new generation grows up that is familiar with it."

MAX KARL ERNST LUDWIG PLANCK

"From my own experience I know that, used correctly, the breath can be truly transformative. My goal is therefore to enable you to take responsibility for your own health, to prevent and significantly reduce a number of common ailments, to help you achieve your goals, and to offer simple, scientifically based ways to change your breathing habits for life."

PATRICK MCKEOWN

# CONTENTS

Foreword . . . . . . . . . . . . . . . . . . . . . . . . . . . . . . . . . . . . . . . . . . ix

Introduction: **Are You Breathing Comfortably?** . . . . . . . . . . . . . . . . . 1

Chapter One: **A New Approach**. . . . . . . . . . . . . . . . . . . . . . . . . . . . 9

Chapter Two: **Exercises for Adults and Children** . . . . . . . . . . . . . 27

    Section One: Functional Breathing . . . . . . . . . . . . . . . . . . . . . 28

    Section Two: Exercises to Stop Symptoms of Asthma,
        Anxiety, Stress, Racing Mind, and Panic Disorder . . . . . . . 55

    Section Three: Tailored Breathing Programs for Specific
        Conditions. . . . . . . . . . . . . . . . . . . . . . . . . . . . . . . . . . 65

    Section Four: Exercises to Improve Focus and Concentration . . . 83

    Section Five: Stress and Relax Body and Mind . . . . . . . . . . . 88

    Section Six: Exercises for Children . . . . . . . . . . . . . . . . . . . . 105

Chapter Three: **How to Breathe** . . . . . . . . . . . . . . . . . . . . . . . . .113

Chapter Four: **The Vagus Nerve and the Heart-Breath-Brain
Connection** . . . . . . . . . . . . . . . . . . . . . . . . . . . . . . . . . . . . . 131

Chapter Five: **Functional Breathing, The Secret of Functional
Movement**. . . . . . . . . . . . . . . . . . . . . . . . . . . . . . . . . . . . . . 163

Chapter Six: **When Breathing Makes You Hurt**. . . . . . . . . . . . . . 185

Chapter Seven: **Sleep-Disordered Breathing** . . . . . . . . . . . . . . . 201

Chapter Eight: **Developing Healthy Airways in Children** . . . . . . . 227

Chapter Nine: **The Breathing Secret for Healthy Blood Pressure** . . . . 255

Chapter Ten: **Freedom From Respiratory Discomfort** . . . . . . . . . . 267

Chapter Eleven: **Sex and Breath, an Intimate Connection**. . . . . . . . 289

Chapter Twelve: **Yes, Breathing Is Different for Women** . . . . . . . . . 323

Chapter Thirteen: **Female Sex Hormones and the Breath** . . . . . . . . 345

Chapter Fourteen: **Sugar, Sugar** . . . . . . . . . . . . . . . . . . . . . . 369

Chapter Fifteen: **Seizure Control and the Breath** . . . . . . . . . . . . . 387

Chapter Sixteen: **Join The Breathing Revolution** . . . . . . . . . . . . . 421

Chapter Seventeen: **Is Nasal Breathing Your First Line
    of Defense Against Coronavirus?** . . . . . . . . . . . . . . . . . . 425

Resources . . . . . . . . . . . . . . . . . . . . . . . . . . . . . . . . . . . . 431

Acknowledgments . . . . . . . . . . . . . . . . . . . . . . . . . . . . . . . 433

# FOREWORD

I'm not sure what first sparked my interest in breathing; whether it was surfing—being held underwater without air—or if I was led to explore my day-to-day breathing practice as part of my journey to maximize my efficiency as a human and become as high performing as I can be. Either way, my quest for correct breathing led me to Patrick McKeown and his clinical work with over 8,000 people, ranging from medical patients to elite athletes. I appreciate the value of "feeling" things and learning through experiencing, but Patrick's scientific explanation of what is happening in the body when I nasal breathe as opposed to mouth breathing truly helped me understand how to use my breath as a tool to support my health and boost my performance.

Patrick's passion for breathing education comes out of his own personal experience. Even though he himself was an extremely dysfunctional breather and an asthmatic—he was told by his doctors that he would be on medication and limited in activities for the rest of his life—he cured himself through breathing practices.

I must admit, I was surprised to learn what a large percentage of us are living with hidden breathing dysfunctions that wreak havoc on our health, sleep, and performance. I truly appreciate that Patrick's teaching empowers people to be proactive in supporting their own good health. Patrick simply explains the importance of nasal breathing and balancing respiratory gases to create better health and mitigate illness, chronic disease, and injuries.

*The Oxygen Advantage* was a game-changing read and is one of the top books we recommend at XPT, not only for health and fitness professionals but for any individual looking to optimize the most important processes in their body.

If breathing and the breath is the essence of life, and it is meant to be intuitive, then how do we find our way back to the basics? Patrick makes this a comprehensive journey that anyone can use and share with their friends and family.

*Laird Hamilton, XPT Extreme Performance Training*™

# INTRODUCTION
## ARE YOU BREATHING COMFORTABLY?

---

I magine a breathing technique that can increase uptake and delivery of oxygen to cells, improve blood circulation, and even unblock the nose. Perhaps it can help open the airways of the lungs, enhance blood flow and oxygen delivery to the brain, improve sleep, and bring calmness to the mind. It might even restore bodily functions disturbed by stress, build greater resilience, and help you live longer. You might think this description sounds far-fetched. But it isn't.

This book will guide you through techniques that are the keys to healthy breathing and healthy living. My goal is to enable you to take responsibility for your own health, to prevent and significantly reduce a number of common ailments, to help you realize your potential, and to offer simple, scientifically based ways to change your breathing habits. On a day-to-day basis, you will experience an increase in energy, better concentration, an enhanced ability to deal with stress, and a better quality of life.

Following on from my work *The Oxygen Advantage*, I'll explore breathing from three dimensions—biochemical, biomechanical, and cadence—with exercises and science to support functional movement of muscles and joints, improve debilitating conditions such as diabetes, epilepsy, lower back pain, PMS, and high blood pressure, and help you enjoy deeper sleep and better sex. The exercises designed to up-regulate and down-regulate the nervous system highlight how powerfully the breath can influence states of the body. Finally, there is a section on the importance of optimal breathing for childhood development. I am not exaggerating when I say that no child will reach their full genetic potential unless nasal breathing and functional breathing are restored.

We enter the world with a breath, and the process of breathing continues automatically for the rest of our lives. Although breathing is an involuntary action and we don't usually give it much thought, the way we breathe has an enormous impact on our health. Because breathing is an innate bodily function that most of us take for granted, it only gets our attention when

1

something goes wrong. However, minute-by-minute, breath fulfills its vital role, providing the body with oxygen, regulating physical mechanisms in the lungs, heart, and blood vessels, and even moderating the stress response.

When breathing is below par, it creates problems throughout the systems of the body. Researchers have listed up to 30 common symptoms and conditions in which poor breathing patterns are a factor.[1, 2] However, because many sufferers breathe normally at least some of the time, it can be hard to know if your breathing patterns are unhealthy.[3]

The rule of thumb I give my students is this: Breathing during rest and light movement such as walking or yoga should be imperceptible, never noticeable. Healthy breathing during rest should be through the nose, driven by the diaphragm. It should be regular, quiet, slow, and almost undetectable. Unhealthy or dysfunctional breathing involves breathing through the mouth, using the upper chest, or breath that is irregular or audible during rest.

There are many forms of dysfunctional breathing, or breathing pattern disorders, at varying levels of severity. The most common is chronic hyperventilation, which involves breathing too fast and taking in too much air. Signs of breathing pattern disorders include the inability to take a satisfying breath, excessive breathlessness during rest or physical exercise, frequent yawning or sighing, and the feeling of just not getting enough air. Other dysfunctions significantly affected by poor breathing patterns include asthma, hay fever, snoring, sleep apnea, and associated psychological conditions like anxiety, insomnia, and panic disorder. Across the board, poor breathing is implicated in poor physical and mental health.

If you were to observe and monitor a random group of people as they sit together in a room, you'd soon start to notice differences in their breathing. Some people breathe through their nose, while others breathe through their mouth. Some will have gentle, slow, quiet breathing, while others will be taking faster, larger, more audible breaths. Some people sigh habitually every few minutes. Others breathe in a nice regular pattern. Some use their diaphragm to breathe abdominally, while others breathe from the upper chest.

Since breathing is a natural process and so vital to life, why do we all breathe so differently?

The answer is that breathing habits are greatly influenced by lifestyle, environment, and genetic predisposition. Everyday habits that may come from choice or necessity (such as sedentary deskwork, watching TV, eating processed foods, and excessive talking) or from psychological conditions (such as stress and anxiety) or hormonal changes that occur during the female monthy cycle can result in persistent faulty breathing, along with all its negative consequences. To get a better sense of this, think of a person who has developed a habit of eating too much. In times of stress, this person may turn to emotional eating, using food as a crutch to help them relax. If they continue to eat this way for weeks or months, their body will soon adapt to habitual overeating and begin to demand more food than they need. In the same way, our breathing patterns can change over time, becoming unhealthy. These unhealthy breathing patterns can form in childhood and even fundamentally alter the way our airways function.

Three fundamental factors have an impact on the way breathing functions:

1. **Biochemical.** The exchange and metabolism of oxygen ($O_2$) and carbon dioxide ($CO_2$).
2. **Biomechanical.** The physical aspects of breathing; the functioning of the respiratory muscles, including the intercostal muscles (which run between the ribs and help form and move the chest wall) and diaphragm (the major breathing muscle, located below the lungs).
3. **Psychological.** The mental and emotional aspects, which may manifest as stress caused by poor breathing or poor breathing caused by stress.

These factors are at the root of breathing pattern disorders, and this is what we'll explore and address in this book.

While the three causes of breathing pattern disorders are biochemical, biomechanical, and psychological, the solutions fall into three parallel categories:

1. **Biochemical.** Addressing blood sensitivity to $CO_2$.
2. **Biomechanical.** Breathing from the diaphragm.
3. **Cadence.** Reducing the respiratory rate to between 4.5 and 6.5 breaths per minute in order to influence the autonomic functioning of the body.

The breathing method I will share in this book forms a straightforward, unique series of exercises that you can easily apply, both during rest and physical exercise. This is no ordinary breathing technique. I would like to introduce you to the Oxygen Advantage®.

## WHAT IS THE OXYGEN ADVANTAGE?

The Oxygen Advantage is a program of simple exercises designed to retrain your breathing. The focus is on light, slow, deep breathing (LSD), which targets the biochemistry and biomechanics of the body and taps into the autonomic nervous system (ANS).

All too often, emphasis is placed only on the biomechanics of breathing—the way it functions muscularly and mechanically. The student is encouraged to take big, full breaths, drawing air deep into the lungs. In the process, the diaphragm is engaged, but the biochemistry is neglected. Taking too big a breath causes blood vessels to narrow, actually reducing oxygen delivery to the cells. In practicing breathing exercises, the biomechanical and biochemical functions and the respiratory rate are inextricably linked—and need to be considered together. Think of the three dimensions of the breath as a three-legged stool. If one leg is missing, the stool will fall over!

Throughout this book, you will find everything you need to understand how breathing impacts your health. Included are 26 breathing exercises, all with different purposes—from breathing retraining to stopping a panic attack, preparing for a presentation or competition to improving sleep, exposing the body to good stress to countering bad stress. Don't worry. You won't need to learn them all. Instead, choose one or two exercises, work with them, and then return to learn more. You will learn how to measure your BOLT (Body Oxygen Level Test) score to assess the health of your breathing, and you will be able to choose the program most suitable for you.

The BOLT is a simple test designed to provide feedback on how well you are breathing. The test involves exhaling normally through the nose, pinching the nose to hold the breath, and timing how long in seconds it takes to reach the first definite physical desire to breathe in. The goal is to reach a BOLT score of 40 seconds. A score of less than 25 seconds strongly suggests a breathing pattern disorder. The BOLT, which will be explained in more detail later, is interchangeable with the three dimensions of breathing as a measure of progress.

As your BOLT score improves, you are likely to find yourself breathing at a slower rate and engaging the diaphragm. I'll share breathing exercises that focus on:

1. Using air hunger to improve biochemistry
2. Using lateral expansion of the lower two ribs to improve biomechanics
3. Achieving the optimal respiratory rate, as understood by scientific study

You can achieve a higher BOLT score by breathing only through the nose and practicing the exercises in this book. I always tell my clients that they will continue to experience asthma, nasal congestion, fatigue, anxiety, and panic attacks until their BOLT score, taken first thing in the morning, is at least 25 seconds. If you have a low BOLT score, changing your breathing patterns can be utterly transformative.

One of the most rewarding things about working with students, even from a distance, is seeing the difference that healthy breathing can make to their lives. I'm lucky that I can experience this in person through coaching, and I can also reach people through the books, videos, and podcasts that I've produced or been involved with. For example, recently, I had an email from Ariella, thanking me for writing my book *The Oxygen Advantage*. Ariella subscribed to my online newsletter and had experienced such good results from practicing the breathing exercises in it that she bought a copy of the book. She said, "Your teachings—in just a few days—have already been life-changing."

Ariella lives with a complex set of rare and chronic conditions that challenge all of her organs. These include dysautonomia (dysfunction of the autonomic nervous system), Ehlers-Danlos Syndrome Hypermobility Type (a connective tissue disorder that impacts the strength and function of connective tissue), and mast cell activation disease (an immune cell disease that causes her body to respond to anything and everything with an allergic reaction). She has struggled with breathing for most of her life, but while her doctors always agreed she didn't have asthma, she was never able to find out why breathing was so difficult. This was complicated by the fact that each of her underlying conditions is known to affect breathing.

Until Ariella found *The Oxygen Advantage*, she struggled tremendously on a daily basis. She was often breathless and constantly felt like she was fighting to get enough air. She had a BOLT score of just eight seconds. This discomfort with breathing often prevented her from sleeping, and once she did get to sleep, her sleep quality was poor. She frequently lost her voice in association with her breathing challenges and often couldn't go outside because her allergy symptoms immediately became worse. Despite consulting with ear, nose, and throat (ENT) doctors, pulmonologists, immunologists, and more, none of her specialists could identify the cause of her breathing problems or help her resolve the issue.

Ariella recalled an incident about a year before she wrote to me, which illustrates just how unwell she was:

> One day, after pushing myself to have a brief conversation through my lost voice and painful breathing, my heart rate spiked, my blood pressure dropped, and I felt like I truly could not get air into my lungs. This episode went on for at least twenty minutes. I texted my husband, who came home to find me crying on the floor, completely exhausted, still trying to gain my breath.

That was Ariella's worst day, but similar experiences had become normal for her.

By the time she wrote to me, although Ariella's underlying conditions were still quite severe, she no longer struggled to breathe on a daily basis. She explained, "Learning how to efficiently and effectively breathe and learning exercises that can help to bring me back to a place of calm breathing has been life changing for me." Ariella still manages symptoms including fatigue, brain fog, and thirst, but improving her breathing has vastly reduced these symptoms. While allergens such as pollen, dust, and mold have always been huge problems for her because of her mast cell disease, those symptoms have improved too. She began taping her mouth at night to ensure nasal breathing while she slept and said: "I feel a noticeable difference when I wake up after sleeping with my mouth closed (the paper tape is so helpful!). When I sleep with my mouth closed, I have more energy, less fatigue, less thirst, and my lips are less chapped."

She also believes that the breathing exercises are beneficial in her struggle with dysautonomia, specifically in stabilizing her low blood pressure.

Simply by integrating the breathing techniques into her daily routine, Ariella not only breathes more comfortably, her fatigue and the functioning of her autonomic nervous system have improved. She describes the breathing work as "incredibly simple, profound, and fundamental to health and wellness." She has been excited to share her discoveries with her healthcare providers and other people suffering with chronic disease—just as I am excited to share them with you.

# CHAPTER ONE
# A NEW APPROACH

## PATRICK'S STORY

In 1998, my life changed forever when I discovered how the poor breathing habits I had developed in early childhood were affecting my body and my quality of life. I was constantly tired, suffering from sleep disorders and respiratory problems, and taking ever-increasing quantities of medication to try to control my asthma. Then I stumbled across the work of the Russian doctor Konstantin Buteyko, and after I made a few changes to my breathing, my symptoms dramatically improved in just a few short weeks. I learned firsthand how effective breathing reeducation can be. Over the past 18 years, after becoming accredited by Doctor Buteyko to teach his method and working to develop my own program of training, I have witnessed life-changing improvements to the health of thousands of women, men, and children.

My story starts when I was a boy, growing up in the small village of Dunboyne on the east coast of Ireland. From a young age, I suffered from asthma, a persistent wheezing and tightness of the chest. My nose was always blocked, so I got into the habit of breathing through my mouth, causing me to snore at night. Sometimes, I even held my breath during my sleep, a potentially dangerous condition known as obstructive sleep apnea. From the age of 14 until my early twenties, I felt constantly exhausted, with little energy to apply in school or university.

In 1994, I had an operation on my nose to relieve 15 years of nasal issues. However, I received no postsurgery advice on the benefits of breathing through my nose or how I might make the change. And so I continued to experience the same problems I'd had before the procedure, including moderate to severe asthma, sleep-disordered breathing, breathlessness, poor concentration, and high stress levels. My dysfunctional breathing patterns were agitating my mind, resulting in excessive overthinking, tension, and fatigue. Despite the countless hours I spent studying, my grades remained just about average. As my conditions became worse, my asthma medications were increased to the point of hospitalization. By my twenties, I was desperate for help.

As chance would have it, my solution was right around the corner. In 1998, I happened to read an article in an Irish newspaper about the work of Doctor Buteyko. At the time, his discovery (later known as the Buteyko method) was relatively new to the Western world. I tried an exercise meant to decongest my nose just by holding my breath. I was so amazed that this simple method worked that I switched to nasal breathing full time. I also worked to slow my breathing to help normalize the volume of air I was taking into my lungs. Within a day or two of paying just a little more attention to how I was breathing, my energy improved, the tension in my head eased, and for the first time in my life, my breathing was easier. During that first week, I experienced what it was like to have a good night's sleep and wake up feeling energized. For the first time in years, I didn't have to drag myself out of bed in the morning and spend hours trying to come round.

The huge improvements to my health, energy, and well-being that I felt in such a short time compelled me to learn more about the method, change my career, and train to teach the Buteyko method to others. In 2002, I received accreditation from Dr. Konstantin Buteyko. Since then, my life has changed for the better in countless ways.

I am now 48 years old. My well-being, focus, and quality of life are immeasurably superior to those of my 16-year-old self. I have brought about massive positive changes in my life simply by learning how to reverse the poor breathing habits I had developed unwittingly in earlier years. Now I hope to share the same information with you.

## A NEW APPROACH

The practice of breath control for health and spiritual progression has been around for millennia in Eastern cultures. For instance, the yogic practice of *Pranayama* is an ancient method of exercising the breath, primarily to vary its speed. It involves things like alternate nostril breathing, abdominal breathing, forceful breathing, and chanting. However, even among yoga practitioners, it is considered, in some of its manifestations, to be an advanced technique.

The methods in this book, which do have a few things in common with yogic breathing, are backed up by decades of scientific research that will help you understand why they work and how to use them. These methods are immediately accessible, take a short time to learn, incorporate easily into your daily routine, whatever your current level of fitness, and will provide you with the tools to continue improving your health for the rest of your life.

## THE TWO PILLARS

The Oxygen Advantage consists of two pillars of breathing—functional breathing pattern training, designed to improve day-to-day breathing, and powerful breath-hold exercises that simulate high-altitude training.

# FUNCTIONAL BREATHING PATTERN TRAINING

Functional breathing helps improve your quality of focus, concentration, posture, and sleep; support the spine; reduce anxiety; and take the hard work out of breathing. It can help you move better, with less risk of injury in sports and day-to-day tasks such as lifting and carrying your child. It can also reduce the onset and duration of breathlessness and exercise-induced asthma (bronchoconstriction). Physiologically, it results in long-term improvements to blood circulation, dilation of the upper airways (nose) and lungs, and oxygen delivery to the cells, optimizing important connections between the respiratory system, heart, and blood pressure.

What we're talking about here is retraining functional breathing habits for daily life. You may have learned breathing exercises in a yoga class, with a personal trainer, or on YouTube. You may have experienced good results, then promptly forgotten about your breathing the minute you stepped outside the studio or gym. Sometimes, we aren't given the context to carry on those exercises as part of a daily routine. In this book, we'll look at that context— how your breathing affects your health and how to use that knowledge to feel better. Every day.

## BREATH-HOLD EXERCISES

High altitude training involves lower air oxygen levels. This causes bodily adaptations to provide a natural advantage when exercising at lower altitudes. By using breath-hold exercises, it is possible to replicate the lower pressure of oxygen while residing at sea level.

Training in this way can produce better aerobic and anaerobic capacity in most athletes. It can allow the body to stimulate anaerobic glycolysis (the process by which blood sugar is broken down to form energy-giving lactate) without risk of injury. It improves the strength of the breathing muscles and tolerance to breathlessness, and it reduces the ventilatory response to hypercapnia and hypoxia (hypercapnia is when $CO_2$ is too high, hypoxia is low blood oxygen). It gives increased $VO_2$ max (the threshold of the body's ability to transport and use oxygen during physical activity) and produces better running economy, better repeated sprint ability for team sports, and better-sustained fitness during rest or injury.

By re-creating the low oxygen pressures coherent with altitude training, it may also be possible to improve disease resistance and general health. In a study that began in 1965 and ran until 1972, scientists examined the effects of high altitude on common diseases in 20,000 soldiers stationed at altitudes of between 3,692 and 5,538 meters. The men had limited access to basic personal hygiene such as baths and changes of underwear, and researchers anticipated that a prolonged stay at high altitudes would result in poor mental and physical health and reduced performance.[1]

Contrary to these expectations, it was found that a two to three years' stay at high altitudes was associated with a statistically significant lower incidence of many physical illnesses, including respiratory infections, high blood pressure, diabetes, asthma, and skin diseases. The number of psychiatric disorders was more than halved at high altitude, despite the monotony of the men's surroundings and their anxiety around isolation from family members.[1]

## UNDERSTANDING THE PROBLEM: SUBOPTIMAL BREATHING

Since breathing is such an intrinsic function, it can be hard to recognize that we could do it better, unless there's an obvious issue that causes regular discomfort. Even then, we might not realize that the problem could be addressed simply by improving our breathing patterns. To grasp the importance of breath training, we need to understand what the problem is.

A breathing pattern disorder, or dysfunctional breathing, is a condition in which breathing is problematic and produces symptoms such as breathlessness. It manifests as a psychologically or physiologically based habit, such as breathing too deeply, breathing too fast (both symptoms of hyperventilation), upper chest breathing during rest, or breathing irregularly with frequent breath holding or sighing.[2] Breathing pattern disorders affect 9.5% of the studied adult population,[2] rising to 29% among people with asthma and 75% of those with anxiety.[3, 4] These figures are not surprising, given that asthma, anxiety, panic attacks, and stress all negatively influence breathing patterns, feeding back to create a vicious cycle of inefficient breathing.

Chronic hyperventilation, the tendency to breathe too much air, is the most common and extensively studied trait in breathing pattern disorders.[5] One typical characteristic is fast breathing, often through an open mouth. This can occur both during waking and sleeping. Other signs include using the upper chest to breathe and having noticeable breathing patterns. Biochemically, it simply means breathing more air than the body needs, causing blood $CO_2$ levels to drop.[6] Although the term *chronic hyperventilation* is often used synonymously with dysfunctional breathing, it is just one type of breathing pattern disorder.

In fact, dysfunctional breathing is not a problem confined to the respiratory system. It has a significant impact on overall health. For example, excessive breathing is closely linked to cardiovascular disease. A research study of a Minneapolis intensive coronary unit found that of 153 heart attack victims, 100% breathed predominantly using their upper chest, 75% were chronic mouth-breathers, and 70% demonstrated open-mouthed breathing during sleep.[7]

Looking at the wider impact on health, a 1998 study reported that patients with just 14 common symptoms were responsible for almost half of all primary healthcare visits in the United States. Of those complaints, which include abdominal pain, chest pain, headache, and back pain, only 10% to 15% were found to be the result of organic illness.[8] At the same time, every one of those ailments can be made worse by disordered breathing. Put simply, the quality of breathing has significant implications for health and longevity.

A comprehensive list of the symptoms and signs of hyperventilation can be found in the book *Behavioral and Psychological Approaches to Breathing Pattern Disorders* by Beverly Timmons and Robert Ley.[9] The following list of symptoms was provided by Dr. L. C. Lum, an Emeritus of the Department of Chest at Papworth and Addenbrooke's Hospitals, Cambridge, United Kingdom in personal communications in 1991. Faulty breathing can affect any organ or system producing symptoms that include:

- **General:** fatigue, poor concentration, poor performance, impaired memory, weakness, disturbed sleep, allergies
- **Respiratory (breathing):** breathlessness after exertion, tight chest, frequent sighing, yawning and sniffing, irritable cough, inability to take a satisfying breath
- **Cardiovascular (the heart and blood vessels):** irregular or fast heart beats and palpitations, Raynaud's Syndrome, chest pain, cold hands and feet
- **Muscles:** muscle pain, cramping, twitching, weakness, stiffness and tetany (muscles that spasm and seize up)
- **Gastrointestinal (the digestion):** heartburn, acid regurgitation or hiatus hernia, flatulence or belching, bloating, difficulty swallowing or feeling of a lump in the throat, abdominal discomfort
- **Neurological (the nervous system):** dizziness, headaches and migraines, paresthesia (tingling or numbness, pins and needles) of the hands, feet, or face, hot flashes
- **Psychological:** anxiety, tension, depersonalization, panic attacks, phobias

L. C. Lum, 1991

Dysfunctional breathing can exist alongside other conditions. For example, patients with chronic obstructive pulmonary disease (COPD) may have coexisting breathing disorders. The exercise-induced breathlessness that people with conditions such as COPD and asthma experience is not always caused by their disease. More often than not, poor breathing patterns also contribute.

## CAUSES OF UNHEALTHY BREATHING PATTERNS

Remember, three main factors are at play in the development of breathing pattern disorders:

1. Biochemical
2. Biomechanical
3. Psychological[10]

While the underlying causes of problem breathing can vary, environmental factors, lifestyle habits, and genetic predisposition are common triggers. Often, these disorders are simply the result of a lack of awareness and a lifelong habit of breathing through an open mouth.

## BIOCHEMICAL TRIGGERS

The biochemical aspect of dysfunctional breathing, which has to do with the balance of oxygen and $CO_2$, is often triggered or exacerbated by a common misunderstanding about deep breathing that, paradoxically, sets off the imbalance. Stress counselors, gym instructors, sports coaches, yoga teachers, Pilates coaches, physiotherapists, and media personalities encourage their clients to "take a deep breath" to bring more oxygen into the body. However, a *deep* breath is often confused with a *big* breath. A *deep* breath is the sort of breath a baby takes naturally, a gentle, quiet inhalation into the belly, using the diaphragm. In contrast, a *big* breath is often taken in loudly through the mouth and generally involves upper chest movement. This results in overbreathing, setting off a biochemical imbalance in $CO_2$ and oxygen levels.

A sedentary lifestyle can also have a huge impact on the way the body processes oxygen. When we move our muscles, we generate $CO_2$, an important gas that helps maintain proper oxygenation of the body. A lack of exercise results in lower production of $CO_2$, and this may contribute to overbreathing. This is essentially a modern affliction. Fifty years ago, people spent an estimated four hours each day doing some sort of physical exercise. Today, as sedentary work has become more common,[11] fewer than 5% of adults manage even half an hour of daily exercise.[12] That means that many people are likely to have biochemically unbalanced breathing patterns.

Even the simple act of talking can cause overbreathing. When we speak, it is normal for both respiratory rate and breathing volume to increase. If we speak at length, we overbreathe. People who work in jobs like retail, telesales, and teaching where they are required to talk all day will know all too well how tired and drained they can feel after work. In addition to its biochemical impact, excessive talking can leave you with a dry throat and a faster heart rate.

## BIOMECHANICAL TRIGGERS

Dysfunctional breathing is often associated with poor coordination of the diaphragm, abdominal muscles, and muscles of the rib cage.[13] This is closely related to posture. The most important breathing muscle is the diaphragm. This thin sheet of muscle is located at the bottom of the ribs, separating the chest from the abdomen. As each breath is drawn into the lungs during rest, the diaphragm moves downward about one or two centimeters. If you regularly slump over your desk at work, you can't breathe effectively, because there simply isn't enough space for the diaphragm to move freely.

Effective diaphragm breathing helps maintain stability of the spine. This means that posture is closely linked to functional breathing patterns. If you breathe well, you will move well. Faulty breathing can result in lower back pain. Conversely, pain in the lower back and neck can affect the way the breathing muscles work, and tension in these areas often results in upper chest breathing by default.[14] If your movement is impaired, either through injury, illness, or lifestyle, your breathing will suffer. Outside of such chronic conditions, poor posture is the major factor in biomechanical breathing dysfunction. Quite simply, if your breathing is abnormal, your movement will be abnormal, and vice versa.

## PSYCHOLOGICAL TRIGGERS

Research has shown that symptoms associated with breathing pattern disorders are strongly influenced by anxiety and other emotional states.[6] In some cases, the psychological influences actually cause the physical symptoms. Some of us may be genetically predisposed to breathe badly. People prone to anxiety, asthma, or panic disorders have a higher risk of dysfunctional breathing because a negative feedback loop develops between the feelings of breathlessness and panic. Deterioration in breathing patterns can trigger the stress response, producing feelings of fear, or worsening anxiety and asthma symptoms. Personality traits such as perfectionism and obsessiveness can also affect breathing patterns.

Stress is a common trigger with serious long-term implications. When the fight-or-flight response is activated, our breathing increases to prepare us for physical activity, just as it did to enable our ancestors to escape a threat. However, in modern society, we rarely have the opportunity to perform the physical exercise necessary to burn off the extra adrenaline. If you have a big work deadline or a nerve-racking call looming, it would be considered inappropriate to address it by sprinting around the office. What's more, the type of stress we experience today is more likely to be chronic, whereas stress for our ancestors was typically short term and immediate.

## THE BIOCHEMICAL ASPECT OF BREATHING

The biochemistry of breathing involves the exchange and metabolism of gases, including the consumption of oxygen and the production of $CO_2$. As the author of one 2017 review into the biochemistry of yoga breathing exercises explains, "We are taught in our medical schools that oxygen is good and carbon dioxide is bad," but the fact is that a certain level of $CO_2$ in the blood is always required for maintaining good health. Most important, "$CO_2$ determines bioavailability of oxygen to the tissues and cells." Oxygen is the prime nutrient required by every cell in the body. Without $CO_2$, the tissues would become starved of oxygen, even when oxygen is available in the blood. In other words, $CO_2$ is not always a waste gas.[15]

### $CO_2$: NOT JUST A WASTE GAS

The reputation of $CO_2$ has been historically rather mixed. The ancient Greeks and Romans used it as a therapeutic aid, by way of the bubbling waters in their natural thermal baths. These baths contained high levels of $CO_2$ in the form of carbonic acid. The Greek physician, Hippocrates, writing in the fourth century BCE, recommended these thermal spas for headaches, gout, asthma, and the healing of wounds.

In the sixteenth century, baths came back into fashion and remained popular for several hundred years. The waters in certain locations were believed to hold a secret life-giving ingredient that we now know to be carbonic acid ($H_2CO_3$). The more $H_2CO_3$ the water contained, the more revitalizing it was considered to be. According to the *History of Industrial Gases*, during a 20-minute $CO_2$ bath, the body absorbs around 6 liters of the gas.[16] Dissolved in water, $CO_2$ causes the skin to tingle as the surface blood vessels dilate. You can get an idea of how this feels by taking a drink of carbonated water. In addition, the baths also release mineral salts.

By the 1800s, the thermal baths in what is now the French town of Royat, attracted thousands of visitors seeking relief from obesity, anxiety, asthma, eczema, and other conditions. In a personal email to me, in July of 2020, James Nestor, author of the best-selling book, *Breath*, explained:

> After a brief soak in the thermal water, bathers would see their skin become rosy and flushed . . . [Those] with asthma reported a sudden clearness in their breathing. Overweight guests would see flab in their stomach or legs began to tighten and disappear.

Even today, in countries such as eastern Hungary, people travel to use the mofettas—dry spas that harness $CO_2$-rich volcanic gas discharge to help with problems from heart and circulatory diseases to gynecological and skin issues, stress relief, and exhaustion. Treatment involves sitting in the healing gas, inhaling it under the supervision of specialist therapists.[17]

Mofetta is an Italian word, listed by the *Oxford Dictionary* as an archaic term for a fumarole—an opening in the earth's crust that emits steam and gases.[18] These volcanic vents are common in areas of France, Romania, and Italy and can be found in the Death Gulch in Yellowstone Park. Mofetta as a treatment for injuries is first mentioned in the work of the sixteenth century Swiss physician and alchemist, Paracelsus.

By the 1930s, physicians in Royat had begun administering $CO_2$ directly to the lungs. Nestor explains that, "this was found to heal respiratory and skin conditions twice as fast as bathing."

Around this time, $CO_2$ therapy made its way across the Atlantic to the United States. Harvard Medical School, and Boston City Hospital ran several innovative studies with the gas, exploring its clinical applications for physical and mental conditions. Disorders of the brain were thought to be caused by low circulation and constricted blood vessels. Trials of $CO_2$ therapy in epilepsy patients found that, after only a few treatments, onset of seizures was reduced. The Yale physiologist, Yandell Henderson, found that a mixture of oxygen and 5% $CO_2$ could generate astonishing results[19] in patients with asthma, stroke, pneumonia, heart attack, asphyxia in newborn babies,[20] and other respiratory disorders, due to the rapid tissue oxygenation it produced. In large quantities, $CO_2$ is also a powerful anesthetic.[21]

The therapy increased its pace during the 1940s and 50s, and much more research was done into its benefits. It was incredibly cheap and easy to administer—a fact that perhaps contributed to its demise. The gas became so popular that circus sideshows would feature public demonstrations of the narcotic effects achieved with high concentrations of $CO_2$ and a campaign began to declare the gas dangerous. Dr. Ralph M. Waters, an Ohio doctor known for professionalizing the practice of anesthesia,[22] made claims about $CO_2$ that included warnings it was a "toxic waste product, like urine."[23] Either he confused potentially dangerous 30% $CO_2$ therapies with highly effective 5% $CO_2$ therapies, was concerned about unregulated treatments, or was motivated by private interest—the treatments Waters specialized in were both expert and expensive.

However, Waters' claims were not without basis. $CO_2$, if administered incorrectly, could kill. One example given was the case of the daughter of famous chemist, James Watt, inventor of the Watt steam engine. Jessie Watt died from tuberculosis after numerous hours of exposure to $CO_2$ therapy. However, according to her physician Thomas Beddoes, who successfully treated many other patients, she was already "too far gone" when she started the treatment. Her father went on to design, with Beddoes, many of the apparatuses and techniques needed to administer various gases to patients.

Whatever Waters's intention, he succeeded in damning the medical use of $CO_2$. The therapy was forced underground, and its purpose became distorted by false claims, lawsuits, and selective scientific studies. A century's worth of medical research showing that $CO_2$ has clinical applications for many conditions was almost entirely forgotten.

In 1904, the Danish biochemist Christian Bohr discovered that $CO_2$ facilitates the release of oxygen to the cells. Oxygen is carried around the body in the hemoglobin in red blood cells. Bohr discovered that $CO_2$ acts as the catalyst for hemoglobin to release its load of oxygen for use by the body. When levels of $CO_2$ in the blood are low, the bond between $O_2$ and hemoglobin increases. This means the body cannot access the oxygen in the blood and it leads to poor body oxygenation.

In 2017, a doctor at Subharti Medical College in India, wrote a detailed review of the benefits of $CO_2$. The paper's author, Dr. Singh, is a yoga practitioner and has dedicated much time to researching how yoga works.[15] Dr. Singh discovered that $CO_2$ stimulates the vagus nerve, an important cranial nerve that you'll read about in Chapter Four. He discovered that increased levels of $CO_2$ in the blood could activate the vagus nerve and slow the heartrate.[15] He describes $CO_2$ as a "natural sedative." It soothes the irritability of the brain's conscious centers, promoting our ability to use logic, reason, and common sense. Without $CO_2$, we can become anxious, depressed, and angry. [15]

$CO_2$ also controls aspects of the homeostasis of blood. You'll read more about homeostasis in Chapter Four, but here it concerns the regulation of blood gases and acidity of the blood to keep everything working within healthy parameters. Singh explains that if $CO_2$ is so good for us, we should work to increase the level of the gas in our bodies. When you practice a breath hold, $CO_2$ gradually builds up in the blood. With practice, you can reduce your sensitivity to $CO_2$, allowing you to tolerate greater concentrations of the gas in your blood to, as Dr. Singh puts it, "supercharge your overall health." Contrary to the alarming claims made by Dr. Waters, Singh cites research that shows increasing $CO_2$ within safe limits in the blood does not cause any harmful effects.[24] He goes so far as to say that "carbon dioxide is truly the breath of life."

## BIOCHEMISTRY OF BREATHING RESTORED

Modern science suggests that the body's sensitivity to $CO_2$ plays a significant role in dysfunctional breathing. When breathing receptors (called chemo-receptors) are overly sensitive to $CO_2$, breathing patterns are more strongly affected as the concentrations of blood $CO_2$ rise and fall. This high "ventilatory response" to blood gas makes breathing harder to control. People who are highly sensitive to $CO_2$ tend to breathe faster than normal, often from the upper chest.

Conversely, people who have developed a higher threshold of tolerance and are less sensitive to $CO_2$ generally breathe in a calm, healthy way. Breathing remains relatively light both during rest and sleep and during more intense and longer periods of exercise. A lower sensitivity to $CO_2$ is beneficial both for sporting performance and for general well-being. In fact, studies have shown that this is one thing that separates outstanding endurance performers from the crowd.[25]

During strenuous physical exercise, the body's consumption of oxygen increases. This slightly reduces the concentration of oxygen in the blood. At the same time, the increased muscle activity and metabolic rate produces more $CO_2$. Normally, as $CO_2$ increases, the respiratory rate accelerates proportionately. This ensures that enough $CO_2$ is exhaled to keep levels of the gas more or less regular in the blood.

A study published in the journal *Medicine & Science in Sports & Exercise* in 1979 concluded that the light breathing typical among endurance athletes might explain the link between low chemoreceptor sensitivity to $CO_2$ and exceptional performanc.[26] In 2007, a trial undertaken by the French biologist and physical education specialist Xavier Woorons showed that lower respiratory rates in trained men at both sea level and high altitudes (where atmospheric oxygen is lower) were linked to reduced blood sensitivity to $CO_2$.[27] Endurance athletes typically have lower ventilatory responses to changes in blood oxygen and $CO_2$ than nonathletes.[28] However, this study put into question the widely held belief that the impulse to breathe (and therefore the feeling of breathlessness) might only be lowered by intense physical training.[25]

Ultimately, the intensity of training required to achieve this result by exercise alone is unrealistic for most people. To address this challenge in an alternative, practical way, the easy techniques offered in this book are designed to reduce the body's ventilatory response to $CO_2$ buildup. As a person increases their BOLT score, their sensitivity to $CO_2$ lessens.

Another important biochemical benefit is offered by nasal breathing as it is taught in this book. Nasal breathing enables the body to make use of nasal nitric oxide (NO), which will be discussed in Chapter Three, and $CO_2$ in the blood. Both chemicals are vasodilators, meaning that they relax blood vessels, causing them to expand. While the importance of $CO_2$ in blood flow and oxygen metabolism has been long understood,[29] the role of nasal nitric oxide in dilating blood vessels in the lungs has only recently been realized.

## BIOMECHANICS OF HEALTHY BREATHING

The movement of air in and out of the airways is achieved by cyclic changes in the volume of the lungs. As the diaphragm and chest wall moves, pressure within the chest varies, causing the inhalation and exhalation of air. Ideally, when we take a deep breath, we should engage the diaphragm to draw the air deep into our lungs. However, if we take in a big gasp of air through the mouth, the air tends to get no farther than the upper chest. It is really only possible to achieve effective long-term diaphragm breathing through the nose.

As well as being central to breathing, the diaphragm plays an important role in controlling posture. During an inhalation, the diaphragm moves downward. As it descends, a positive pressure is generated in the abdomen, which contributes to posture control and stability. The pressure acts like an inflating balloon, supporting the front of the spine and the pelvis.[30] Conversely, good posture improves breathing.

Breathing from the diaphragm accomplishes several important things. It will:

- Slow respiration
- Calm the mind
- Draw air deep into the lungs
- Improve gas exchange
- Support functional breathing for functional movement
- Generate intra-abdominal pressure (IAP) for control of posture and spinal stability

## THE PSYCHOLOGY OF BREATHING

In our modern world, it may not seem possible to live in a stress-free environment, but simply by breathing correctly, the worries and pressures of daily life can become manageable. Scientists have studied contemplative breathing practices, the connections between breath and the fight-or-flight reaction, the ways that breathing affects cognition, and even how types of social interaction interact with the respiratory system to affect our mental and physical well-being. We'll look at these in detail later. Suffice it to say, the breath has a significant impact on our mental state, just as our mental state can have a positive or negative effect on our ability to breathe well.

## TOWARD A SOLUTION FOR DYSFUNCTIONAL BREATHING

The causes of breathing pattern disorders fall into the three categories we have just explored: biochemical, biomechanical, and psychological. In training, I offer solutions for dysfunctional breathing by working on the biochemistry, biomechanics, and cadence of breathing. Cadence refers to the practice of reducing the respiratory rate to between 4.6 and 6 breaths per minute.

### THE CADENCE OF BREATHING

The term "cadence breathing" is often used in sports like running to describe a method of controlled breathing where the athlete coordinates the breath with physical movement. For example, a runner might breathe out with the heel-strike of the dominant foot. This is not what I mean by cadence breathing. I use "cadence" to refer to the practice of controlling the respiratory rate, specifically by slowing down breathing so that inspirations and expirations occur at a rate of 6 breaths per minute (bpm).

Exercises designed to slow breathing on a long-term basis can reduce breathlessness and improve performance during intensive physical training.[31] It also benefits overall physical and mental health. Countless studies have demonstrated that reducing the cadence of the breath to 6 bpm optimizes oxygenation, stimulates blood pressure receptors, reduces dead space in the lungs, curbs the onset of inflammation, increases heart rate variability, and builds vagal tone (we'll look at those last two in Chapter Four).

Dead space is the volume of a breath that is inhaled but does not participate in gas exchange. At the end of each inhalation, the space in the upper and lower airways fills with air. This space includes the nasal cavity, throat, and trachea or windpipe. Around 150 milliliters of this inhaled air leaves the body unchanged, having failed to reach the alveoli, the small air sacs in the lungs where gas exchange takes place. Slowing the respiratory rate reduces the air lost to dead space, and provides more time for more oxygen to diffuse from the lungs into the blood.

Let's do the math:

- **Tidal volume ($V_T$).** The normal volume of air entering the lungs during one inhalation while at rest
- **Respiratory rate (RR).** The number of breaths per minute (bpm)
- **Minute ventilation (MV).** The volume of air that enters the lungs during one minute (respiratory rate multiplied by tidal volume) **RR x $V_T$ = MV**[32]

The following calculations clearly show what happens when the respiratory rate is reduced from 12 breaths per minute to 6 breaths per minute. The first calculation uses a tidal volume of 500 milliliters per inspiration, which represents the average for a healthy young adult at rest.[33] The second uses a tidal volume of 1,000 milliliters, representing the doubled breathing volume when the breath is slowed by half. Both scenarios use the equation $RR \times V_T = MV$ to calculate the volume of air breathed in through the nose. To calculate the air that reaches the alveoli, the 150 milliliters of dead space is taken into account.

### Breathing at 12 breaths per minute:
Air entering the nose: 12 bpm × 500 mL = 6 liters
Air reaching the alveoli: 12 bpm × (500 mL – 150 mL) = 4.2 liters

### Breathing at 6 breaths per minute:
Air entering the nose: 6 bpm × 1000ml = 6 liters
Air reaching the alveoli: 6 bpm × (1,000 mL – 150 mL) = 5.1 liters

At 12 breaths per minute, the volume of air that reaches the alveoli is 4.2 liters. At 6 breaths per minute, it increases to 5.1 liters. This represents a 20% increase in breathing efficiency.

These figures are backed up by research, which has confirmed that the increase in blood oxygenation in slow breathing is due to a proportionately greater volume of air reaching the alveoli instead of remaining in dead space.[34] This has implications for sports, climbing altitude, endurance, and performance. It also has applications for respiratory disorders and heart disease.

According to a 2008 paper, respiratory rate is a crucial "vital sign" when it comes to identifying serious illness.[35] Vital signs are the measurements that doctors monitor at least once a day in patients on acute wards. Those include pulse rate, temperature, blood pressure, and respiratory rate. Unfortunately, multicenter reviews have found that documentation in many hospitals is poor.

Respiratory rate is often not recorded, even in cases where the patient's primary illness is a respiratory condition. This is despite the fact that fast breathing has been shown to predict heart attack and admission to intensive care.[35]

Crucially, research shows that a respiratory rate of more than 27 bpm is the most important predictor of heart attack in hospital wards, and that in medically unstable patients, fluctuations in the speed of breathing are much greater than changes in systolic blood pressure or heart rate. This has led to the conclusion that respiratory rate could provide a more accurate measure of at-risk patients than other vital signs. A 2005 study reported that 21% of ward patients who breathed at between 25 and 29 bpm died in hospital.[36] Another paper from 2007 showed that just over half of the patients on general wards who suffered cardiac arrest or needed to be admitted to intensive care had a respiratory rate of more than 24 bpm.[35] In 95% of cases, these people could have been identified as high risk as many as 24 hours before they became seriously unwell.

As we will discover throughout this book, while most of us will not fall into these high-risk categories, there are huge benefits to be gained from slowing down the breath.

## IS YOUR BREATHING "HEALTHY" BREATHING?

Considering the importance of breathing and its role in regulating and delivering oxygen to every single cell in the body, it's surprising to find that few people understand the basic rules. The common advice to "take a deep breath" inevitably results in more air in the lungs but less oxygen reaching vital systems. So why are the benefits of light, undetectable breathing so little known? First, while it is difficult to know the exact reason, the Western human pschye typically leans towards the idea that louder and bigger is better. Second, the practice of taking noticeable, full breaths as often espoused in yoga—a technique that contradicts the original intention of yoga masters—may have contributed to the wrongly held idea that bigger is better in terms of the breath.

There are two possible ways to usefully measure the breath. The first is to count the number of breaths per minute. The second is to determine the size of each breath. The normal breathing rate for a grown adult at rest can be anywhere between 9 and 16 breaths per minute,[37] but most people take 10 to 12 breaths, inhaling around half a liter (500 milliliters) of air per breath. Therefore, the average air volume is around 6 liters per minute.

If you want to determine if you are overbreathing, you won't find the answer just by counting the number of breaths you take per minute. You must also take the size of each breath into account. When I look at a person's breathing, I observe them from the moment they walk into the room, checking whether they breathe through their nose or mouth, observing the size of each breath, noting whether breathing movements are from the upper chest or from the abdomen, estimating the number of breaths per minute, and seeing if there is a natural pause between breaths. Healthy people breathe gently, quietly, calmly, and effortlessly with a natural pause on the exhalation. Each breath is taken in and out through the nose, even during light physical exercise such as walking. There should be no feeling of breathlessness during rest. If you are breathing in a healthy manner, you should not even be aware of your breath.

Observing your own breathing habits is a worthwhile exercise. Find a quiet place to sit calmly for a few minutes, and follow the movements of your breathing:

- Are you breathing through your nose or mouth?
- Is your breathing abdominal or from the upper chest?
- How big is the "wave" of each breath?
- As soon as you breathe out, do you need to breathe back in immediately, or is there a natural pause between your breaths?
- Is it easy for you to see the movements of your breathing?

If your breathing is noticeable and requires effort during rest, it is likely your breathing has room to improve.

Throughout the rest of this book, I will help you look at your everyday breathing habits and help you understand how your breathing patterns influence the way you breathe during sleep, rest, exercise, and even sex. As you practice each exercise, you will learn how it will impact the biochemistry, biomechanics, or cadence of your breath. You will discover how light, slow, deep (LSD) breathing improves all three dimensions of functional breathing, separately and simultaneously. Ultimately, nasal breathing will provide the foundation for you to achieve healthy breathing patterns, gain control over your autonomic nervous system, and build a better relationship with your diaphragm.

# CHAPTER TWO
# EXERCISES FOR ADULTS AND CHILDREN

---

I n this chapter, you will find all the breathing exercises you need to develop a personalized program suitable for your own needs and level of fitness. Beginning with your BOLT score, these exercises are categorized so you can easily identify what you can and should practice, depending on your specific health condition and goals.

The second part of this book contains detailed explorations of the science of breathing as it pertains to various health conditions and some case studies describing how real people just like you have benefited from these exercises. However, if you are anything like me, you will want to get into it right away and maybe read up on the research later, which is why I decided to get to the point and begin the book with the exercises. Also, since we each begin life with a breath, it seems fitting to start the process of introducing you to the Oxygen Advantage by addressing the practical matter of breathing.

The following exercises can be powerful. If you are pregnant and in your first trimester, please do not practice any of the breathing exercises. In your second trimester, you can practice gentle nose breathing and slow, low breathing with relaxation. If you have any serious medical condition(s), please get the all-clear from your medical doctor before practicing the exercises in this book. Do not practice any exercises involving holding of the breath to create a strong air hunger.

I hope you find this new experience with the breath inspiring, and I urge you to commit to daily practice of the exercises. For a little effort, I know you will experience significant rewards in health, fitness, and mental well-being.

## SECTION ONE: **FUNCTIONAL BREATHING**

### THE BOLT

Before we begin, it's time to test your breathing. I use a measurement called the BOLT, or Body Oxygen Level Test. It's a simple exercise that serves as a useful way to appraise breathing patterns. You can use it as you work through the exercises in this book, and indeed for the rest of your life, to understand where you are now and track your progress.

When we are told to hold our breath, the natural instinct from child-hood is to take in a big breath and hold it until we feel ready to burst. This is not what we mean by "breath holding" in this context. Indeed, breath holding tests that focus on the maximum time you can hold an inhalation are unreliable because they can be subject to differences in lung volume and even to personality traits like competitiveness. On the other hand, breath holding *after* exhaling ensures a more consistent lung volume, both for the individual and measured across a group of individuals.

The BOLT involves holding the breath after exhaling until the first invol-untary movements of the breathing muscles or the first definite desire to breathe. Scientists have proven that holding the breath in this way cannot be influenced by training or will power.[1] This means that the reading is less subjective and more accurate.

Your BOLT score provides effective feedback on functional breathing as well as on exercise tolerance, and as such can be a good indicator of fitness. It is also an excellent objective measure of breathlessness.

The BOLT score is influenced by several factors. These include:

- Chemosensitivity to carbon dioxide (CO)
- Bronchoconstriction in the lungs or airways (narrowing of the airways affects breath-hold time)
- Level of discomfort felt in the diaphragm during the breath hold
- Anxiety and other psychological or emotional influences.

Since 1975, scientists have demonstrated that breath-hold time offers a useful index of sensitivity to $CO_2$ due to the relationship between the respi-ratory impulse and the pressure of $CO_2$. When we hold our breath, our lungs are not able to get rid of $CO_2$, and so it accumulates in the blood. The length of time it takes for our brain to react to this increase of blood $CO_2$ is directly related to our body's sensitivity to $CO_2$ (respiratory chemosensitivity). Because $CO_2$ provides the primary stimulus to breathe in, breath holding is a powerful method for inducing the sensation of breathlessness. Research has proven that the breath hold test provides a great deal of information about the onset and duration of dyspnea (shortness of breath).[1] The length of time you are able to voluntarily hold your breath during the BOLT provides an indirect indicator of sensitivity to $CO_2$ buildup in the blood.

In his 2010 book *Exercise Physiology*, the author William D. McArdle claims that for a person with normal breathing patterns, the breath-hold time after exhalation, before the desire to breathe triggers inhalation, is about 40 seconds.[3] However, in my experience, while many athletes who attend the Oxygen Advantage training do eventually achieve a BOLT score of 40 seconds, very few people have a BOLT score of 40 seconds on their first day. The normal score to expect from an athlete is around 20 seconds. People with asthma, childhood asthma, rhinitis, or anxiety and panic disorders often have a BOLT score of just 10 to 15 seconds.

The breath hold time in indivudals with breathing pattern disorders, including chronic hyperventilation, tends to be lower.[4] As the BOLT score increases, respiratory rate decreases, and the natural pause following exhalation increases. When the BOLT score is 40 seconds, the typical respiratory rate is eight to ten breaths per minute. Slowing the respiratory rate of breathing provides numerous benefits, including better breathing efficiency.

## CHECKING YOUR BOLT SCORE

To measure your BOLT score, you will need some sort of timing device that counts in seconds. The stopwatch on your smartphone or tablet is ideal.

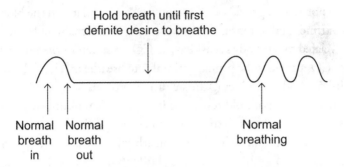

THE BOLT:

- Take a normal, silent breath in through your nose.
- Allow a normal, silent breath out through your nose.
- Hold your nose with your fingers to prevent air from entering your lungs.
- Count the number of seconds until you feel the first distinct desire to breathe in.

A low breath-hold time in seconds indicates a greater tendency toward faster, upper chest breathing with no natural pause between breaths.

Be aware that people with asthma and COPD demonstrate significantly lower breath-hold times than those with normal breathing. This is because breathhold time is related to measures of lung function.

The best way to get an accurate representation of your breathing is to measure your BOLT score in the morning just after waking. When you are fast asleep, breathing continues subconsciously and without interference. For this reason, the morning BOLT score gives a truer measure because it indicates how well you breathe when you can't possibly be thinking about your breathing.

During your first few weeks with the breathing exercises, you should notice an improvement of three to four seconds in your BOLT score each week. After that, progress will continue at a slightly slower pace. Physical exercise can be gradually introduced to increase the BOLT score above 20 seconds.

When the breathing exercises are practiced correctly, your breathing pattern can be retrained. If your very first BOLT score is 10 seconds, it will take at least three weeks to reach a BOLT score of 20 seconds and six months to reach a BOLT score of 40 seconds. Improvement will depend on the severity of your symptoms and on how much attention you bring to reducing your breathing. The more focus you give to your breathing each day, the better.

At the same time, there is no need to become obsessed with your breathing. Allow the changes to gradually occur. The breath cannot be forced into compliance. Many of the exercises involve breathing less air for periods of time during the day. Allow the breath to gradually reduce by paying attention to the airflow entering and leaving the nostrils, slowing it down without tensing up the breathing muscles.

Practice the breathing exercises formally for the first few weeks and then incorporate them into your way of life. Your progress will be reflected in a higher BOLT score. You will also have lighter breathing and begin to feel better.

The BOLT measures the number of seconds you can comfortably hold your breath after an exhalation. You must not try to push beyond the first distinct urges to breathe. This isn't a competitive challenge. Nor is it a measure of willpower. Continually practicing the BOLT will not change the result either. Your BOLT score will only increase when you use the exercises and begin to reduce your breathing volume toward normal.

## THREE DIMENSIONS OF FUNCTIONAL BREATHING TRAINING

Throughout this book you will read about addressing breathing pattern disorders in three ways. Those three approaches encompass the biochemistry, biomechanics, and cadence of the breath. In simple terms, they refer to the relative level of $CO_2$ in the blood, the function of the diaphragm, and the speed at which you breathe. In the following exercises, we'll look at each of those aspects in turn. The focus is on breathing that is *light, slow, and deep*. This is easy to remember if you use the acronym *LSD*.

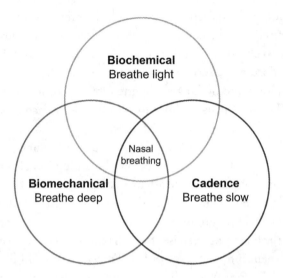

## Breathe light, slow and deep

| Breathe Light (Biochemistry) | Breathe Slow (Cadence) | Breathe Deep (Biomechanics) |
| --- | --- | --- |
| Reduces breathlessness | Stimulates vagus nerve | Enables slow breathing |
| Regulates breathing patterns | Improves alveolar ventilation | Improves lung volume |
| Normalizes ventilation | Stimulates baroreceptors | Increases $O_2$ uptake in blood |
| Enables slow breathing | Improves heart rate variability | Increases ventilation perfusion |
| Reduces negative pressure in upper airways during sleep | Improves respiratory sinus arrhythmia | Improves spinal stabilization |
| Improves blood circulation | Optimizes parasympathetic/ sympathetic balance | Improves functional movement |
| Improves $O_2$ delivery to cells (Bohr effect) | Helps restore functioning of the autonomic nervous system (ANS) | Increases lymphatic drainage |
| Harnesses higher concentration of nitric oxide | Reduces negative pressure in upper airways during sleep | Dilates throat during sleep (reduces risk of sleep apnea) |
| Achieves calmer mind | Achieves calmer mind | Achieves calmer mind |

## BREATHE LIGHT, SLOW, AND DEEP—THE EXERCISES

### #1. Breathe Light (Biochemistry)

This exercise helps normalize breathing biochemistry, resulting in improved oxygen uptake and delivery and reduced sensitivity to $CO_2$, while working toward normalizing breathing volume. It is suitable for everyone, except those with serious health concerns or those in the first trimester of pregnancy.

The *Breathe Light* exercise involves reducing the volume of air you are taking into your body to create a tolerable hunger for air. *Air hunger* is the feeling that you would like to take a slightly bigger breath or that you are not getting quite enough air.

Achieving a slight or tolerable air hunger signifies that $CO_2$ has accumulated in the blood. One of the functions of $CO_2$ is to act as a catalyst for the release of oxygen from the red blood cells. With gentle, light, and soft breathing, the blood vessels open, and more oxygen is released from the red blood cells to feed the tissues and organs.

Breathing *light and slow* also enables nitric oxide to accumulate in the nasal cavity and travel to the lungs where it helps sterilize the air and open the airways and blood vessels in the lungs. This means that better oxygen transfer to the blood can take place.

During this exercise, concentrate on achieving and maintaining a feeling of air hunger. The feeling of air hunger should be on both the inhalation and the exhalation. Don't be overly concerned about breathing using the diaphragm. It doesn't matter at this point. If you are already doing so, then great. If not, that's fine too. Your focus will be on slowing down the breath, quietening the breath, and softening the breath. If the air hunger becomes too much, take a rest for 20 seconds before returning to the exercise.

As you reduce the volume of air you breathe, it is normal to feel a slight tension in your diaphragm breathing muscle. If you find you are experiencing involuntary contractions of the diaphragm, then the need for air is too much. With practice, the goal is to maintain a tolerable air hunger for four to five minutes. If your breathing feels shallow during this exercise, that's okay for the duration of the exercise. Focus on the air hunger not on the biomechanics.

The goal of this exercise is to feel a "hunger" for air, to feel that you would like to take in a slightly bigger breath. After a short while practicing the exercise, $CO_2$ will accumulate in your blood, creating the feeling that you would like to take in more air. This is valuable feedback that you are performing the exercise correctly and reducing your breathing volume toward normal.

The air hunger you feel during this exercise should be tolerable. If you notice that your breathing rhythm is becoming fast or chaotic, the need for air is too much. If this happens, stop the exercise and breathe normally for half a minute, then resume gentle, light breathing to create a tolerable need for air once more.

Don't deliberately interfere with your breathing muscles, hold your breath, or freeze your breathing. Instead, allow your breathing to soften using relaxation—a slow breath in and a gentle slow breath out.

Continue practicing the exercise for around four minutes.

### Breathe Light, Variation One

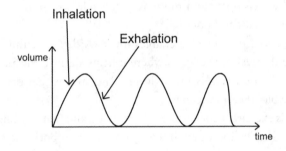

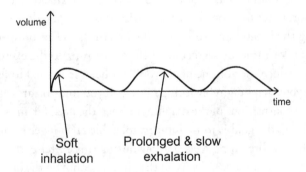

Directions:

- Sit up straight in a chair or cross-legged on the floor or lie down on your back.
- If sitting, imagine a piece of string gently pulling you upward toward the ceiling from the crown of your head.
- Place your hands on your chest and tummy, or in your lap.
- Observe your breath as it enters and leaves your nose. Feel the slightly colder air entering your nose and feel the slightly warmer air leaving your nose.
- Begin to reduce the speed of each breath as it enters and leaves your nose. Breathing should be light, quiet, and calm.
- Slow down your breathing so that you feel hardly any air entering and leaving your nostrils. Your breathing should be so quiet that the fine hairs in the nostrils do not move.
- The goal is to create a feeling that you would like to take in more air. To create air hunger, your breathing now should be "less" than it was when you started.
- If you feel stressed or lose control of your breathing, the air hunger is too strong. When this happens, take a rest for 20 or 30 seconds and start again. It is normal at the beginning to take a rest a few times during the exercise.
- Continue practicing the exercise for around four minutes.

## Breathe Light, Variation Two

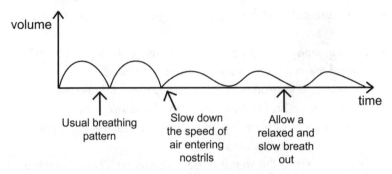

Directions:

- Sit up straight in a chair or cross-legged on the floor or lie down on your back.
- If sitting, imagine a piece of string gently pulling you upward toward the ceiling from the crown of your head.
- Place your finger underneath your nose so you can monitor the airflow from your nose.
- Bring your attention to the airflow on your finger.
- As you feel the warm air on your finger, gently slow down your breathing.
- Take a soft breath in through your nose and allow a gentle and prolonged breath out.
- Breathe so softly that you feel hardly any air blowing onto your finger. Imagine that your finger is a feather and that your breathing is so soft that the feather doesn't even flutter.
- There is no need to hold your breath or try to restrict your breathing. The more warm air you feel, the harder you are breathing. Can you quieten and soften your breathing to the point where you feel hardly any air on your finger?
- You are doing the exercise correctly if you feel a tolerable need for air. I need you to feel like you want to breathe in more air.
- Continue practicing the exercise for around four minutes.

## Breathe Light, Variation Three

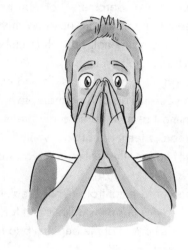

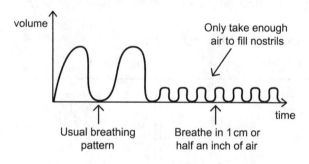

Directions:

- Sit up straight in a chair or cross-legged on the floor or lie down on your back.
- If sitting, imagine a piece of string gently pulling you upward toward the ceiling from the crown of your head.
- Cup your hands against your face. Have hardly any gaps between your fingers. This serves two purposes. First, the hands provide good feedback of your breathing volume. Second, exhaled air

pools in the hands so that you rebreathe a higher concentration of $CO_2$. Use the hands as a "barometer" of your breathing.

- Take a short breath in through your nose. With your hands cupping your face, only breathe half an inch (1 cm) of air into your nose. Then breathe out half an inch.
- Breathe just enough air to fill your nostrils and no more. Take a flicker of air into your nostrils and no more. Exhale calmly through your nose. It is almost as if you are hardly breathing at all.
- The goal is to create a feeling that you would like to take in more air, to feel an air hunger—the feeling that you would like to take in a deeper breath.
- If you feel stressed or lose control of your breathing, the air hunger is too strong. When this happens, take a rest for 20 to 30 seconds and start again. It is normal at the beginning to take a rest a few times during the exercise.
- Continue practicing the exercise for around four minutes.

## #2. Breathe Deep (Biomechanics)

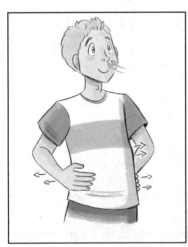 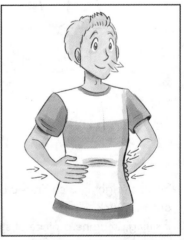

Breathe in, lower ribs move outwards          Breathe out, lower ribs move inwards

This exercise helps practice diaphragmatic breathing, which in turn enables slow breathing, calms the mind, improves oxygenation within the body, and has many positive effects on posture and breathing mechanics in general. The diaphragm is the main breathing muscle and is important for postural control as well as helping foster functional breathing habits.

**The emphasis here is on improving the biomechanics of breathing. Try not to overbreathe.**

Directions:

- Sit up straight in a chair or cross-legged on the floor.
- Imagine a piece of string gently pulling you upward toward the ceiling from the crown of your head.
- Place your hands at either side of your lower ribs.
- Silently breathe in, bringing the air deep into your lungs. As you inhale, feel your ribs expanding outward. As you exhale, feel your ribs moving inward.
- Take fuller breaths but fewer of them. As you breathe in, feel your lower ribs moving outward, and, as you breathe out, feel your lower ribs moving inward.
- There is no need to hear your breathing during this exercise.
- Continue practicing the exercise for approximately four minutes.
- During the inhalation, as the diaphragm moves downward, expansion is generated to the front, sides, and back of the trunk. Your diaphragm is producing intra-abdominal pressure, which causes the ribs to move outward.

### #3. Breathe Slow (Cadence)

This exercise involves changing the cadence (speed) of your breathing to six breaths per minute.

As we will see later in the book, this kind of reduced breathing has many benefits, including improved breathing efficiency and oxygenation, reduced chemosensitivity to $CO_2$, better vagal tone, and a higher BOLT score.

As your BOLT score increases, your respiratory rate will decrease and the natural pause following exhalation will increase. When breathing is slower, a larger volume of air per breath is delivered to the alveoli (the small air sacs in the lungs where gas exchange takes place). This is because less volume of air per minute is lost to "dead space." (There's an equation that illustrates this in Chapter One if you want to understand it better.)

*Breathe Slow* may be a helpful exercise for you if you have a strong fear of suffocation, because the increase in $CO_2$ during this technique is better tolerated by the body. This can actually help regulate your fear response. *Breathe Slow* also helps maintain the balance between the parasympathetic and sympathetic nervous systems, improving both mental and physical resilience.

**The emphasis here is on achieving a respiratory rate of six breaths per minute. Biomechanics is incorporated through lateral expansion and contraction of the lower ribs. There is no need to deliberately breathe harder to breathe deep. As respiratory rate reduces, the size of each breath will increase. This is normal. However, try not to allow the size of each breath to increase disproportionately. This is a common mistake.**

By breathing light and slow with focused attention on breathing slow, the goal is to feel the slightest hunger for air. This signifies that you are not overbreathing during the exercise.

If your BOLT score is less than 15 seconds, slowing the breathing rate to 6 breaths per minute may be challenging. In this situation, begin by slowing down the breathing to 10 breaths per minute by breathing in "light and slow" for 3 seconds, and out "light and slow" for 3 seconds. As your BOLT score improves, reduce the breathing rate to 6 breaths per minute as described in the following exercise.

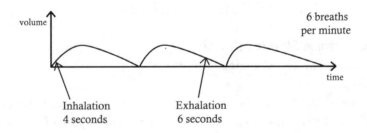

Directions:

To reach a cadence of approximately six breaths per minute, this exercise encourages you to reduce your breathing so that each inhale measures four seconds and each exhale measures six seconds:

- Sit up straight on a chair or cross-legged on the floor. Place your hands on either side of your abdomen, on your lower two ribs.
- As you breathe in, feel your ribs moving outward, and, as you breathe out, feel your ribs moving inward.
- To pace your breathing, inhale for a count of four seconds and exhale for a count of six seconds.
- Breathe in, 1, 2, 3, 4, breathe out, 1, 2, 3, 4, 5, 6. (If your BOLT score is less than 15 seconds, breathe in 1,2,3, breathe out, 1, 2, 3).
- As you breathe in, feel your ribs moving outward, and, as you breathe out, feel your ribs moving inward.
- Breathe in for a count of four seconds and breathe out for a count of six seconds.
- Continue the exercise for approximately four minutes.

Alternatively, you can breathe in for a count of five seconds and breathe out for a count of five. *Breathe in, 1, 2, 3, 4, 5, breathe out, 1, 2, 3, 4, 5.*

Both options result in a breathing rate of six breaths per minute and work well in helping improve the automatic functioning of the body—those processes that occur during every waking minute without you having to think about it or consciously direct them.

## A Question of Air Hunger

I had the following question from a student:

When practicing to achieve air hunger and cadence breathing, is the whole point to minimize the volume of air during this time? The reason I ask is that you say to breathe LSD (light, slow, and deep), but when I try to breathe light and slow during the 4 seconds in, 6 seconds out, it seems like I cannot take as deep a breath. I don't feel as much movement of the first two ribs.

I was wondering if changing to a count of 6 or 7 seconds in and 8 or 9 seconds out would be a good idea where I can still breathe really light/slow, achieve air hunger, and take a much deeper breath (really feel the expansion of the first two ribs)? Any thoughts on doing this?

The answer is that these are three different exercises. You should focus on each one separately at first. Then bring all three together.

- *Breathe Light* (biochemistry)—the focus is on air hunger.
- *Breathe Slow* (cadence)—the focus is on six breaths per minute.
- *Breathe Deep* (biomechanics)—the focus is on breathing with greater use of the diaphragm.
- *Breathe Light, Slow, Deep* (LSD)—biochemistry, biomechanics, cadence—brings all three together, breathing light, slow, and deep.

The main thing to remember is that when practicing for biomechanics and cadence, you should not overbreathe. This is a common problem. People breathe low, but in the process take full big breaths, disrupting the biochemistry. While you don't specifically need to feel air hunger to practice biomechanics and cadence, a light air hunger ensures that you are not overbreathing. The priority, when practicing cadence breathing, is on a breathing rate of between 4.5 and 6.5 breaths per minute. The secondary aim is to avoid overbreathing.

### #4. Breathe Light, Slow, and Deep (LSD)

This exercise brings all three dimensions of functional breathing together to encourage you to *Breathe Light, Slow, and Deep*:

**Light:** Create a light air hunger by taking in slightly less air with each breath.

**Slow:** Reduce your breathing cadence to take fewer breaths. Pace your breathing to six breaths per minute.

**Deep:** Practice diaphragmatic breathing so that you can feel the lower ribs expanding and contracting with each breath.

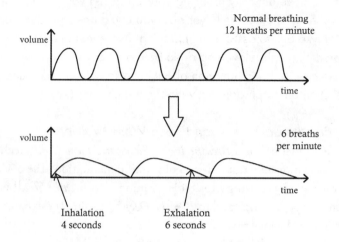

Normal breathing
12 breaths per minute

volume

time

6 breaths
per minute

volume

time

Inhalation          Exhalation
4 seconds          6 seconds

Breathe light, slow and deep

Directions:

- Sit up straight in a chair or cross-legged on the floor. Place your hands on either side of your abdomen, on your lower two ribs.
- Slow down the speed of air as it enters and leaves your nose. Your breathing should be light, quiet, and still.
- At the top of each inhale, bring a feeling of relaxation throughout your body, and allow a slow, soft, relaxed breath out. The air should leave your body slowly and effortlessly.
- Gently soften the breath to generate the feeling that you would like to take in a bigger breath.
- With each inhalation, take the air deep into your lungs. As you breathe in, feel your ribs expanding outward. As you breathe out, feel your ribs moving inward.
- Gradually reduce your breathing rhythm so that you are breathing in for four seconds and out for six seconds.
- Breathe in, 1, 2, 3, 4, and breathe out, 1, 2, 3, 4, 5, 6.
- Breathe light, slow, and deep.
- Continue this exercise for approximately four minutes.

- If you have difficulty reducing your breathing volume with lateral expansion of the lower ribs, you could use a product called Buteyko Belt to assist with improving awareness and practice of breathing light, slow, and deep both during rest and physical exercise. More information about Buteyko Belt can be found in the section on diaphragm activation in this chapter (#8).

### #5. Breathe Light, Slow, and Deep While Walking

This exercise incorporates *Breathe Light, Slow, and Deep (LSD)* techniques with physical movement. It is a kind of walking meditation. The objective is to *Breathe Light* by creating a tolerable air hunger, to *Breathe Slow* by taking fewer breaths per minute, and to *Breathe Deep* by feeling the expansion and contraction of the lower two ribs.

Breathing light allows $CO_2$ to accumulate in the blood, and that allows the release of more oxygen to the cells. However, $CO_2$ is also generated through increased metabolic activity. Combining the *Breathe Light, Slow, and Deep* exercise with walking is an effective way to improve your BOLT score and reduce breathing volume.

If you want to, you can wear the SportsMask for this exercise. This will assist in reducing your breathing volume and create added resistance to generate the feeling of air hunger. To help counter the feeling of air hunger while wearing the mask, breathe slow and deep through your nose. You can find out more about the SportsMask and purchase a mask at SportsMask.com.

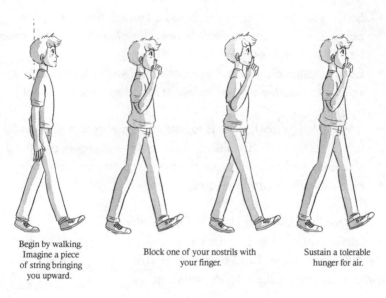

Begin by walking. Imagine a piece of string bringing you upward.

Block one of your nostrils with your finger.

Sustain a tolerable hunger for air.

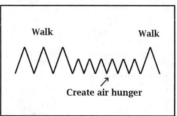

Walk          Walk

Create air hunger

## Directions:

*If you are using a SportsMask, continue straight on to exercise 6.*

The objectives here are to breathe lightly during your walk, to breathe less air than you normally would, and to feel a hunger for more air. Remember to bring your focused awareness to the breath, just as you did for *Breathe Light*. This exercise is to be done while walking at a gentle pace.

- As you continue to walk, block one of your nostrils (it doesn't matter which) with your finger. This will concentrate the air entering and leaving your nostrils.

- Soften your breathing as you breathe through one nostril. The objective is to create a tolerable need for air, to feel slightly breathless, to want to take in more air.
- Concentrating air flow through one nostril will reduce breathing volume to create a hunger for air. Try to sustain the feeling of air hunger.
- If the feeling of air hunger is too strong, then breathe slow and low. Breathing less breaths but fuller breaths improves breathing efficiency and helps alleviate the feeling of air hunger.
- Practice the exercise for five minutes.

### #6. Breathe Slow and Deep While Walking

This variation is also to be practiced at a steady, comfortable walking pace. You should remove your hand from your nostril at this point. Also, ensure that you are breathing light during walking.

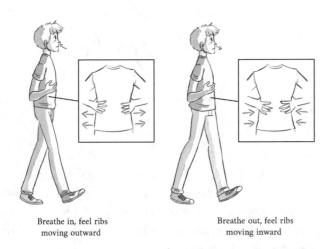

Breathe in, feel ribs
moving outward

Breathe out, feel ribs
moving inward

### Directions:

- Place your hands on your sides to feel your lower two ribs.
- As you breathe in, feel your ribs moving outward.
- As you breathe out, feel your ribs moving inward.

- Breathe light, slow, and deep.
- Reduce the number of breaths per minute, and allow the size of each breath to be deeper, taking fuller breaths but fewer of them. Take fuller breaths but try to make sure that you don't breathe in too much air.
- As you breathe in, feel your lower ribs moving outwards, and, as you breathe out, feel your lower ribs moving inwards.
- Continue this exercise for five minutes.

The objectives here are to breathe light, slow, and deep (LSD) during your walk, to breathe less than you normally would, and to feel air hunger.

### #7. Breathe Light, Slow, and Deep While Jogging

This exercise involves jogging or fast walking with the mouth closed for one minute, followed by normal walking for one minute. Combining metabolic activity with reduced nasal breathing offers several benefits, including lower sensitivity to $CO_2$, improved breathing efficiency during physical activity, less breathlessness, and stronger breathing muscles.

While this exercise is a challenge, it should not be stressful. The objective is to push yourself but not to lose control of your breathing. For those unable to jog, fast walking will suffice. You can practice this exercise by continuing straight on from *Breathe Light, Slow, and Deep During Walking*. Simply increase your pace to a fast walk or jog.

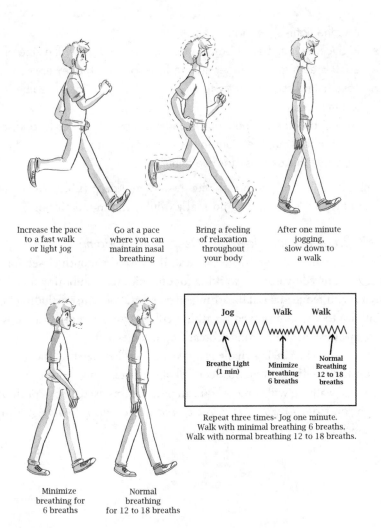

Increase the pace to a fast walk or light jog

Go at a pace where you can maintain nasal breathing

Bring a feeling of relaxation throughout your body

After one minute jogging, slow down to a walk

Minimize breathing for 6 breaths

Normal breathing for 12 to 18 breaths

Repeat three times- Jog one minute.
Walk with minimal breathing 6 breaths.
Walk with normal breathing 12 to 18 breaths.

## Directions:

- Increase your pace to a fast walk or jog. Continue to jog for one minute at a pace where you can maintain nasal breathing.
- Remember, this should be a slight challenge but not stressful.
- Continue to breathe in and out through your nose. Don't hold your breath or freeze your breathing. Just breathe gently in and out through your nose.

- *Breathe Light*: Soften your breathing, taking in just the amount of air that you need.
- *Breathe Slow*: Slow down the speed of your breathing.
- *Breathe Deep*: Bring the air into the lower regions of the lungs and allow a complete and normal exhalation.
- After one minute of fast walking or jogging, slow down your pace to a walk. Walk for one minute, minimizing your breathing for 6 breaths. There is no need to minimize breathing if you are wearing SportsMask.
- Take very small breaths in and out through your nose. Just take a flicker of air in and a flicker of air out. Bring enough air to fill your nostrils and no more. This will involve breathing less than you normally would.

Now restore your normal breathing for 12 to 18 breaths . . .

- Next, as you breathe in, feel your lower two ribs move outward, and as you breathe out, feel your lower two ribs move inward.
- As you walk or jog, take your attention out of your mind and direct it to your breath.
- Concentrate on your breathing. Focus on your breathing. Make your walk or jog a breathing meditation.
- Feel the air coming into your nose, and feel the air leaving your nose.
- It is normal for the mind to wander. If your mind wanders, gently bring your attention back to your breathing.
- Follow your breath. Feel your breathing. Take your attention out of your head and onto your breathing. Feel the air coming into your nose, and feel the air leaving your nose.

The objectives are to breathe light, slow, and deep (LSD) during physical movement, to breathe less than you normally would, and to feel a hunger for air.

- **Light:** Breathe softly to produce a nonstressful air hunger (wearing a SportsMask will naturally create a resistance to breathing and cause air hunger).

- **Slow:** Breathe fewer breaths, but fuller breaths. Take the air deep into the lungs.
- **Deep:** As you breathe in, feel your lower two ribs move outwards, and, as you breathe out, feel your lower two ribs move inwards.

If the feeling of air hunger is too strong with the SportsMask, adjust the setting on your mask to increase airflow.

### Quick Summary of the Exercise:

This exercise incorporates the techniques from *Breathe LSD* and adds a metabolic challenge in the form of a fast walk or jog.

1. Jog for one minute, breathe LSD.
2. Walk for one minute—practice minimal breathing for 6 breaths, then recover with normal breathing for 12 to 18 breaths.
3. Repeat the exercise three times.

## DIAPHRAGM ACTIVATION

### #8. Buteyko Belt

The Buteyko Belt is specifically designed as an aid to enhance and support your practice of functional breathing. It will assist you in activating the diaphragm and breathing lightly with a minimum of effort as you go about your daily activities. The light tension of the belt against your body helps bring awareness to the movement of the lower ribs and abdomen. It applies gentle resistance to help train and strengthen breathing muscles, and it slows the breathing, helping you *Breathe Light*.

The belt can be worn around the midriff to direct attention to this area or across the chest to help reduce the movements of the upper chest.

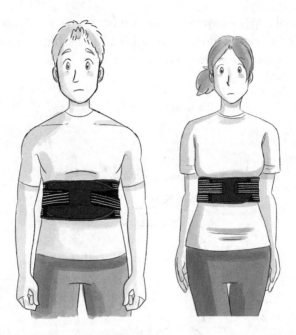

**Wearing the belt:**

Wrap the belt around your diaphragm so that it sits midway between your navel and your chest. Tighten or loosen the straps on each side of the belt to achieve the optimum resistance to your breathing. If you feel no air hunger, then tighten the straps until a tolerable air hunger is achieved. If the air hunger is uncomfortable, loosen the straps to achieve the optimum air hunger.

Directions:
-----------

- As you slowly inhale, feel your lower ribs and abdomen pushing against the belt.
- As you slowly exhale, feel the belt pushing against your lower ribs and abdomen.
- Breathe light, slow, and deep (LSD).

In addition to wearing the Buteyko Belt to practice your breathing exercises, it can be worn while you are on the computer, driving your car, watching TV, or doing any other activity where you are relatively sedentary. Wear the belt for up to 20 minutes at a time, two to three times per day.

## #9. Diaphragm Activation Lying on Back

It is easier to activate abdominal breathing when lying on your back in a semi-supine position or when lying on your front.

Breathe in softly–book gently rises

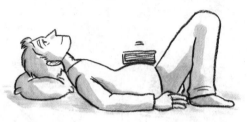

Breathe out softly–book gently falls

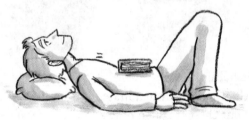

## Directions:

- Lie on a mat with a small pillow under your head and knees bent, as shown above.
- Place a book just above your navel.
- Concentrate on breathing into your abdomen.
- Breathe in, gently guiding the book upward.
- Breathe out, gently guiding the book downward.
- While breathing in, imagine inflating your belly with a light amount of air, and watch your book rise. While breathing out, imagine a balloon slowly deflating of its own accord.
- Continue the exercise for five minutes

## #10. Diaphragm Activation Lying on Front

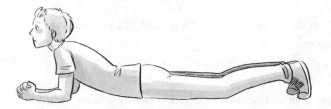

Inhale—push abdomen towards the floor

Exhale—abdomen moves to resting position

### Directions:

- Lie face down on the floor, resting on your elbows.
- Push off the floor, resting on your elbows so that your tummy is not touching the floor.
- As you breathe in, gently push your abdomen toward the floor.
- As you exhale, gently draw your abdomen inward.

The floor and gravity can help activate movement of the diaphragm. Continue this exercise for three to five minutes.

## #11. Breath Hold Activation

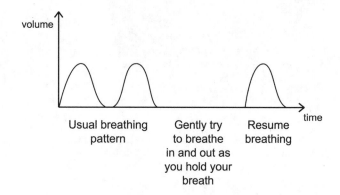

Directions:

- Take a soft silent breath in through your nose.
- Allow a soft silent breath out through your nose.
- Pinch your nose with your fingers to hold your breath for about 10 seconds or so.
- As you pinch your nose to hold your breath, gently try to breathe in and out.
- Feel your abdomen move in and out as you try to breathe.
- After 10 seconds or so, release your nose, and resume breathing through the nose.
- Rest for one minute with normal breathing and repeat again.
- Repeat three to five times.

# SECTION TWO: **EXERCISES TO STOP SYMPTOMS OF ASTHMA, ANXIETY, STRESS, RACING MIND, AND PANIC DISORDER**

## #12. Breathing Recovery, Sitting

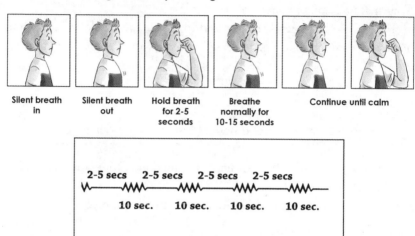

| Silent breath in | Silent breath out | Hold breath for 2-5 seconds | Breathe normally for 10-15 seconds | Continue until calm |
|---|---|---|---|---|

This exercise is suitable for everyone and can be practiced throughout the day.

The practice of many small breath holds helps calm down the breathing. Over the years, I have used this exercise with clients to very good effect to stop asthma symptoms such as wheezing and coughing, to reduce stress levels, and to help control breathing during a hyperventilation or anxiety attack. For people who have experienced severe trauma in their lives, frequent practice of this exercise throughout the day offers considerable relief.

I consider this exercise to be an "emergency" exercise. It is very hard to slow your breathing down when it is out of control, because the air hunger or sense of suffocation during an asthma or panic attack can be quite strong. Instead of trying to slow your breathing, calm it using this exercise.

As you repeat the small breath holds, it is important not to try holding your breath for longer that 2 to 5 seconds. Longer breath holds in these circumstances may destabilize your breathing. For the purposes of this exercise, your maximum breath hold should be no longer than **half your BOLT score at the time.**

Between the breath holds, try to avoid shallow, fast breathing as this will only intensify the feeling of air hunger and breathlessness. It is much more efficient to breathe low and slow to optimize the amount of air that reaches the small air sacs in the lungs. This allows more oxygen to reach the blood.

Start by getting yourself into a comfortable seated position. In this emergency exercise, we'll begin by holding the breath for up to 5 seconds, followed by normal breathing for around 10 seconds.

The exercise helps gently calm breathing, open up the blood vessels, and increase the amount of oxygen released to tissues and organs, including the brain.

Directions:
---

- Sit up straight and take a normal breath in and out through your nose.
- Pinch your nose with your fingers to hold the breath for up to five seconds. Count: 5, 4, 3, 2, 1.
- Let go of your nose and breathe normally through your nose for 10 seconds.
- Repeat the sequence for as long as symptoms are present.

If you have asthma and your symptoms continue for as long as five minutes, take your medication. If you are having a severe attack, take your rescue medication immediately. If your symptoms do not respond to your medication within a few minutes, seek medical attention.

Additional exercises and instruction to help with asthma and panic disorder can be found in exercise #16 in this chapter and in Chapter Ten.

## #13. Breathing Recovery, Walking

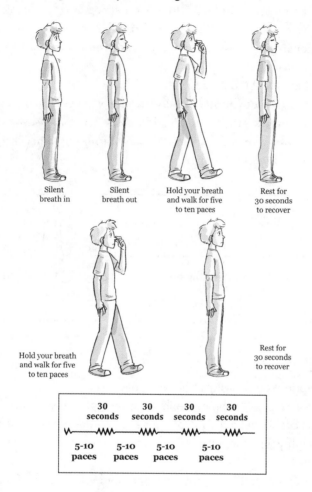

Silent
breath in

Silent
breath out

Hold your breath
and walk for five
to ten paces

Rest for
30 seconds
to recover

Hold your breath
and walk for five
to ten paces

Rest for
30 seconds
to recover

| 30 seconds | 30 seconds | 30 seconds | 30 seconds |
|---|---|---|---|
| 5-10 paces | 5-10 paces | 5-10 paces | 5-10 paces |

## Directions:

- Exhale through your nose.
- Pinch your nose with your fingers to hold your breath, and walk for 5 to 10 paces, holding your breath.
- Stop walking.
- Breathe in through your nose, and rest for about 30 seconds while standing still.
- Repeat up to 10 times.

If you are practicing at home, you can repeat this exercise six times, five times per day. Holding the breath for up to 10 paces is very suitable for anyone with severe asthma, COPD, or panic disorder. It is also ideal if you have disproportionate breathlessness, anxiety, racing mind, or a low BOLT score.

### #14. Decongest the Nose

If you find it difficult to breathe nasally because of congestion or obstruction in your nose, this exercise is very effective. *Please note that holding the breath to generate a strong hunger for air is not suitable during pregnancy or if you have serious medical conditions.*

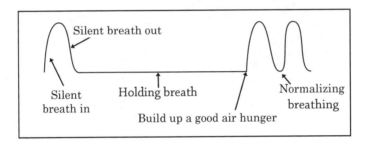

Directions:
_____

- Sit upright on a straight-backed chair.
- Take a small, light breath in through your nose if you can and a small breath out through your nose. If you are unable to inhale through your nose, take a tiny breath in through the corner of your mouth.
- After exhaling, pinch your nose and hold your breath. Keep your lips sealed.
- Gently nod your head or rock your body until you feel that you cannot hold your breath for any longer. You should feel a relatively strong need for air.
- At this point, let go of your nose, and breathe in gently through it. Breathe gently in and out with your mouth closed. When you first breathe in, try to avoid taking a deep breath. Instead, keep your breathing calm and focus on relaxation. Use the mantra: "Relax and breathe less," if it helps.

Directions:

This exercise can help ease the diaphragm back to its resting position.

- Slowly exhale through your nose. Do not force the breath in any way.
- As you exhale, gently suck your stomach inward, almost as if you are "squeezing the air out of your stomach."
- Continue to exhale slowly until you have breathed out all the remaining air from the lungs.
- As you exhale, imagine that your diaphragm is moving back up to its resting position.
- Allow the inhalation to happen naturally.
- Repeat several times over the course of 10 minutes.

This exercise can be used at any time—whether you are suffering from breathing difficulties or not—and it will help improve functioning of the diaphragm breathing muscle.

## #16. Three Exercises to Help Stop a Panic Attack

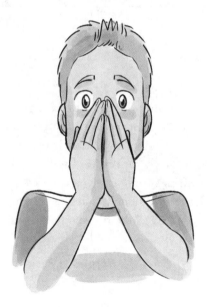

## 1. Breathing into Cupped Hands

At the first sign of a panic attack, cup your hands across your mouth and nose, and gently slow down your breathing. If you can breathe slow and low with lateral expansion and contraction of the lower ribs, then great. Otherwise, just concentrate on breathing slow. Cupping the hands will pool $CO_2$ from the exhaled breath, allowing you to rebreathe the $CO_2$ back into your lungs. This will increase $CO_2$ in the blood, which will improve blood flow and oxygen delivery to your brain. This is like the "brown paper bag" technique, but it is safer because it allows a plentiful supply of oxygen while increasing $CO_2$.

**OR**

## 2. Breathe Slow and Deep

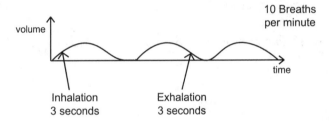

Fast and shallow breathing will feed into feelings of suffocation and air hunger. To help alleviate air hunger, slow down your breathing with lateral expansion and contraction of the lower ribs. If the feeling of air hunger is quite strong, breathe in slowly for two to three seconds and out slowly for three to four seconds. If this feels okay, you can slow down your breathing a little more, inhaling for five seconds and exhaling for five seconds. Place your hands on your sides to feel the ribs gently expanding and contracting as you breathe.

**OR**

## 3. Breathing Recovery, Sitting

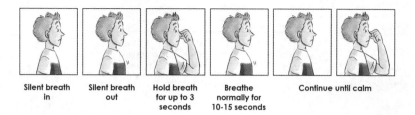

Silent breath in | Silent breath out | Hold breath for up to 3 seconds | Breathe normally for 10-15 seconds | Continue until calm

- Sit up straight and take a normal breath in and out through your nose.
- Pinch your nose with your fingers to hold your breath for up to three seconds. Count: 3, 2, 1 . . .
- Let go of your nose and breathe through your nose for 10 to 15 seconds.
- Repeat the sequence for as long as symptoms are present.

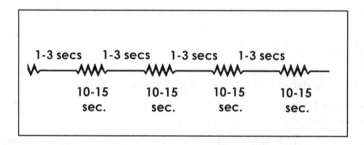

### #17. Achieve Deeper Sleep

This exercise can be practiced before you go to sleep. (The procedure and evidence for nose breathing during sleep is described in detail in Chapter Seven on sleep and in the Children's Exercises section of this chapter.)

The following Breathe Light practice is an excellent way to help with sleep-disordered breathing. It also promotes relaxation and enables you to fall asleep more easily.

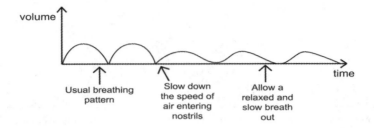

## Directions:

- Place one hand on your chest and one hand on your abdomen.
- Gently soften and slow down your breathing to create a slight hunger for air.
- Slow down the speed of air as it enters your nostrils.
- Allow the breath out to be slow and relaxed.
- The goal is to breathe softly so that about 30% less air enters your lungs.
- You are doing it correctly when you feel a tolerable air hunger.
- If the air hunger is too much, take a rest for 15 seconds and start again.
- Continue the practice for approximately 15 minutes.

### #18. Alleviate the Feeling of Suffocation or Air Hunger

The normal response to the feeling of air hunger or suffocation is to begin breathing fast through an open mouth. This kind of breathing is shallow and will only feed into your discomfort and fear. This is because a considerable volume of inhaled air remains in the airways and upper chest instead of reaching the small air sacs deep in the lungs where oxygen transfers to the blood.

If you have a low BOLT score of less than 15 seconds, it is likely that you frequently feel air hunger during everyday breathing. One of the most commonly reported symptoms is the feeling of not being able to take a deep breath. In the long term, a BOLT score of over 20 seconds is necessary to alleviate this feeling.

Some people might only experience air hunger during asthma, anxiety, or panic related symptoms. Others may feel breathless as a matter of course. To reduce the everyday feeling of air hunger, practice the breathing program specific to your condition or BOLT score, as described in the next section.

# SECTION THREE: **TAILORED BREATHING PROGRAMS FOR SPECIFIC CONDITIONS**

## BASED ON BOLT SCORE

Each of the conditions listed here is covered in significant detail in the second part of this book. This section is intended as a practical guide to help you develop a breathing program. The suggestions for each condition include numbered exercises that you will find in the previous section.

If you have any of the conditions listed here, I recommend that you spend some time reading the relevant chapters to find out more about the way dysfunctional breathing and breathing exercises impact your symptoms. (Also, consult your qualified medical practitioners.)

**Topics covered here are:**

- Asthma and respiratory issues, including post-COVID-19 care
- Activities based on BOLT score
- Hormone fluctuations in women (PMS, pregnancy, and menopause)
- Diabetes
- Epilepsy
- Heart rate variability
- Sleep disorders (sleep apnea, snoring, and insomnia)
- Panic disorder, anxiety, and a racing mind
- Detoxification

## ASTHMA AND RESPIRATORY ISSUES (INCLUDING POST-COVID CARE)

Over the past 18 years, I have seen many people with asthma experience a 50% reduction in their asthma symptoms within two weeks of attending my workshops and applying the exercises. More recently, people have reported significant improvements to breathing control post-Covid. The benefits of functional breathing for asthma and post-Covid include a significant reduction in symptoms such as:

- Nasal congestion
- Coughing
- Wheezing
- Breathlessness
- Colds

Symptoms will noticeably lessen each time the BOLT score improves by five seconds.

### Daily Practice

Nasal breathing during wakefulness slows and deepens the breath. This may help maintain the strength and function of the breathing muscles and reduce breathlessness. Nasal breathing also harnesses a gas called nitric oxide, which is produced in the nasal cavity. Nitric oxide has antiviral and antibacterial qualities, so it protects against infection.

Regardless of your current BOLT score, you should breathe only through your nose during rest, physical exercise, and sleep. Alongside your practice of full-time nasal breathing, follow the program suitable for your BOLT. As your BOLT score improves, progress to the next level.

### BOLT Score of Less Than 10 Seconds

Nasal breathe during rest, exercise, and sleep.

Practice *Breathing Recovery, Sitting* (exercise #12) for 10 minutes every hour.

**OR**

Practice *Breathing Recovery, Walking* (exercise #13) following the instructions below.

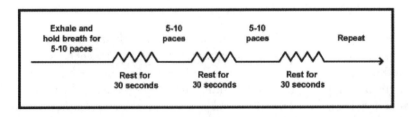

Directions:

- In a standing position, make sure you have space to walk freely.
- Exhale gently through your nose.
- Pinch your nose with your fingers to hold your breath.
- Walk for 5 to 10 paces while holding your breath. Take small paces, not great big strides. The aim is not to see how far you can walk.
- Release your nose and breathe in through it.
- Rest for 30 to 60 seconds.
- When breathing is comfortable, repeat.
- Practice 5 to 10 repetitions two times per hour during the day.

## BOLT Score Between 10 and 15 Seconds

- Nasal breathe during rest, exercise, and sleep.
- Practice *Breathing Recovery, Sitting* (exercise #12) for 10 minutes, two times per day (and if you experience symptoms such as wheezing, coughing, or chest tightness).
- Or *Breathing Recovery, Walking* (exercise #13) as described above. Complete five repetitions of this exercise three times per day.
- *Breathe Light* (exercise #1) for 10 minutes, three times daily.
- *Breathe Slow and Deep While Walking* (exercise #6) for 10 minutes, daily.

## BOLT Score Greater Than 15 Seconds

- Nasal breathe during rest, exercise, and sleep.
- Practise breath holds after an exhalation during your warm-up for 10 to 15 minutes prior to physical exercise. (If you are pregnant or have a serious medical condition, please don't practice breath holding. Follow the guidelines below.) To help decongest the nose, open the airways and improve oxygen delivery to the brain, exhale and hold the breath to create a medium air hunger (a tolerable feeling that you would like to breathe more air). Then resume breathing in and out through your nose during continuous movement. Repeat a breath hold after an exhalation five times during the warm-up.

- *Breathe Light* (exercise #1) for 10 minutes, three times per day.
- *Breathe Slow and Deep While Walking* (exercise #6) for 10 minutes, daily.

If you have symptoms such as wheezing, coughing, or chest tightness, return to the first two exercises and practice the small breath holds in *Breathing Recovery, Sitting (exercise #12)* for 10 minutes every hour.

**OR**

- Practice *Breathing Recovery, Walking* (exercise #13) for 5 to 10 repetitions two times per hour during the day.

## BREATHING FOR FEMALES

There is a strong connection between respiratory chemistry and cyclical fluctuations in sex hormones. This means that, if you are female, the way you breathe is strongly affected by the way your hormone levels change during your monthly menstrual cycle.

After menopause, these changes are no longer present, but postmenopausal women can be more vulnerable to respiratory illness and infection, and to osteoporosis, which is connected to breathing biochemistry.

Breathing exercises are beneficial in moderating these changes and can help:

- Reduce pain, especially cyclical pain exacerbations in chronic pain conditions like fibromyalgia
- Alleviate symptoms of PMS
- Improve autonomic balance
- Reduce hot flashes
- Better regulate mood
- Improve sexual functio
- Reduce headaches and menstrual migraines
- Support bone mineral density

As your BOLT score increases, you will experience less cyclical hyperventilation—and a reduction in associated symptoms. You can also use the exercises to ease your body's transition through menopause as the relationship between sex hormones and the breath changes.

## Daily Practice

- Make sure you breathe only through your nose during rest, physical exercise, and sleep.
- Track your BOLT score during your monthly cycle. This will give you clues as to how (and why) your breathing is changing.
- Is your BOLT score lower during days 10 to 22 of your monthly cycle (between ovulation and menstruation)? This may indicate breathing pattern changes due to hormonal fluctuations, most notably, an increase in progesterone which is a respiratory stimulant.
- Work to improve your BOLT score to above 25 seconds.

**If your BOLT score is less than 15 seconds, or you experience a fear reaction to the feeling of air hunger, then practice both of the following:**

- *Breathing Recovery, Sitting* (exercise #12 or #16) for 10 minutes, four times daily.
- *Breathe Light* (exercise #1) for 15 to 30 seconds, followed by a rest of 1 minute. Practice this for 10 minutes, three times per day.

**If your BOLT score is greater than 15 seconds, practice:**

- *Breathe Light* (exercise #1) to create air hunger for 10 minutes, four times daily.
- *Breathe Slow and Deep While Walking* (exercise #6) for 10 minutes, once per day.

## After Menopause

Postmenopausal women are at higher risk of sleep disorders, including obstructive sleep apnea. To maintain lung health, support breathing biochemistry (which is essential for healthy bone mineral density), and reduce risk of respiratory infection and sleep disorders, make sure to breathe only through your nose during rest, physical exercise, and sleep.

Practice the following exercises every day to improve your BOLT score and support general health and resilience:

- *Breathe Light* (exercise #1) for 10 minutes, two times daily.
- *Breathe Slow* (exercise #3) for 10 minutes, two times daily.
- *Breathe Deep* (exercise #2) for 10 minutes, two times daily.
- Physical exercise with mouth closed.

## *During Pregnancy*

Functional breathing can help with abdominal muscle strength, hyperventilation, and anxiety, and even support you during labor. As your baby grows, you will discover breathing is not always so easy. Hormonally mediated changes occur in breathing early on in pregnancy, and it's normal for pregnant women to hyperventilate.

Breathing exercises are beneficial during pregnancy. As your pregnancy progresses, your body needs more oxygen to function, and your baby needs oxygen too. By preventing hyperventilation, you will lessen feelings of pain in your muscles and joints. Pregnancy can cause anxiety, and slow breathing is a great way to destress. Sleep apnea is a risk factor for expectant mothers, so it is worth paying attention to how you breathe during sleep.

Most pregnant women are anxious about labor, but if you develop a regular breathing practice, labor will be less traumatic for you and your baby, both in terms of pain and oxygen desaturation. Breathing exercises help you learn to stay present, meaning you will feel more in control during your pregnancy and your labor. You will also be better able to recover after the birth.

### First Trimester

During your first trimester, do not practice any reduced breathing exercises. Instead, work to prevent hyperventilation with the following steps:

- Avoid overeating,
- Avoid overheated environments, and
- Use mindfulness meditations or similar practices to reduce stress.

During this first three-month period, your BOLT score should not increase by more than 2 seconds per week. Progress must be very gentle.

### Second Trimester

During your second trimester, you may practice a number of breathing exercises. *Breathe Deep* (exercise #2) will help strengthen your pelvic floor muscles and *Breathe Slow* (exercise #3) will help relax your mind and body. You will benefit from practicing the exercises while lying down on your back with your head on a pillow and your knees raised. As your pregnancy progresses, you may find it easier to lie on your side.

Go gently with the air shortage at this time, focusing on relaxation and slow breathing instead. Continue with a gentle practice after your baby arrives. Diaphragm breathing will help your pelvic floor to recover.

## DIABETES

Functional breathing is helpful for people with both types of diabetes because it improves blood glucose control. There is a link between diabetes and asthma, and there is an important correlation between sleep quality and diabetes control. Sleep is strongly influenced by the breath, as is the health of the heart—another important concern for people with diabetes.

- If you have type 1 or type 2 diabetes, it is vital that you breathe only through your nose during rest, physical exercise, and sleep.
- Speak with your medical doctor before undertaking any of the breathing exercises in this book.
- Breathing exercises can cause blood sugar to drop. It is therefore important that you monitor your blood glucose levels during any breathing practice.

### Daily Practice
- *Breathe Light* (exercise #1) for 10 minutes, two times daily.
- *Breathe Slow* (exercise #3) for 10 minutes, three times daily.
- *Breathe Deep* (exercise #2) for 10 minutes, once daily.
- If you have a racing mind, practice the small breath holds exercise, *Breathing Recovery* (exercise #12 or #13).
- Breathe nasally during rest, exercise, and sleep.
- When you exercise, keep your mouth closed.

Remember, you must monitor your blood sugar levels more frequently. *Breathe Light* (exercise #1) to create air hunger may reduce blood sugar levels. If you feel hypoglycemic, stop the exercises immediately and take a snack.

When your BOLT score increases beyond 20 seconds, or if it increases by more than 5 seconds from your starting point, please consult with your medical doctor as you may require adjustments to your medication. Never stop taking your medication suddenly or without medical advice.

## EPILEPSY

Hyperventilation is a known seizure trigger. There is a strong link between blood $CO_2$ levels and vulnerability to some types of seizures.

In terms of general health, epilepsy frequently exists alongside other conditions, especially depression, which may also be characterized by breathing pattern disorders. People with epilepsy are more likely to suffer with respiratory and cardiovascular problems, obesity, and other disorders, including diabetes.

If you suffer from epilepsy, it is important to restore full-time nasal breathing. Make sure that you breathe only through your nose during rest, physical exercise, and sleep, to reverse and prevent chronic hyperventilation.

### Daily Practice
- *Breathe Light* (exercise #1) for 10 minutes, three times daily.
- *Breathe Slow* (exercise #3) for 10 minutes, twice daily.
- *Breathe Deep* (exercise #2) for 10 minutes, once daily.
- If you have a racing mind, practice *Breathing Recovery, Sitting or Walking* (exercise #12 or #13).
- Breathe nasally during rest, exercise, and sleep.
- When you exercise, keep your mouth closed.
- Breathe nasally during sleep. If you use a lip tape to help ensure nasal breathing during sleep, do not place the tape directly across your lips. Instead, use a support like MyoTape which surrounds the lips, gently keeping the lips together and reminding your mouth to close. This provides a safe way to ensure nasal breathing during the night, when you cannot consciously control your breathing.

## IMPROVE HEART RATE VARIABILITY

Heart rate variability (HRV) is a useful index of well-being and resilience. Good HRV indicates a healthy balance in the autonomic nervous system and is indicative of good health.

It is possible to access the benefits of optimal HRV using the breath. Numerous studies have shown that breathing at a rate of six breaths per minute optimizes HRV and produces lasting positive effects.

The first adjustment you must make to improve your HRV is to switch to full-time nasal breathing. Breathing only through the nose during rest, physical exercise, and sleep slows the breath, activates the diaphragm and stimulates the vagus nerve. You can read about this in detail later in the book in Chapter Four.

### Daily Practice

- Slow breathing to an average of six breaths per minute.
- *Breathe Light* (exercise #1) to create air hunger, for 10 minutes, twice daily.
- *Breathe Light, Breathe Slow, Breathe Deep* (exercises #1–3) for 10 minutes four times daily, or 20 minutes twice daily.

## IMPROVE SLEEP QUALITY, INSOMNIA, SNORING, AND SLEEP APNEA

If your breathing during the day is less than optimal, your breathing during sleep will be dysfunctional too. If you suffer with snoring, insomnia, or sleep apnea, breathing exercises can help significantly reduce your symptoms. Above all, it is vital to restore nasal breathing during sleep, because breathing through an open mouth activates the stress response, and it leaves the airway more vulnerable to collapse, which can trigger snoring and even cause the breathing to periodically stop altogether.

### Tips for Better Sleep Hygiene

To enjoy a restful night's sleep, it is important to practice good sleep hygiene. Most of us know that this involves less screen time and alcohol just before bed, but many of us resist the idea, because watching the TV with a glass of wine is a nice way to wind down. Unfortunately, this habit doesn't really help you relax. In reality, it stimulates the nervous system, preventing you from sleeping well.

- Avoid blue light. If you must use your smart phone, TV, or laptop before bed, it is a good idea to wear blue light filtering glasses for at least two hours before sleep. For a good brand, seek out OwlEye glasses.

- If you spend all day in front of a computer screen, you may find that wearing blue light filtering glasses throughout your working day helps you sleep and relieves eyestrain and headaches.
- If you use your mobile phone as your alarm clock, switch it to flight mode in the settings before you sleep.
- Your bedroom should be cool, airy, silent, and dark.
- Don't eat or drink alcohol late in the evening. Enjoy a glass with dinner, but then set it aside to give your body time to digest. If you regularly drink late into the evening, you will feel noticeably less groggy in the morning if you give it a miss.

## Insomnia

A racing mind and breathing irregularities both contribute to insomnia. When you find yourself lying awake in the middle of the night, this can be partly due to dysfunctional breathing during sleep. However, the hyper-arousal caused by poor daytime breathing patterns is also to blame. To tackle insomnia, it is necessary to activate the body's relaxation response. It is also essential to improve breathing patterns during sleep so that the airway can function without causing the breath to stop or adding resistance to breathing.

**If you have difficulty falling asleep:**

- Make sure you breathe only through your nose during rest, physical exercise, and sleep.
- *Breathe Light* (exercise #1) to achieve air hunger for 15 minutes before sleep.
- *Breathe Light* (exercise #1) for 10 minutes, three times daily.
- *Breathe Slow* (exercise #3) for 10 minutes, twice daily.
- *Breathe Deep* (exercise #2) for 10 minutes, once daily.

**If you frequently wake up after four or five hours of sleep:**

Waking up after a few hours of sleep is challenging—not quite fully alert to get up and start the day, yet not tired enough to fall back asleep easily. Disturbances to breathing during sleep, including partial or total collapse of the throat, can cause awakening.

- Bring attention to your breathing to help calm racing thoughts.
- *Breathe Light and Slow* to help activate your body's relaxation response (exercise #1).
- Once your BOLT score is greater than 20 seconds, air turbulence in your nose and throat will reduce. You will sleep more deeply and be less likely to wake during the night.

## Snoring

Mouth snoring is the result of a large volume of air passing through a collapsible airway, causing the soft palate to vibrate. It stops when the mouth is closed during sleep.

Nose snoring is caused by turbulent airflow in the nasal airway, where the nose meets the throat (the nasopharynx). Obstruction of the nose caused by nasal stuffiness, deviated septum, or an anatomically smaller nose can increase resistance to breathing. However, hard fast breathing also contributes to nose snoring.

To illustrate the impact of faster and harder breathing during nasal snoring, I often ask my students to make the sound of a snore through the nose. To do this, it is normal to tighten the throat at the back of the nose and speed up breathing. Now, begin to slow down the speed of your breathing, in and out through the nose. Slow down your breathing until it is almost imperceptible. Breathe hardly any air in and out of the nose. Now, try and snore when your breathing is light and slow. You will find it more difficult.

Snoring is not solely due to a compromised nasal airway. Breathing patterns can also play a role. Having a low BOLT score with a faster respiratory rate and increased volume of air per minute contributes to turbulence in the upper airway. While most interventions target the airway, the missing piece of the puzzle is flow. Any engineer investigating resistance to flow in a pipe will not only consider the diameter of the pipe but will also take into account the speed and volume of the flow.

To stop mouth snoring, use MyoTape to keep the mouth closed during sleep. You simply cannot snore through the mouth when breathing is through the nose.

**To significantly reduce nasal snoring:**

- Decongest your nose using the nose unblocking exercise (exercise #14).
- Restore nasal breathing during wakefulness and sleep.
- Reduce the flow of breathing by using *Breathe Light* (exercise #1) for 10 minutes, four times a day.
- Increase your BOLT score to above 20 seconds.

For many people, nasal snoring can be eliminated altogether. For others, particularly those with a narrow airway, nasal snoring will continue but at a lower intensity, meaning it won't be so loud and problematic.

## OBSTRUCTIVE SLEEP APNEA

If you suffer with obstructive sleep apnea (OSA), I recommend that you read Chapter Seven on sleep-disordered breathing and see bonus Chapter 18 online at www.HumanixBooks.com/The Breathing Cure, which describes the phenotypes or physiological causes of obstructive sleep apnea and the ways in which breathing exercises can help.

OSA has serious implications for long-term health and well-being. It is associated with cardiovascular disease, mortality in pregnant women, sexual dysfunction, depression, and sudden cardiac death. If you have this condition, it is worth learning more about how you can reduce its symptoms and severity.

The first step in addressing OSA is to make the switch to nasal breathing during sleep. This is just as important even if you use CPAP to treat your sleep apnea. Mouth breathing is a common factor for CPAP noncompliance, because air that is meant to keep the airways open leaks out through your open mouth instead.

The good news is that breathing exercises improve sleep apnea symptoms as well as supporting general health. Follow the next exercise protocol to reduce your symptoms and enjoy better sleep.

*Daily Practice*

- Breathe only through your nose during rest, physical exercise, and sleep.
- Adopt the correct tongue resting posture. Three quarters of your tongue should rest in the roof of your mouth, with the tip of your tongue placed behind, but not touching, your top front teeth. For supports on correct tongue resting posture, check out MyoSpots.com.
- Achieve a minimum BOLT score of 25 seconds.
- Practice *Breathe Light* (exercise #1) for 15 minutes, twice daily. Schedule one session just after waking and another session before sleep.
- *Breathe Slow and Deep While Walking* (exercise #6) for 20 minutes, once per day.
- Tape your mouth closed to sleep using MyoTape. If you feel anxious about wearing tape around your mouth, wear the tape for 20 minutes before sleep to become comfortable with it.
- If your mouth is naturally moist in the morning, there is no need for the tape. A dry mouth signifies open mouth breathing during sleep.

## PANIC DISORDER, ANXIETY, AND RACING MIND

Panic disorder is often characterized by feelings of breathlessness and fear of suffocation. For this reason, one of the things most likely to trigger a panic attack can be fear of having a panic attack. However, while anxiety, racing thoughts, and panic are categorized as psychological problems, scientists have found a strong biochemical link. People with panic disorder often have a strong sensitivity to the accumulation of $CO_2$, and the feeling of suffocation can be alleviated by normalizing breathing patterns.

When you regularly expose your body to controlled mild air hunger for a short duration, which is the objective of the *Breathe Light* exercises, your body begins to become less sensitive to the feelings of suffocation and to the chemical changes that trigger those feelings. As a result of the connections between the biochemistry of breathing and the functioning of the nervous system, slow breathing can be used to calm the mind. Functional breathing improves blood flow and oxygen delivery to the brain, allowing you to think more clearly and calmly.

The diaphragm is connected to the vagus nerve, which releases a calming neurotransmitter that slows the heart rate. This is why breathing deeply calms the mind. Breathing at a rate of 4.5 to 6.5 breaths per minute activates your body's relaxation response and balances your nervous system, as well as optimizing heart rate variability and blood pressure.

## Emergency Practice
If you feel a panic attack coming on, there are three exercises you can use to help stop it in its tracks. These exercises are also helpful in calming a racing mind:

1. *Breathing Recovery* (exercise #12 or #16).
2. Cup your hands over your face to rebreathe $CO_2$. This is safer than breathing into a paper bag as it maintains inhaled oxygen at a sufficiently high level.
3. Switch your breathing from fast and shallow to slow and deep. You can do this by placing your hands on your trunk either side of your lower ribs so that you can feel the expansion and contraction of your ribs as you breathe in and out through the nose:
   • Breathe in for three seconds.
   • Breathe out for three seconds.
   • Repeat until panic symptoms have subsided.

## Daily Practice
If the feeling of air hunger brings on a strong fear response, regular practice of the following short exercises will help desensitize your body's reaction to the feeling of air hunger:
*Breathing Recovery, Sitting* (exercise #12) for 10 minutes, six times daily.

**OR**

*Breathe Light* (exercise #1) to create air hunger for 15 to 30 seconds, followed by rest for 1 minute. Repeat for 5 to 10 minutes, six times a day.

**OR**

*Breathing Recovery, Walking* (exercise #13) Walk for 5 to 10 paces while holding the breath. Practice five repetitions, six times a day.

**If you are comfortable with the feeling of air hunger:**

- *Breathe Light* (exercise #1) for 10 minutes, three times daily.
- *Breathe Slow* (exercise #3) for 10 minutes, two times daily. If your BOLT score is less than 15 seconds, practice a 3-second inhale and a 3-second exhale. If your BOLT score is greater than 15 seconds, practice a 5-second inhale and a 5-second exhale.
- *Breathe Deep* (exercise #2) for 10 minutes, once per day.

## POST-COVID-19 CARE

I had an email from a colleague recently asking me for some advice about COVID-19. She wrote:

> I have a patient who was diagnosed with COVID-19 in April 2020. When I first met her, she couldn't say one sentence without becoming breathless. When we started working together in October 2020, her BOLT score was just 3 seconds. Now, two months later, her BOLT score is around 10 or 11. She can't do much exercise, because it is difficult enough to breathe through her mouth. She wears MyoTape throughout the day and she can do small breath holds and *Breathe Light*, but the other exercises are too difficult. We did the exercise to decongest the nose and she immediately got a severe headache. She is also experiencing headaches during the other exercises. Her BOLT score after the breathing exercises goes up to around 20 seconds, but her morning BOLT score stays around 10. What else can I do? What causes the severe headache she experiences during the exercise?

Many people with COVID-19 are experiencing severe breathlessness. BOLT scores as low as three seconds have been reported. When the BOLT score is this low, it will be difficult to say a complete sentence without becoming breathless.

To improve the breathing, the objective is to increase the BOLT score gently and consistently. With such a low BOLT score, the risk with any breathing exercise is that it could contribute to unstable breathing.

*Exercise Protocol*

1. *Breathing Recovery, Sitting* (#12) for 10 minutes every hour. Also practice this exercise if the nose feels congested. It is important to hold your breath for no longer than half your BOLT score at that time—so if your BOLT score is just 3 seconds, you will hold your breath for a maximum of 1.5 seconds.
2. Practice slow breathing with lateral expansion and contraction of the lower ribs to improve alveolar ventilation.
   - Inhale slowly through your nose for 3 seconds.
   - Exhale slowly through your nose for 3 seconds.
   - If you are comfortable with this, inhale slowly through your nose for 5 seconds.
   - Exhale slowly through your nose for 5 seconds.
   - As you breathe in, feel your lower ribs gently moving outward.
   - As you breathe out, feel your lower ribs gently moving inward.
   - Practice for 5 minutes, 5 times a day.
3. Breathe only through your nose, day and night. Wear MyoTape to keep your mouth closed during sleep. MyoTape is particularly suitable in this instance as it does not cover the lips.

It is unusual to suffer severe headaches when practicing the exercises. If you practice intensive breath holds, headaches can occur due to increased $CO_2$ in the blood. Generally, the headache will subside fairly quicky.

If you do experience a headache, reduce the intensity of the exercises. Go even more gently as you practice *Breathe Light* and *Breathing Recovery, Sitting*.

## OTHER CONDITIONS

**For people with:**
Schizophrenia
Uncontrolled hyperthyroidism
Chest pains
Heart problems within the past six months
Sickle cell anemia
Cancer

Arterial aneurysm
Kidney disease

Make sure you breathe only through your nose during the day, during exercise and at night. You can practice the *Breathe Slow* exercise (#3) or walking with nasal breathing and listen to the free MP3 download available from OxygenAdvantage.com/breathe-light.

**For older people and people with:**
Second and third trimester pregnancy
High blood pressure
Diabetes
Epilepsy
Panic disorder and anxiety
Sleep apnea
Cardiovascular issues
Serious medical conditions

Only practice breathing recovery exercises and breathing light, slow, and deep through the nose during rest and physical exercise. Refrain from practicing any breathing exercise that involves holding of the breath to generate a strong air hunger.

## A WORD ABOUT DETOXIFICATION

As your BOLT score increases, you may experience the effects of detoxification. The exercises in this chapter are designed to help normalize metabolic activity, improving the body's ability to get rid of waste and clearing the system of toxins.

During the detoxification period, it is very important to continue with your breathing exercises. If you stop, detoxification might not be completed. It is also beneficial to drink a glass of warm water with a quarter teaspoon of good-quality sea salt dissolved in it each day.

You may find that the symptoms experienced during a cleansing involve a brief aggravation of your condition. For example, if you have asthma, you may experience excess mucus production in the nose and airways, especially during physical activity with nasal breathing. You may also experience other mild side-effects such as a slight headache, diarrhea, increased yawning, a head cold, insomnia, a bad taste in the mouth, and reduced appetite. These are all just signs that your body is readjusting to a healthier way of life. In general, symptoms should not be disruptive to normal life and will pass in one or two days. Like any detoxification process, there is always a short adjustment phase.

If the idea of a "breathing detox" is new to you, you may be interested to know that toxins, including alcohol, leave the body via the lungs.[7] To illustrate this, there was a woman in my hometown of Galway, Ireland, who had some knowledge about breathing. She was arrested on suspicion of drunk driving. The woman failed the Breathalyzer test and was taken to the police station for blood tests. While in the back of the police car, she deliberately hyperventilated for several minutes. I can only imagine what the officers must have thought.

Despite the Breathalyzer results, blood results at the station showed low alcohol levels and she was allowed to go. I am in no way encouraging or condoning drunk driving. I do, however, find it fascinating that it is possible to get rid of alcohol from the blood through the breath. Recent research in Canada even suggests that hyperventilation could provide a lifesaving therapeutic intervention in cases of alcohol poisoning.[8]

# SECTION FOUR: **EXERCISES TO IMPROVE FOCUS AND CONCENTRATION**

One question I'm often asked by my students is "What is the difference between breathing techniques designed as 'stressors' and breathing techniques that are meant as 'relaxers'?"

The answer is that breathing exercises that focus on increasing the speed or duration of the inhalation are "stressors." So are breath holds involving strong air hunger. These include Oxygen Advantage exercises that use breath holding to create a strong air hunger, and they include some of the techniques used by Wim Hof.

Breathing exercises designed to slow the speed and/or lengthen the duration of the exhalation are "relaxers." Breath holds involving light air hunger are relaxers. *Breathe Light* (exercise #1), with its emphasis on relaxation and light air hunger, is a relaxer. So is slow breathing, because the vagus nerve, which drives the parasympathetic nervous system (the "rest and digest" branch of the autonomic nervous system), is only activated on exhalation. This means that spending longer in the exhalation phase is beneficial to relaxation. You can read about this in detail in Chapter Four.

**Important:** Hyperventilation and breath holding are very powerful exercises designed to temporarily disrupt the body's balance to trigger adaptations. They are not suitable during pregnancy or for anyone with serious health conditions, including diabetes, sleep apnea, epilepsy, anxiety, panic disorder, or cardiovascular issues.

### #19. Box Breathing

This exercise can be used as an alternative to *Breathing Recovery, Sitting* (exercise #12). *Box Breathing* is traditionally practiced by military personnel to balance the autonomic nervous system (ANS). It is designed to create a state of relaxed alertness, getting you "in the zone." There are different versions of the exercise depending on your BOLT score.

**If your BOLT score is less than 15 seconds:**

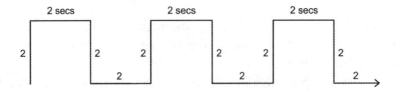

- Breathe in for 2 seconds.
- Hold for 2 seconds.
- Exhale for 2 seconds.
- Hold for 2 seconds.
- Breathe in for 2 seconds.
- And so on . . .
- Practice for 5 minutes.

**If your BOLT score is 15 seconds or more:**

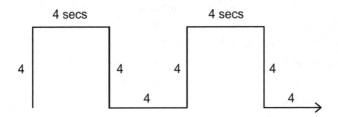

- Breathe in for 4 seconds.
- Hold for 4 seconds.
- Exhale for 4 seconds.
- Hold for 4 seconds.
- Breathe in for 4 seconds.
- And so on . . .
- Practice for 5 minutes.

### #20. Preparation for Public Speaking or Performance

You can use breathing exercises to achieve a state of flow in which your mind is relaxed and alert at the same time. I personally use the following sequence for public speaking, to enter a flow state, focus attention, and stay present.

The same exercises can be used for interviews, presentations, performance, and sport events.

Good quality sleep is imperative. Your ability to focus the mind under pressure very much begins the night before.

**To prepare the night before:**

- *Breathe Light* (exercise #1) to create air hunger for 15 minutes before sleep.
- Nasal breathe only during sleep (use MyoTape to close the lips).

**In the 30 minutes pre-speech/performance:**

## 1. Relax your mind

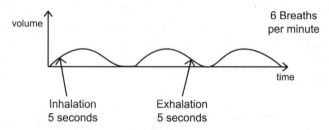

- Sit down and place your hands either side of your lower ribs.
- Close your eyes and bring your attention inward. This will also helps reenergize.
- *Breathe Light, Slow, and Deep* (exercise #4) for 5 to 10 minutes. Ideally, practice for 10 minutes.

## 2. Increase alertness

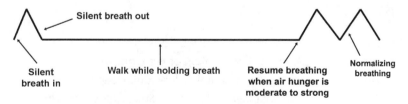

- Exhale through your nose.
- Pinch your nose with your fingers to hold your breath and walk for 10 to 50 paces while holding your breath to generate a moderate to strong air hunger.

- Stop walking.
- Breathe in through your nose and rest for 30 seconds or so while standing still.
- Repeat five times.

**This practice will allow you to move your attention out of your mind and away from racing thoughts.**

As you walk into the room to make your presentation, disperse your attention throughout your body. Take your attention out of your head. Walk into the room with every cell of your body.

During the presentation, direct some of your attention to your body, instead of having all your attention stuck inside your head.

Be aware that the feelings of breathlessness, depersonalization, and being "out of your body" that sometimes accompany performance anxiety are all just symptoms of chronic hyperventilation, not a sign that you are not up to the job!

Perform with every cell of your body.

### #21. Warm-Up for Physical Exercise

This warm-up exercise is not restricted to walking or jogging. It can be used for any sport and can be applied during continuous movement. Breath holding on the exhalation until a moderate air hunger is achieved can be incorporated into most warm-up routines. Perform five breath holds during the warm-up, with a minute or two rest in between each. It makes sense to open the airways and blood vessels, harness nasal nitric oxide, and increase oxygen delivery to the cells prior to physical exercise.

Directions:

- Move at a moderate pace for 10 to 15 minutes.
- Nose breathe only for the duration of the warm-up.
- During the warm-up, breathe light, slow, and deep.
- Take fuller breaths but fewer of them, with lateral expansion and contraction of the lower ribs.
- Exhale through your nose and pinch your nose with your fingers to hold your breath.
- Continue moving during the breath hold.

- When the feeling of air hunger is moderate, let go of your nose, and breathe through it.
- Minimize your breathing taking half of a normal breath in and out through your nose for six breaths.
- Resume normal breathing for a minute or two.
- Repeat the breath hold five times during your warm-up.

# SECTION FIVE: **STRESS AND RELAX BODY AND MIND**

## IS BREATHING TO STRESS THE BODY A GOOD IDEA?

Some of what you read in this book might seem to contradict information you may have heard in relation to other popular breathing methods. There is currently an explosion in breathwork, and several techniques have received significant coverage. This global "breath revolution" is a positive thing. The breath is a vital tool for health, performance, and self-mastery.

The interest in various kinds of breathwork is also a good thing because there is a widespread lack of knowledge about the basic principles of breathing. This is reflected in the fact 60% to 80% of adults have dysfunctional breathing patterns.[9] It is therefore worth looking at the ideas behind several types of breathing exercises to understand how they affect the body and why they may be ideal for some people but not for others.

My main purpose in addressing this subject is not to raise arguments about which breathing method is best. I am interested in discussing the importance of balance and helping you understand your options. Some breathing techniques use deliberate hyperventilation, and since the focus of this book is on reversing the harmful effects of chronic hyperventilation, I want to offer some explanation as to why these exercises can be helpful. It is my opinion that when conscious hyperventilation is practiced, it is important to balance its effect with reduced volume breathing exercises. In other words, if you up-regulate the body, it is also necessary to down-regulate. This produces the best long-term results in terms of breathing biochemistry and the function of the autonomic nervous system.

### #22. Prepare for Simulation of Altitude Training
This exercise is to be performed to a comfortable air hunger only.

The objectives are to experience a light to medium hunger for air (depending on your BOLT score) and to prepare for stronger breath holds.

#### Directions:

- Take a normal breath in and out through your nose.
- Pinch your nose to hold your breath, and walk for 10 to 15 paces.

- Stop walking and release your nose. Breathe in through your nose and resume gentle breathing in and out of your nose.
- Wait for 30 to 60 seconds and repeat.
- And again, take a normal breath in and out through your nose. Pinch your nose with your fingers and walk 10 to 15 paces while holding your breath.
- Stop walking and release your nose. Breathe in through your nose and resume gentle breathing in and out of your nose.
- Wait for 30 to 60 seconds and repeat.
- Repeat the exercise five times.

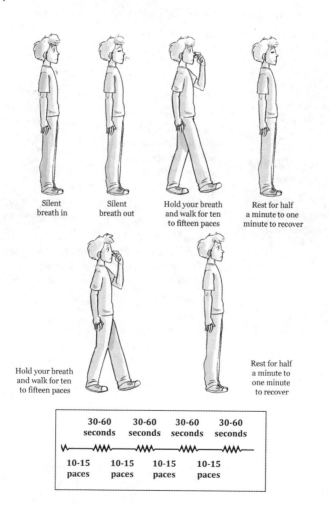

Silent breath in

Silent breath out

Hold your breath and walk for ten to fifteen paces

Rest for half a minute to one minute to recover

Hold your breath and walk for ten to fifteen paces

Rest for half a minute to one minute to recover

| 30-60 seconds | 30-60 seconds | 30-60 seconds | 30-60 seconds |
|---|---|---|---|
| 10-15 paces | 10-15 paces | 10-15 paces | 10-15 paces |

| Exercise #23:<br>Simulation of<br>Altitude Training | Exercise #24:<br>Get out of Your<br>Head | Exercise #25:<br>Rapid Fire Breaths |
|---|---|---|
| Normal Breathing, Breath Holding, Minimal Breathing | Hard Hyperventilation, Breath Holding, *Breathe Light* | Light Hyperventilation, Breath Holding, *Breathe Light* |
| Low Oxygen, High $CO_2$ | Low Oxygen, Low $CO_2$ | Low Oxygen, Normal to High $CO_2$ |
| Blood $CO_2$ increases.<br><br>Blood flow to the brain improves.<br><br>Oxygen delivery to the brain increases.<br><br>The exercises:<br>• Stress the body, reducing blood pH<br>• Stimulate the vagus nerve to increase vagal tone<br><br>*Minimal breathing* is needed for the body to recover breathing after breath holding. | Blood $CO_2$ decreases.<br><br>Because $CO_2$ drives breathing, lowering $CO_2$ in the blood means the breath can be held much longer.<br><br>As the breath is held for a significant length of time, blood oxygen saturation can drop to very low levels.<br><br>The exercises:<br>• Increase blood pH to stress the body<br>• Exercise the breathing muscles<br>• Stimulate the vagus nerve to increase vagal tone<br><br>*Breathe Light* is needed to recover and normalize blood pH after hyperventilation and breath holding | Blood $CO_2$ may decrease if breathing is fast and hard with increased minute ventilation.<br><br>During the breath hold, $CO_2$ in the blood increases, causing blood flow and oxygen delivery to the brain to increase.<br><br>The exercises:<br>• Stimulate the vagus nerve to increase vagal tone<br><br>*Breathe Light* is needed for recovery after fast breathing and breath holding. |

### #23. Simulation of Altitude Training

When you hold your breath to create a strong air hunger following a passive exhalation, several things happen.

**1. The breath hold causes a disturbance to the blood's acid-base balance.**
As the breath is held, the cells continue to extract oxygen from your blood. Meanwhile, excess $CO_2$ cannot leave the blood through your lungs. Regular practice of breath holding exposes the body to increased acidosis. This causes the body to adapt. The result is less acidity of the blood during intense exercise and a delay in the onset of fatigue.

**2. The breath hold strengthens the breathing muscles.**
This combination of high $CO_2$ (hypercapnia) and low blood oxygen saturation (hypoxia), along with the sensation of discomfort in the diaphragm, causes the respiratory center in the brain to send impulses to the breathing muscles to resume breathing to restore blood gases to normal. As the breath hold continues, these impulses increase in intensity, causing the diaphragm to contract repeatedly. In essence, the diaphragm receives a workout as it continues to contract throughout the breath hold.

**3. The body experiences "good" stress.**
When you hold your breath until a strong air hunger is experienced, you expose your body to short-term stress. This is beneficial because it causes the body to make adaptations that improve the functioning of the immune system. Breath holding also boosts mental preparedness and willpower. For athletes, it can help develop tolerance for strong feelings of breathlessness and can significantly reduce exercise-induced asthma.

When practicing this exercise, it can be motivating to wear a handheld pulse oximeter to observe your blood oxygen saturation as it lowers to between 80% and 87%. This low blood oxygen level simulates training at an altitude of 4,000 to 5,000 meters (13,000 to 16,400 feet) above sea level where the pressure of atmospheric oxygen is much less.

In my experience, most students can achieve simulation of altitude training within three to four days of practice. Progress will depend on your BOLT score, your level of fitness, and your genetic predisposition. Many students manage to simulate altitude training on their first day of practice.

The exercise causes the following effects:

- Creates a medium to strong hunger for air
- Activates the diaphragm
- Improves respiratory muscle strength
- Improves immune function
- Reduces the perception of breathlessness
- Greatly disturbs blood gases (hypoxic/hypercapnic response) to improve aerobic and anaerobic capacity
- Generates anaerobic glycolysis without the need to perform intense physical exercise
- Reduces chemosensitivity to $CO_2$
- Quietens the mind (the mind stops thinking during a stronger breath hold)
- Acts as a measure of the upper limit of breathlessness

This exercise is ONLY SUITABLE for those in good health.

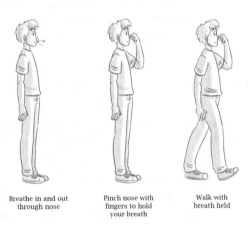

Breathe in and out
through nose

Pinch nose with
fingers to hold
your breath

Walk with
breath held

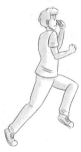

When you feel
a medium
hunger for air,
increase your pace
to a fast walk
or jog

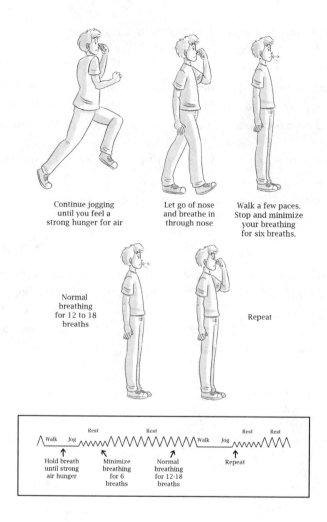

Continue jogging until you feel a strong hunger for air

Let go of nose and breathe in through nose

Walk a few paces. Stop and minimize your breathing for six breaths.

Normal breathing for 12 to 18 breaths

Repeat

## Directions:

- Take a normal breath in and out through your nose.
- Pinch your nose with your fingers to hold your breath.
- Start walking with your breath held.
- Walk faster.
- Jog.
- Jog faster.
- Relax into the muscle contractions.

- When the air hunger is moderate to strong, let go of your nose, and breathe in through the nose.
- Walk a few paces and stop.
- Practice minimal breathing for six breaths. Take very short breaths in and out of the nose. Just breathe in enough air to fill the nostrils and no more. Take hardly any air into your lungs for six breaths or so.
- And now breathe normally for 12 to 18 breaths. Allow your breathing to recover.
- Following 18 normal breaths, repeat the exercise.
- Repeat five times.

### #24. Get out of Your Head

This exercise activates the sympathetic and parasympathetic nervous system—the body's stress-balancing relaxation response. It also exercises the breathing muscles. It is to be practiced while sitting or lying down. Each set consists of three steps. **This exercise is ONLY SUITABLE for those not pregnant and in good health.**

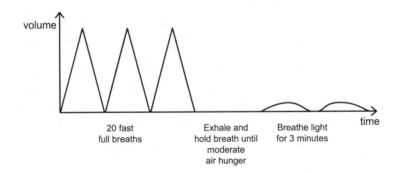

### Directions:

**Step 1:**
- Breathe a fast, full breath in and a fast, full breath out through your nose. Fill your lungs with air and exhale fast.
- Repeat 20 full breaths in and out.

**Step 2:**
- Exhale and hold the breath until you experience a medium to strong air hunger. You may want to pinch your nose with your fingers to hold the breath.

**Step 3:**
- Breathe light with air hunger for three minutes. Slow down the speed of your breathing. During the inhalation, feel hardly any air entering your nose. Allow the exhalation to be slow, prolonged, and relaxed.
- Repeat the exercise two to three times from Step 1.

### #25. Rapid Fire Breaths

This morning, while working on this chapter, I had a telephone call with Yasin Seiwasser. Yasin has been practicing martial arts and meditation for over 35 years and is a former German MMA Champion. He holds the world record for the fastest knockout of three seconds in an MMA title fight, has trained US special forces and marines, and has worked as a bodyguard for the King of Saudi Arabia. Needless to say, he knows a thing or two about self-control.

We discussed an exercise that can disrupt homeostasis (the body's state of healthy equilibrium) to "shake" the autonomic nervous system. This exercise changes the acidity of the blood by altering the concentration of blood $CO_2$. $CO_2$ fluctuates from normal to low to high (normocapnic/hypocapnic/hypercapnic). The exercise activates the two branches of the autonomic nervous system alternately and repeatedly, stimulating sympathetic, parasympathetic, sympathetic, parasympathetic (stress, relax, stress, relax), and so on. It also brings attention to the breathing and gives the respiratory muscles a workout. **This exercise is ONLY SUITABLE for those not pregnant and in good health.**

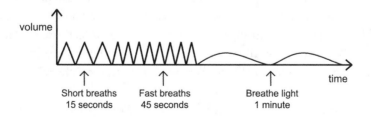

Directions:
_____

- Place your hand on your belly. Begin slowly by taking a short breath in and out through the nose. As you take each short breath in, push your belly outward. As you take each short breath out, pull your belly inward. Do this for 15 seconds.

**THEN**

- Increase the speed to a respiratory rate of up to three breaths per second. Continue breathing using the belly. Breathe as fast as you comfortably can. Do this for 45 seconds.

**THEN**

- Practice *Breathe Light* (exercise #1) with prolonged exhalations, developing the feeling of air hunger. Do this for 1 minute.

Practice three rounds of the fast breathing for one minute followed by light breathing for one minute.

Then sit still for three minutes and let the energy flow. Observe your breath and thoughts without interference. This will help activate your parasympathetic nervous system.

Recap: One minute fast breathing, one minute light breathing, one minute fast breathing, one minute light breathing, one minute fast breathing, one minute light breathing. Sit still for three minutes.

## THE HEALTH BENEFITS OF HORMETIC STRESS

In much of this book you will find practices to reduce stress, reduce stress hormones, and relax the body and mind. You will also find many descriptions of the potential negative effects stress can have on the body in terms of health, inflammation, cardiovascular disease, and even how long you live.

However, some breathing exercises are designed to activate the body's stress response for the purposes of good health. To understand this, it is necessary to examine the benefits of these methods and the difference between "types" of stress.

First, let's clarify what stress is. Stress is the disruption of equilibrium (homeostasis) in the body. It is something that puts your systems off-balance.

The type of stress involved in these breathing techniques is called *hormetic stress*, or *hormesis*. Hormesis is a way of using stress to your advantage because stress triggers adaptations in the body, and this can be harnessed for positive effect. For instance, when you work out, you need to "damage" your muscles so that your body will rebuild them. Over time, this causes your muscles to become stronger.

Hormetic stress can be introduced using breathing techniques. Although breathing techniques using this concept have recently become popular, this is not a new idea. Ancient breathing practices have a lot to teach us when it comes to stimulating adaptations in the body via the disruption of homeostasis.

### The Balance of Opposites

One concept universally found in traditional yoga breathing (Pranayama and Tibetan yoga breathing) is the balance of opposites.

This ancient principle is relevant today. These are breathing techniques that:

- Use large, slow, full breaths.
- Involve very fast mouth breathing.
- Focus on keeping the breath to a minimum.
- Involve not breathing at all for periods of time.

As with different strands of yoga, these methods can attract followers who are almost evangelical in their approach. This can make it hard to work out which method is "right." The answer is, used correctly, they all are.

This book is not about yoga breathing, but it is relevant. Traditional Pranayama, which is the yogic practice of breath control, teaches that to master our breathing, we must develop great flexibility and adaptability. This means being able to switch from small to large breaths, very fast or very slow, using the mouth or the nose. For example, some breathing techniques limit us to a very small amount of air, reducing the normal volume of air inhaled by as much as 10 times. Others require that we breathe a volume of air almost 20 times greater than normal.

To illustrate these differences, let's take a look at two ancient breathing techniques. One is from traditional Pranayama and the other from Tibet. These exercises use hyperventilation balanced with breath holds and slow breathing. This moderates the impact on the levels of $CO_2$ in the blood and maximizes the oxygenation of cells and organs.

### 1. Bhastrika (Indian Yogic Breathing)

*Bhastrika* is a classic Pranayama technique also known as the *Bellows Breath* and sometimes called the *Breath of Fire*. It uses complete, full breaths in rapid succession (as many as 60 breaths per minute for a total of 100 breaths),[10] which means it is a hyperventilation technique. After one minute of hyperventilation, the student holds the breath on a full inhale for as long as possible to balance the discharge of $CO_2$ that occurs during the fast breathing. This extended breath hold is followed by a long, slow exhalation, which is repeated several times before returning to the start of the exercise with the fast breathing. The whole practice is completed using only nasal breathing. The hyperventilation phase of this breathing practice works on biochemistry, reducing $CO_2$ and alkalizing the body. It also works on biomechanics, massaging the internal organs in the abdomen with the diaphragm. Perhaps more important, it affects the autonomic nervous system, activating both the sympathetic and parasympathetic branches, stress balanced by relaxation. In this way, the practice triggers adaptations in the body that allow the body to better maintain balance in its systems under stress.[11]

### 2. Tum-mo Breathing (Tibetan Pranayama)

Tum-mo breathing is based on slow breathing and breath holds. Reduced slow breathing following hyperventilation is also used. The practice is characterized by a technique called "vase breathing," which is accompanied by static contraction of the muscles in the abdomen and pelvis during a breath hold after inhalation. Today a variation of this practice has been made popular by the work of the Iceman, Wim Hof, and his Wim Hof Method.

There are at least two types of Tum-mo practice, *Forceful Breath* and *Gentle Breath*. These two types differ in terms of the breathing technique involved and in their goals. Although both are based on vase breathing, one is forceful and vigorous while the other is gentle and without strain.

Scientists have proven that Tum-mo breathing produces heat in the body[12-14] (a process called thermogenesis), a side effect of the practice that is useful in colder climates like that of Tibet. The goal of *Forceful Breath* is to raise "psychic heat" while *Gentle Breath* is designed to maintain it.

It is physically difficult to use the complex *Forceful Breath* technique for extended periods or while walking around. In Tibetan monasteries, *Gentle Breath* is used during a ceremony that involves drying wet sheets. The sheets are draped around the bodies of the monks who practice Tum-mo to raise their body temperature, sometimes by as much as 17° Fahrenheit, causing the sheets to dry.[15, 16] Like *Bhastrika*, Tum-mo breathing is practiced using only nasal breathing.

## HORMETIC BREATHING PRACTICE FOR MODERN LIFE

Leonardo Pelagotti is an Oxygen Advantage instructor based in Paris, France. He was a national-level gymnast for 15 years and achieved a black belt in Kung-fu Shaolin after just five years of practice. Since 2017, he has been an instructor of the Wim Hof method, a practice that combines meditation, breathing exercises, and exposure to cold to regulate stress levels. He works closely with the method's founder, Wim Hof, and has trained hundreds of people to overcome their fears and mental limitations. Leonardo is also an Oxygen Advantage Master Instructor. He has a scientific background that enables him to understand and teach the processes behind these hormetic breathing techniques and to apply them to modern living.

One of the fundamental principles in this book is the reduction of sensitivity to $CO_2$ in the blood. This is achieved by means of exercises that down-regulate breathing to counteract hyperventilation. If you use techniques that involve deliberate hyperventilation, the secret is to balance your breathing practice. Leo explains:

> Exercises to elevate carbon dioxide and balance breathing are especially important for anyone who practices deliberate hyperventilation techniques. If this is not done, you will experience an increase in sensitivity to $CO_2$, which is the opposite of what we want to achieve.
>
> In exercises involving hard and fast breathing, such as Wim Hof breathing, for instance, if you don't practice any exercises to raise levels of carbon dioxide (reduced breathing and breath holds), sensitivity to $CO_2$ increases and the result is a faster breathing rate and an increased responsiveness to $CO_2$, which manifests as breathlessness.

To create and maintain physiological balance, different breathing techniques must be used to move within the full spectrum of breathing. This means that you become able to manipulate levels of oxygen and $CO_2$ in your blood so that they are high, low, or normal.

In Pranayama, many exercises exist and these all have different purposes and benefits.[10] In the same way, the reduced breathing techniques in the Oxygen Advantage can be integrated with well-known hypercapnic/hyperventilation techniques like Sudarshan Kriya, Holotropic Breathwork®, Tum-mo breathing, and the Wim Hof method.

The Oxygen Advantage provides a way to "dose" the activation of the stress and relaxation responses correctly to benefit from both without potentially causing tolerance to $CO_2$ to suffer. This allows for the perfect balance in your breathing practice, in which you can up-regulate and down-regulate your autonomic nervous system and breathing biochemistry at will.

## THE PRACTICE

What Leo suggests is a concept linked to hormetic stress using breathing exercises that work along the three dimensions of breathing patterns:[17]

1. The biochemical dimension—alters $CO_2$ levels in the blood from normal to low to high (normocapnic to hypocapnic to hypercapnic).
2. The psychological dimension—activates both the sympathetic and parasympathetic nervous systems.
3. The biomechanical dimension—practices both deep and shallow breathing.

### #26. Hormetic Exercise 1: CATANA Breathing

This breathing exercise takes its name from its dual action on the metabolism—catabolic (CAT) and anabolic (ANA). It isn't necessary to understand what these terms mean, only that the practice is a form of hormetic breathing. Its objective is to disrupt homeostasis to promote adaptations in the body that, in turn, will lead to a stronger physiological balance. CATANA is a breathwork training based on a hypo/hyperventilation equilibrium—a balancing of underbreathing and overbreathing. This technique fosters physical regeneration and mental calmness.

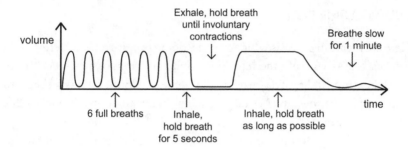

### Directions:

- First, perform six full breaths, inhaling slow and deep from the diaphragm, up through the ribs, and finally to the chest. Inhale only through the nose, without friction or force. After each inhalation, exhale through your nose. Begin each exhalation by simply relaxing your belly, then your chest.
- After these six breaths, inhale and hold your breath for five seconds with full lungs. Release on the exhalation, naturally letting the exhaled breath out.
- Hold your breath after the exhale. At the first diaphragmatic contractions, resume breathing as follows . . .
- Take a deep and slow inhale, and, at the top, hold your breath again for as long as possible. During this phase, contract your pelvic floor muscles and bring your navel in toward your spine.
- When you can't hold your breath any longer, exhale as slowly as possible and resume breathing as slowly as you can for about one minute.
- Repeat the entire exercise up to five times.
- When you are comfortable with the exercise, you can add a final element to finish. This element integrates the exercise on a psycho-physiological level. As you breathe in and out in a natural and

uncontrolled way, imagine energy entering and recharging your body on each inhalation and imagine debris leaving your body for each exhalation.

## FINDING YOUR PACE

There are breathing exercises for everyone. Some people feel a lot better when they practice Wim Hof's method. Some find a program of hyperventilation, breath holding, and recovery exercises extremely helpful. Others feel benefit from slow breathing exercises or practicing many small breath holds while sitting or walking.

Ultimately, the foundation of breathwork is restoring functional breathing patterns with normal biochemistry and biomechanics. Without this, a crucial piece is missing from the puzzle. Regardless of the breathing method you prefer, always remember that healthy breathing for humans, whatever your age or state of health, is in and out through the nose, Light, Slow, and Deep.

This story from a fellow Irishman Niall Donnelly, who lives in California, illustrates the point that sometimes the people who are most driven to succeed and achieve are the very same people who find the greatest relief from slowing down and reducing the breath.

Niall has a full, demanding life. He's the CEO of a tech company and has children to keep him busy. He began meditating four or five years ago to stave off stress, but found his mental chatter made it difficult. Instead, he doubled up his daily physical exercise and, with a little meditation thrown in, that kept him feeling good for a couple of years. But, as life happened and stress levels grew, he found his anxiety ramping up to the point where he began experiencing panic attacks. He was determined not to go down the route of medicating and decided to study and test as many methods as he could to see what did and did not work for him. He tried many breathing techniques, from Pranayama to Wim Hof, Kundalini, Tum-mo, and more besides. He says:

> I for one was more enamored with the more "glamorous" techniques in my early days. It's like the whole yoga community worldwide following their guru's and not questioning whether the breathing

techniques are good for them or not, it doesn't make sense. I found them all very interesting and they all brought pretty deep experiential and emotional release experiences. Especially the more mouth-driven hyperventilation ones, which I initially spent most of the time doing. But something deep inside me kept saying, "Something's not right here." I started to feel like the techniques couldn't be good for my heart or my brain, and the fact my fingers and toes were getting cold indicated that the practice was doing the reverse of everything I thought I knew about taking deep breaths to oxygenate my body. At this stage, I began to experience more panic again. So one day I just stopped the harder breathing. I listened to my heart and my gut and then just lay in my meditation room and did six breaths a minute for 40 minutes. Then I came out and said to my wife: "This feels good. Something is telling me to slow my life down and slow my breath down and I need to listen to this." I then started bringing six breaths a minute into my day as much as I could and within days, I could feel a change. I'm a very energetic guy with a lot of demands, but everything started to slow down. I'm convinced that light breathing and $CO_2$ tolerance training have the power to shift humanity because overbreathing is making us all physically and mentally ill.

The lesson in this story is simple. You may find that hyperventilation breathing techniques work for you, especially if you balance them with light breathing. But, if they don't, don't push yourself to practice them. Focus instead on exercises that make you feel well, even if they seem less glamorous and exciting. Listen to your body and it will thank you.

Niall and I talked again recently as I was preparing the final manuscript for this book. He told me he had been practicing a humming technique and noticed positive changes to his sleep and his heart rate variability.

I've been testing all sorts of things sleep related for a few months, but the best thing I've found is breathing light mixed with humming before sleep. In bed, before sleep, I take a small breath in through my nose (around 60% or 70% of my normal breathing volume) and then hum the exhale out. I repeat this cycle for 10 minutes. On every third or fourth breath, I hold my breath for 3 seconds at the end of the exhalation. I wear an Oura Ring at night (see Chapter Four), and this past week it's showing very clear signs of increased HRV, lower resting heart rate and reduced respiratory rate overnight. I am also getting more deep sleep, better REM cycles, and around 15% more sleep. I'm falling asleep faster and staying asleep throughout the night in a better way.

Humming has been part of my meditations for a few years, but I only tried it before sleep about a week ago. I'm pretty blown away by how helpful it is. I even have fewer crazy, vivid dreams when I hum, where normally I'm a jumpy, nightmarish person.

The other great thing I find with humming is it helps me extend my nasal exhalation. Otherwise, I kind of struggle with this after doing a small inhalation. Maybe the extra nitric oxide from humming has something to do with a better sleep? Interesting to think about.

Niall is quite right. It is now widely understood that nitric oxide facilitates sleep, particularly non-rapid eye movement sleep, and is intimately connected to sleep homeostasis.

## SECTION SIX: **EXERCISES FOR CHILDREN**

These children's exercises provide excellent tools with which to restore healthy breathing patterns in even quite small children. Information about identifying dysfunctional breathing in your child and ideas to motivate young people to engage with the practice can be found in Chapter Eight on children's breathing.

## 1. MOUSE BREATHING

Children sometimes find it difficult to understand the concept of reduced breathing exercises, so breathing reeducation in children requires a creative, playful approach. The last thing you want is for breathing practice to become a stressful chore. Teaching through stories is generally an excellent way to ensure that children engage with and remember the techniques. I find the following story about a cat and mouse works well, especially when it's necessary to remind your child to reduce their breathing throughout the day.

Sit quietly with your child, somewhere you won't be disturbed. Ask the child to relax and to drop their shoulders. Next, ask the child to pretend to be a little mouse. You get to play at being a big, hungry cat. This hungry cat has very good hearing and is listening carefully for the mouse's breathing. Your child (the mouse) must see how quietly they can breathe so the cat doesn't hear them. This is not a breath-holding exercise. The little mouse must be clever and continue to breathe. If the cat cannot hear the mouse's breathing, the mouse will be left alone, but if the cat hears so much as a sniff, it will chase the mouse.

Using the cat and mouse story, follow these instructions with your child:

- Ask your child to sit down with good posture.
- Now, it's time to relax and become as soft and wobbly as jelly.
- Place a finger under your child's nose to monitor airflow.
- Next, the child should try to breathe so gently that the breathing is silent, with no movement from the chest or tummy.
- This reduction in breathing will create a feeling of air hunger. Your child will experience an urge to take big breaths. Encourage them

to keep their breathing soft (so the cat does not hear them), maintaining the air shortage for the duration of the exercise.

- Perform the exercise several times, for one to two minutes each time.

## 2. STEPS EXERCISE FOR CHILDREN

Children and teenagers can get a lot from the *Steps Exercise*. It can also be used to measure progress. The *Steps Exercise* is simple and requires the child to hold the breath during walking, jogging, or running.

**Precautions:** If the child, teen, or adult has pulmonary hypertension, epilepsy, or any serious medical condition, you **must not** practice the *Steps Exercise*. People with pulmonary hypertension should not practice this exercise because holding the breath to reach a strong air hunger will cause a temporary increase in blood pressure.

If you or your child has diabetes, be aware that breath-hold exercises can lower blood sugar levels. Take a snack before practicing the exercise and monitor blood sugar levels frequently during the *Steps*.

If your child is wheezy or coughing, limit the *Steps Exercise* to between 10 and 20 paces. The *Steps Exercise* will help improve asthma and reduce the child's symptoms, but it is important that breathing at the end of the exercise remains controlled. Heavy breathing after a breath hold can exacerbate symptoms.

### BEGINNERS' STEPS

Small children (four to six years) can be introduced to the *Steps Exercise* by walking a short distance of only five paces or so with the breath held. It can be useful to ask another adult or an older sibling to help. You can then stand at either end of the walking distance so that the child can walk back and forth from one helper to the other.

Adult one   →   Distance of five paces   →   Adult two

Before your child begins the exercise, place a piece of paper tape across his or her lips. This will ensure that the child breathes nasally. Alternatively,

I have designed a special tape called MyoTape which is a great tool for teaching nasal breathing. It is suitable and specifically sized for children and is available from MyoTape.com. The tape does not cover the lips. Instead, it safely surrounds the mouth, eliminating any anxiety that may come from taping the mouth and allowing the child to talk and take a sip of water whenever they need to.

### Here's how to do the Steps:

- To begin the exercise, breathe in and out gently through your nose.
- After an exhalation, pinch your nostrils closed with your fingers to hold the breath.
- With the breath held, walk the five-pace distance between your two helpers.
- Let go of the nose and resume gentle nasal breathing.
- Wait for between 30 and 60 seconds and repeat the exercise.

## ADVANCED STEPS

When you have established that the child is able to hold his or her breath over a short distance, gradually increase the number of paces. You can do this by lengthening the distance between the two helpers. Or you can keep the five-pace distance and have the child walk back and forth several times before releasing the breath, like swimming laps underwater. It is important to find out how many steps the child can achieve. This is determined by asking the child to gradually take more steps with the breath held until a strong air hunger is felt.

After the breath hold, the breath must be taken in through the nose. The breathing must also be calmed immediately. The first breath after the exercise will usually be bigger than normal. Make sure that your child reduces or suppresses the second and third breaths to keep the breathing gentle. You can combine this exercise with the cat and mouse story, reminding the child to breathe like a little mouse so that the big cat cannot hear them when they release the breath hold.

The *Steps Exercise* should be performed six times per set, with about 30 seconds or a minute's rest between each repetition. Sets of *Steps* are to be practiced two to three times per day. Count the *Steps* out loud and record your child's score so that progress can be monitored from week to week. Compare each week's *Steps* with the previous scores to evaluate improvement, and encourage your child to increase the number of *Steps* they take. You could work this into a star chart and motivate your child with rewards. The *Steps Exercise* can also be incorporated into other activities such as skipping or running.

## IMPORTANT INFORMATION

Young children have a relatively strong response to the buildup of $CO_2$ in the blood, although this will lessen as they get older. With this in mind, the *Steps Exercise* should be adapted according to the child's age. Children aged between five and seven should aim to achieve 50 to 60 paces during *Steps*. For children aged between eight and nine years, the goal is to reach 60 to 70 paces. And for children aged ten and over, 80 paces is optimal.

Be mindful of your child's breathing throughout the day. If at any time you can hear your child breathing, or see them breathing with their mouth open, remind them to breathe gently through the nose with their tongue in the roof of the mouth. Ensure that your child does not let any air sneak in through the mouth. This too can be made into a game, reinforcing the importance of keeping the mouth closed by telling off the "sneaky" air for trying to get in.

Children have short attention spans, so games can really help. If your child becomes bored with practicing the exercises, you can replace the *Steps* with breath holding while playing, jogging, running, hopscotch, performing jumping jacks, or jumping on a trampoline.

Breath-hold exercises such as the *Steps* can be very effective for decongesting the nose. However, if your child continues to feel an air hunger after six repetitions of the *Steps Exercise*, there may be an obstruction at the back of the nose due to enlarged adenoids. There is much detailed information about this in Chapter Eight on children's breathing.

## USING MOUTH TAPE TO RESTORE NASAL BREATHING

It may be useful to place tape across the child's lips during the *Steps Exercise*. This will help you ascertain how comfortable nasal breathing is for the child after doing the exercise. Holding the breath to achieve a strong air hunger has no reported risks for healthy children, and, as I discovered in the course of my teaching, taping to bring the lips together is an invaluable tool in breathing reeducation.

During my work with children and parents, I occasionally encountered a child who persistently breathed through an open mouth, no matter how many times we emphasized the importance of nose breathing. In most cases, these children were able to unblock their noses by practicing the *Steps*, so it became apparent that their habit of mouth breathing was not due to a nasal obstruction. The parents would feel as if they were constantly nagging to no avail, the child would become frustrated and upset by the constant pressure to breathe through the nose, and I couldn't figure out why this mouth breathing habit continued despite all our combined efforts. Then I began working much more with lip tape, ensuring that the children wore paper tape across their lips for periods during the day. This simple but profoundly effective technique was a game changer, resulting in an immediate improvement in nasal breathing habits for those children.

If the idea of taping your child's mouth seems profoundly alien to you, it's worth looking at the research. A new study published in 2020 explored the effectiveness of lip tape as an objective tool to assess nasal breathing.[19] The study was to find out if tolerance to lip taping could be used to identify people at risk of mouth breathing. The test involved having participants breathe nasally for three minutes with the mouth taped. Researchers wanted to find out whether mouth taping could be used to discover if the cause of mouth breathing was anatomical or habitual. This is not possible with traditional methods, especially when the patient is unaware of problems with nasal breathing. It is particularly challenging in children who may not be able to articulate that they are struggling to breathe through the nose.

As the study's authors state, the establishment of full-time nasal breathing is now appreciated as "the single most important objective in securing adequate craniofacial and airway development in children."

The study involved 633 participants, including 315 children aged between 3 and 11 years. Researchers discovered something interesting. Most participants with self-reported mouth breathing or moderate to severe difficulty nasal breathing were still able to comfortably breathe through the nose for at least three minutes. More than 80% of participants who mouth breathed almost all of the time while awake were able to pass the lip-taping test.[19] This is consistent with earlier studies, which indicate that mouth breathing can persist after a nasal obstruction has been removed. That underlines the importance of breathing reeducation in reestablishing nasal breathing.

An easy way to ensure consistent and ongoing nasal breathing is to ask your child to wear medical grade paper tape or MyoTape around their lips for at least half an hour each day. It is helpful to combine this with an activity that distracts the child, such as reading, watching TV, or playing on a tablet or phone. You may also have to engage in some good old-fashioned bargaining. For example, you may find it helpful to allow screen time on the condition that your child wears the MyoTape.

If you still have reservations, you can see for yourself how MyoTape works, still allowing the child to speak. Simply search for my free children's breathing program on YouTube where you will find my daughter, Lauren, modeling the lip tape.

The best approach when helping children to improve their breathing habits is to be consistent and patient. The idea that it takes 21 days to form or change a habit is unrealistic and outdated. Scientists have found that, on average, a new habit takes 66 days to build, and it can even take as long as 254 days[20]. This time is necessary for new neural connections to establish and for breathing behavior to change. If you are trying to change your own breathing habits, you will need to be equally patient.

If you would like to explore further ways to explain the concept of breathing light and the *Steps Exercise* to your child, many people have found my book *Buteyko Meets Dr. Mew* to be a useful aid in teaching children and teenagers about breathing through full-color comic book storytelling.

- Ask your child to wear MyoTape across the lips for at least half an hour each day. It is best to do this when the child is distracted.
- Use games to introduce the techniques to small children. Be as creative as you like!
- Start by practicing the *Steps Exercise* for beginners.
- Practice the *Steps* while walking, jogging, or running. Do this for six repetitions, two to three times a day.

As you will discover in Chapter Eight on children's breathing, children can benefit enormously from breathing exercises that promote nasal breathing and help prevent sleep-disordered breathing. I believe passionately that this is absolutely vital for each child to reach their full potential. This is why my children's breathing program will always be free of charge. You can find a wealth of free tutorial videos on YouTube by searching for "*Patrick McKeown Children.*"

# CHAPTER THREE
# HOW TO BREATHE

---

In texts about the anatomy and physiology of breathing, the respiratory tract is described as the path[14] for air to travel from the nose to the lungs. The mouth doesn't get a mention for one simple reason: despite common habits and preconceptions, our bodies are designed for nasal breathing. It has been said that breathing through the mouth is like eating through the nose.

I was a habitual mouth-breather throughout my childhood and into my early twenties. For all that time, I completely bypassed my nose. Little did I know that the development of the lower half of the face and jaw is largely influenced by whether the mouth is open or closed during the formative years of childhood. Prolonged mouth breathing even altered the structure of my face, resulting in a smaller nasal airway, high upper palate, underdeveloped jaw, and crooked teeth.

Although mouth breathing is a distortion of an intrinsic bodily function, it is incredibly common. A 2008 study of 370 randomly selected children between three and nine years old, all from Abaeté, Brazil, found that 55% were mouth breathers.[1] In 2010, a Portuguese study examined the incidence of mouth breathing in children aged between six and nine. The results of 496 parental questionnaires revealed that nearly 57% of the children breathed through their mouths.[2] The frequency of mouth breathing among adults receives less attention, but one 2016 paper of more than 9,000 people from a town in Japan reported that 17% breathed through their mouths.[3]

As we'll see, mouth breathing doesn't just disrupt the growth of the face and teeth. It is also a significant factor in a variety of problems, ranging from obstructive sleep apnea to high blood pressure, a reduced quality of life and fatigue.[4–9]

## WHAT'S SO GREAT ABOUT
## BREATHING THROUGH THE NOSE?

Nasal breathing performs at least 30 functions on behalf of the body.[10] One of the most important of these is oxygenating the blood, organs, and cells. Because the nostrils are significantly smaller than the mouth, nose breathing while awake creates about 50% more resistance to airflow than mouth breathing. This results in a 10% to 20% greater oxygen uptake in the blood.[11, 12] Breathing through the nose filters and warms the air before it enters the lungs, and the resistance created by nasal breathing makes the breathing slower and deeper, engaging the diaphragm and calming the mind.[13]

Contrary to the advice of many sports coaches, it is not a good idea to breathe in through the nose and out through the mouth. In one study where subjects were instructed to breathe that way, nasal stuffiness increased by 200%. What's more, congestion persisted for 10 minutes after the challenge ended.[14] Even during only exhaling, mouth breathing causes the loss of heat and water. To be precise, 42% more water is lost when exhaling through the mouth than through the nose.[15] This loss of moisture and warmth causes inflammation, stuffiness, and dehydration—which makes breathing more difficult. Once your nose is blocked, you can find yourself needing to breathe through your mouth, and so mouth breathing can become a habit.

It is best to breathe both in and out through the nose. This not only facilitates oxygenation, it also helps prevent nasal congestion. When your nose is clear, breathing is easier during both rest and exercise. It may sound contradictory that nasal breathing helps clear your nose. After all, most people breathe through their mouth because their nose is blocked. However, when your nose is blocked, the counterintuitive act of breathing through the nostrils helps keep the airways clear, prevents dehydration, and improves breathing volume.

When you inhale or exhale through the nose, breathing is slower due to the extra resistance created by the smaller airway. This resistance to exhaling in nasal breathing helps maintain lung volume.[16] Even after maximum exhalation, there is always some air left in the lungs. This air is called residual volume. When the nose is blocked, forcing mouth breathing, total lung capacity and residual volume both decrease significantly.

To understand why this residual volume is important, think about inflating a balloon.[17] The most difficult part is blowing the initial volume of air to get the balloon going. However, if you allow an inflated balloon to deflate just partway, it is much easier to reinflate it than when you let all of the air escape.

In the same way, if your lungs were completely emptied of air after every exhalation, breathing would require more effort, the lungs would collapse, and strenuous activity would be impossible. Every time you exhale through your mouth, you may breathe out more air than necessary. That means that every inhalation takes extra effort. Breathing becomes much harder work than it needs to be.

During nasal breathing, several things happen differently than they do during mouth breathing:

- When breathing through the nose, the lungs can extract oxygen from the air during *both* exhalation and inhalation.[18] Although the oxygen supply to the air sacs in the lungs is renewed during the inhalation, oxygen diffuses continuously into the blood,[18] because the small size of the nostrils helps create a flow of air back into the lungs even during nasal exhalation.
- The slower nasal exhalation gives the lungs more time to extract the oxygen. When this optimal blood gas exchange occurs, carbon dioxide ($CO_2$) is processed properly, and blood pH remains balanced.
- Air inhaled through the nose passes through the nasal mucosa. This stimulates reflex nerves that control regular breathing.[19, 20] (One reason mouth breathing can lead to snoring, sleep apnea, and irregular breathing patterns is that it bypasses this nasal mucosa.)
- The air passes through the nose, which houses the olfactory bulbs. Those are connected to the hypothalamus, the part of the brain linked to many automatic functions such as heartbeat, blood pressure, appetite, thirst, and homeostasis.
- In nasal breathing, the sinuses produce nitric oxide (NO), which is necessary for regulating inflammation in the airways and in the body's defense against airborne pathogens, viruses, and bacteria.

## NASAL NITRIC OXIDE: THE WINNING ELEMENT

While the link between $CO_2$ and blood oxygenation was demonstrated as far back as 1904 in the research of the Danish biochemist Christian Bohr, it was not until much later that the role of nitric oxide was fully understood. In fact, NO was considered a toxic gas. This small and simple molecule[22] was associated, along with nitrogen dioxide, with environmental pollution, acid rain, car exhaust fumes, and the smog found in overpopulated industrial cities. The presence of NO in the exhaled breath of humans[23] was not shown until 1991. In 1992, nitric oxide was named "Molecule of the Year" by *Science* magazine,[24] and in 1995, it was discovered that the gas is produced in the nasal cavity and paranasal sinuses, a group of four air-filled spaces surrounding the nose. The concentration of NO originating from the nose is 100 times higher than in the lower airways.[25]

The paranasal sinuses have a variety of important functions. They humidify and warm inhaled air and make our speech more resonant. They also lighten the head and protect vital structures in the event of facial trauma. These sinuses are positioned around the nose and release nitric oxide[26] into the nasal airways as we inhale through the nose.[27] According to Jon Lundberg, a professor of NO Pharmacologics at Sweden's Karolinska Institute, large amounts of NO are constantly being released into the nasal airways as we breathe. Every time a breath is taken in through the nose, NO follows the airflow down into the lungs, where it opens the airways[28] and increases oxygen uptake by the blood.

When we breathe, air travels into the lungs, reaching the alveoli—the small air sacs where gas exchange occurs and oxygen is absorbed from the air into the blood. The ratio of air-to-blood that reaches the alveoli every minute is called the *ventilation-perfusion ratio*. Ventilation refers to the air we breathe, perfusion to the flow of blood to the small air sacs in the lungs. Ideally, enough oxygen should reach the bloodstream to fully saturate the blood. However, two factors can cause an imbalance where the upper parts of the lungs receive more air while the lower parts receive more blood. These are mouth breathing and gravity. When this ventilation-perfusion mismatch occurs, the body is less able to use the oxygen in the lungs, resulting in poor oxygenation.

NO facilitates a significantly more efficient balance of perfusion to ventilation, as shown in the diagram.

How does it do this? Nitric oxide has vasodilatory properties; that is, it prompts the blood vessels in the lungs (and other places) to relax, opening them up for stronger blood flow. When you inhale through the nose, NO is carried down into the lungs where it helps redistribute the blood more evenly. This counteracts the negative effect that gravity can have on blood flow in the lungs.[29] Mouth breathing not only causes the shallow, fast breathing shown in the first picture (below), it also bypasses nasal nitric oxide altogether.

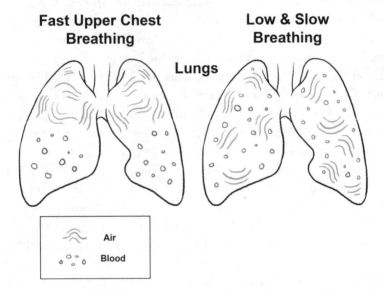

A 2017 article concluded that nitric oxide is instrumental in many additional aspects of respiratory function, including bronchial smooth muscle tone, pulmonary blood flow, mucus output, and other processes, such as antioxidant homeostasis, lung development,[22] and local host defense.

In particular, NO is key to the production of a vital substance called surfactant. Pulmonary surfactant, produced in the lungs, is a complex mixture of specific lipids, proteins, and carbohydrates. It decreases surface tension in the alveoli, facilitates the uptake of oxygen into the blood, prevents lung collapse and edema, and is vital to the elasticity of the lungs. This is often illustrated by a comparison with washing-up liquid between two panes of glass. The soap allows the two panes to move freely over each other. In the lungs, surfactant allows easier breathing with less friction and is fundamental to our ability to breathe air.[22, 30] Nitric oxide controls the production of surfactants and maintains surfactant function. That is why the gas is often used in treating premature babies.[31]

## A FIRST LINE OF DEFENSE

In 1999, Lundberg and Weitzberg reported that nitric oxide inhibits the growth of various pathogens, including bacteria and viruses. This suggests that NO in the nasal airways could serve to help protect the body from infection.[27] As the world battles the unprecedented global pandemic caused by the COVID-19 coronavirus, the relationship between NO and respiratory infection takes on new relevance. Research in the wake of the first SARS virus had found that NO acts to keep the sinuses sterile.[32] It is also thought that the very low levels of nasal nitric oxide in people with cystic fibrosis and Kartagener's syndrome might play a part in their increased vulnerability to respiratory infections.

A 2013 paper, "Evidence for the Cure of Flu through Nose Breathing," reported that nasal breathing benefits patients with flu.[33] This is consistent with previous studies that showed NO has "opposing effects" in infections including pneumonia and flu.[34] A 2009 laboratory experiment found that NO inhibited the replication of SARS in two ways. In fact, NO inhibits the replication of a variety of viruses.[35] While the 2009 study didn't specifically use nasal nitric oxide, earlier research into the common cold had found that we produce more NO in the nose and airways when the human rhinovirus is present, which suggested that NO may be the body's way to help clear viruses.[36]

A wave of clinical trials during the 2020 pandemic has continued to explore the antiviral properties of nitric oxide. Research teams all over the world have studied inhaled NO for the treatment of COVID-19.[37-39] Scientists theorized that high concentrations of inhaled NO, when administered in the early stages of the infection, would have a viricidal effect and prevent progression to a more severe form of the illness. Research also hypothesized that NO might reduce the severity of the illness and patients' recovery time.

In June 2020, a company in Canada began phase II clinical trials of a nitric oxide nasal spray in the fight against COVID-19.[40] Speaking to the *Globe and Mail* in April 2020, Dr. Chris Miller, chief science officer at SaNOtize Research and Development Corp. said the product is, "Much like hand sanitizer for the nose." Before the pandemic, Dr. Miller and his colleagues had been developing the spray as a treatment for chronic sinusitis, but research indicating that NO prevents the novel coronavirus from replicating caused them to redirect their efforts.[41] The spray is intended to limit the spread of the virus, especially among healthcare workers treating patients with COVID-19.

One scientific article suggests that therapies designed to increase the levels of NO, such as gas inhalation, could improve oxygenation and boost overall health in patients with COVID-19. Significantly, this article also points to lifestyle factors that reduce NO in the airways, especially mouth breathing and smoking. The researchers argue that combining nasal breathing and good quality sleep with a healthy lifestyle could help decrease viral load.[39]

The same article mentions anecdotal evidence that taping the mouth during sleep reduces common colds. This may be due to the humidifying and filtering effects of the nose. It is also thought that the increase in NO in the airways may reduce viral load during sleep and give the immune system a boost. The article reports that mouth breathing, whether constant or intermittent, may reduce the benefits of NO, leading to "unobstructed viral replication." It concluded that "mouth breathing during sleep may therefore worsen the symptoms of COVID-19."[39]

COVID-19 presents a serious challenge. Apart from the fact that humans have no immunity to this virus, it behaves very differently from flu, has a high viral load, and is poorly understood. What is known is that it attacks a specific type of cell known as a type 2 pneumocyte.[42] Type 2 pneumocyte cells are responsible for the production and secretion of surfactant. (If you recall, NO plays an important role in production of surfactant.) This is one reason why the virus can be deadly, even in young, healthy patients.

It is important to remember that nasal nitric oxide cannot do its job (or protect you from disease) unless you breathe through your nose. Nasal breathing alone will increase the amount of NO in the airways, but research has found that humming can produce even higher levels of nitric oxide.[43] One 2015 study reports that humming produces seven times more NO than normal exhalation.[44] It is believed that oscillations in the air accelerate the exchange of gases between the nasal cavity and sinuses.[45] Another paper discovered that "strong" humming was effective in treating chronic rhinosinusitis, a fungal condition that causes inflammation and infection in the nasal passages. Again, NO was identified, this time as an antifungal agent.[46] Other research has found that the concentration of nasal nitric oxide also increases during breath holding. One study comparing scuba divers to breath-holding divers reported higher levels of circulating NO in the breath-holding group.[47]

## BREATHING WITH A FACE MASK

During the 2020 coronavirus outbreak, debate has raged over the wearing of protective face masks—whether masks lessen viral spread, protect the wearer, or prevent the wearer from passing the virus to others. Many people argue that the measure is ineffective. Others complain that they find it difficult to breathe when wearing a mask. Whatever the arguments, studies have definitively proven that masks prevent infected people from making others sick.[48]

A 2020 article in the *Harvard Business Review* suggests that better masks are needed to fully protect against virus-containing particles.[49] A study from 2003 explores the use of nasal plugs instead of face masks but points out that it is necessary to "only breathe through the nostrils, as breathing through the mouth will nullify the protection offered by the nasal plug."[50] Unfortunately, despite research clearly demonstrating that mouth breathing contributes to high viral load, poor immune defense, and more severe forms of the novel coronavirus,[39] nobody is talking about the fact that many people are mouth breathing inside their protective face masks.

In July 2020, as the UK government enforced mask-wearing in shops, I received an email from my friend, a medical doctor. He wondered how many people were aware of the way they breathe when wearing a mask. He shared the following example: "I went to the barber on Sunday. The barber had a mask on. All I could hear was fast breathing through the mouth while he wore the mask." My friend explained his concerns:

> Since April, I have tried to convince everyone I meet to breathe only
> through the nose, with or without a mask. Many older people are

surprised when I stop them and ask how they breathe when they have a mask on. Some said they didn't know or didn't pay attention. And more than 90% said they had to breathe through their mouth because they couldn't breathe nasally with the mask on!

My friend is adamant that nasal breathing will help prevent the spread of viruses and the subsequent fatalities. He says, "When we mouth breathe, any virus has a direct route to our lungs. Masks plus nasal breathing will help keep the virus from entering the patient's respiratory system."

An article in the *Independent*, "Learning how to breathe again in the new normal," looks at breathing with and without a face mask in a post-COVID environment[51]. The author describes the prevalence of unhealthy breathing habits and calls on experts to define the problems of breathing with a face mask. The article quotes breathing expert Paul DiTuro, who suggests that respiratory training will help. DiTuro describes a simple exercise to make mask-wearing more comfortable:

> Just before putting on your mask, take five "quality" breaths. With each breath, inhale through the nose for four seconds, exhale through the mouth for six seconds, then rest for two seconds. Repeat these five breaths as soon as you put on the mask, and again after you remove it.[51]

The concepts here are good. Inhaling for four seconds and exhaling for six equates to a breathing rate of six breaths per minute, which maximizes many important physiological functions, as well as activating the relaxation centers of the nervous system.

Unfortunately, as we discussed earlier, breathing in through the nose and out through the mouth is not a good idea. It causes nasal congestion and inhibits gas exchange in the lungs. The importance of breathing only through the nose, awake or asleep, with or without a face mask, cannot be underlined too strongly.

## BEATING NASAL CONGESTION

Mask or no mask, if you suffer from a constantly blocked nose, nasal breathing may seem impossible or even frightening. However, breath holding and physical exercise can actually help open the nasal airways.[52] In a few pages, you'll find a breath-holding exercise for decongesting the nose. Exactly how this works remains a matter of debate, but holding the breath increases $CO_2$ in the blood, pools nitric oxide within the nose, and activates the body's sympathetic stress response. While long-term sympathetic activation is damaging to health, the stress response plays a necessary and beneficial role[53] in the immune system[54] and in regulating inflammation.[55]

As far back as 1923, an article in the *American Journal of Physiology* reported that holding the breath could ease nasal stuffiness.[56] If this information had been made public at the time, millions of children and adults suffering from rhinitis could have found relief simply by holding their breath whenever their nose was bunged up. Decades later, in 1977, researchers showed that rebreathing exhaled air decreased nasal congestion. Even holding the breath for just 30 seconds made breathing easier for most of the subjects tested.[57] The main stimulus for this result? Carbon dioxide.[58]

According to Dr. James Bartley, an ear, nose, and throat surgeon, nasal resistance is inversely related to end-tidal $CO_2$.[59] End-tidal $CO_2$ is the concentration of $CO_2$ in the air at the end of an exhaled breath. It is a direct measure of how much $CO_2$ there is in the lungs, and under normal circumstances, an indirect measure of the pressure of $CO_2$ in the blood. Bartley's finding means that as levels of $CO_2$ reduce in the lungs and blood, the nose becomes more congested. Studies have shown that a reduction of $CO_2$ in the lungs (from normal pressure of 40 mmHg to 35 mmHg) corresponds with a 10% increase in nasal congestion.[52] Anxiety also typically corresponds with lower end-tidal $CO_2$ levels.[60]

This is also relevant in a complaint known as empty nose syndrome (ENS)—where a patient with clear nasal airways experiences a variety of symptoms, including sensations of nasal obstruction, dryness and crusting, and feelings of breathlessness[61] and drowning. ENS can result from major or minor surgical procedures including turbinate surgery, laser therapy, and submucosal resection, even when surgery and medical support is successful. At present, its existence, diagnosis, and management are all controversial, with discussion raging as to whether neurological or psychosomatic factors may contribute.[61]

ENS can be caused by the removal of the turbinates. The turbinates are small structures inside the nose that filter and humidify the air as it passes through the nostrils into the airways and lungs. They are made up of a bony structure surrounded by vascular tissue and a mucus membrane. They can become inflamed and swollen when allergy, infection, or irritation is present, producing an excessive amount of mucus, which causes the nose to block.

ENT Jim Bartley also explored the feeling of nasal stuffiness in hyperventilation.[62] In 2005, Bartley examined 14 patients who complained of nasal congestion after surgery and of feeling unable to breathe nasally, despite having an apparently adequate nasal airway with no collapsed tissue inside the nose, and a surgical success rate between 63% and 85%. Some had tried nasal steroids and oral antihistamines without relief. Bartley noted that some were breathing rapidly, predominantly into their upper chest. He assessed each for hyperventilation syndrome and discovered that all displayed a heightened respiratory rate of around 18 breaths per minute with an upper chest breathing pattern. On a subjective breathing questionnaire, 12 of the 14 participants had scores indicative of hyperventilation. Three patients had an end-tidal $CO_2$ reading of 35 mmHg, which indicates low blood $CO_2$. Five had breath retraining; this successfully relieved nasal congestion for two of them.[62]

Bartley concluded that patients who suffer from constant feelings of nasal congestion, particularly after failed nasal surgery, should be assessed for hyperventilation syndrome. The primary issue in those patients may actually be poor breathing patterns. Even slightly fast and/or hard breathing causes a feeling of air hunger that patients often interpret as nasal stuffiness. While the functioning of the physical airway is a relevant concern, air flow must also be considered.

If someone with chronic hyperventilation complains of nasal obstruction, with no identifiable anatomical reason, surgery may not be the answer.[62] Breathing reeducation may be. If you have undergone nasal surgery and still feel as if your nose is constantly blocked, your breathing pattern is likely to be at the root of the problem. If you do have nasal congestion, rhinitis or asthma, try the exercises in this book first. Decongest your nose using the following breath-holding exercise, switch to nasal breathing, and improve your BOLT score. I have used these techniques with thousands of people who have attended my workshops over the years and found that many destined for nasal surgery did not require it.

Because the nose is designed to regulate air intake,[63] switching to nasal breathing significantly improves the symptoms of nasal stuffiness and will dramatically reduce your symptoms in the long term.

## EXERCISE TO UNBLOCK THE NOSE

Before you read any further, try this exercise to see just how effective it is for clearing your nose. The exercise is the same for adults and children. *This exercise is not suitable for women who are pregnant.*

- Sit upright on a straight-backed chair.
- Normalize your breathing and breathe calmly. Take a small, light breath in through your nose if you can and a small breath out through your nose. If you are unable to inhale through your nose, take a tiny breath in through the corner of your mouth.
- After exhaling, pinch your nose and hold your breath. Keep your lips sealed.
- Gently nod your head or rock your body until you feel that you cannot hold your breath any longer. You should feel a relatively strong need for air.
- At this point, let go of your nose, and breathe in gently through the nose. Breathe gently in and out with your mouth closed. When you first breathe in, avoid taking a deep breath. Instead, keep your breathing calm and focus on relaxation. Use the mantra "relax and breathe less" if it helps.
- Repeat the exercise until you can breathe easily through your nose. If your nose does not become fully unblocked, wait around one minute, and practice the same steps again. You may need to do the exercise several times.

After you have completed the exercise, your nose will be unblocked. However, until you have improved your BOLT score to over 25 seconds, the exercise will decongest your nose onlny temporarily. Once your BOLT score is 25 or more, your nose will stay unblocked for much longer periods. I always explain to my students, especially the teenagers, that you have two options. You can improve your BOLT score to 25 seconds, or you can experience nasal congestion for the rest of your life. When you consider all of the negative consequences of mouth breathing for sleep, stress, and other health concerns, the choice is obvious.

Remember, until you have changed the underlying breathing patterns that contribute to nasal stuffiness, it is quite normal for the nose to block again. With regular practice of the exercises in this book, your body will adapt, and your nose will start to remain clear. Practice this exercise whenever your nose feels congested. Even if you have a heavy cold, this exercise can help you maintain nasal breathing.

## MAKING THE SWITCH

The first step in addressing poor breathing patterns and increasing your BOLT score is to switch from mouth to nose breathing. Even though its primary function is respiratory, the nose is often underused for the essential task of breathing. While total mouth breathing is rare, as most people tend to switch from mouth to nose breathing and vice versa, it is incredibly common for children and adults to mouth breathe some of the time, either out of habit or due to nasal obstruction.

When you first switch from mouth to nasal breathing, the volume of air you inhale with each breath may immediately reduce. This is likely to feel a little strange to begin with. You will probably experience a slight air shortage since the volume of air inhaled through the nose is less than you are used to inhaling through the mouth. Don't worry. Air hunger is a good sign of progress. Any discomfort will diminish in a few days. Your body may try to trick you into breathing more by yawning, sighing, or sneaking in the odd mouth breath. Try not to increase your breathing in those ways. When you feel the need to breathe big—for example, if you experience the impulse to sigh—hold your breath for 5 to 10 seconds following the sigh.

One thing to be aware of that may seem odd, even unfair, as you make the switch from mouth to nasal breathing, is that the size of the nose is actually an important factor in breathing habits. People with a small nasal airway are much more likely to breathe through an open mouth than those with an adequate nasal size. Mouth breathing is a very normal reaction to a small nasal airway. The smaller the nose, the greater the resistance to breathing, and the more air hunger is experienced in breathing through the nose.

## HOW TO BREATHE DURING EXERCISE

A spacious nasal cavity and large nostrils are definitely useful for breathing through the nose during physical exercise. If your nasal airway is small, the resistance to breathing and the resulting air hunger may be too much during exercise. To help open the nasal passages, you can use the exercise-specific NasalDilator, which I have designed specifically for this purpose.

Earlier, we talked about how $CO_2$ creates the primary stimulus to breathe and is instrumental in oxygenation. Nose breathing during physical exercise slows the breath and reduces breathing volume, which influences the levels of $CO_2$ in the blood. However, most of us will not spontaneously choose to breathe through the nose during heavy exercise.[64] Without proper training for at least six to eight weeks, the air hunger caused by nose breathing can become quite pronounced as exercise intensifies.

Breathing through the nose is usually only comfortable during gentle exercise, when the total volume of air entering the lungs every minute (called *minute ventilation*) is less than 35 liters. Once minute ventilation has increased to between 35 and 41 liters,[65] the tendency is to start mouth breathing. The exact switching point from nose to mouth breathing is highly personal, influenced by individual sensitivity to $CO_2$, metabolism, and the size of the nose.

Mouth breathing is faster than nose breathing. It feels preferable under certain conditions because the shallow, fast breaths result in a greater volume of air entering the lungs. This causes blood $CO_2$ to drop, which reduces the feeling of air hunger.[66] However, breathing through the nose is actually more efficient because it allows the lungs to extract more oxygen from the air. The percentage of oxygen in expired air decreases when nasal breathing during exercise, indicating that more of the oxygen is being used.[67] Continuing nasal breathing practice over a period of six to eight weeks will encourage your body to adapt, delaying the onset of breathlessness. Whether or not you currently include physical exercise in your weekly routine, this applies to you. We all have a threshold at which mouth breathing feels necessary. Whatever your starting point, whether you start to wheeze during your workout or when you just try to get up off the couch, you can begin to improve your fitness by restoring nasal breathing.

The importance of breathing through the nose rather than the mouth should not be underestimated. It encourages functional breathing and larger oscillations of the diaphragm, supporting functional movement, and preventing injury. It is an important element of getting "in the zone"—that state of peak focus when everything flows and you can perform at your best. (Chapter Five looks more deeply at the connection between breathing and movement.)

It is also important to remember that nasal breathing helps retain heat and moisture in the body. During exercise, this can make a big difference as to whether you experience a dry mouth. It can protect your airways from trauma, including exercise-induced asthma and cyclist's cough.

Nasally restricted breathing can be used during exercise to improve performance.[68] This has implications for nonathletes too. In a 2018 paper, professor of exercise science and Olympic triathlon coach, Dr. George Dallam looked in detail at the breathing of athletes.[66] Five male and five female recreational runners trained and raced using only nasal breathing for six months. Dallam recorded comparative results when the participants breathed only through the nose and only through the mouth, wearing a swimming nose clip to close the nostrils. The trial used a graded exercise test to examine performance, breathing rate, oxygen uptake, and breathing efficiency at $VO_2$ max. $VO_2$ max is maximum oxygen consumption during intense exercise. It is used to measure cardiovascular fitness and aerobic endurance in athletes.

Dallam's study produced the following results:

- Respiratory rate was much slower in nasal breathing than in oral breathing (39.2 bpm vs 49.4 bpm).
- End-tidal $CO_2$ was significantly higher in nose breathing than mouth breathing (44.7 mmHg vs 40.2 mmHg).
- Ventilation (volume of breathing) was reduced by 22% in nasal breathing.
- Nose breathing resulted in lower end-tidal oxygen pressure and a lower percentage of oxygen in expired air, indicating that more oxygen was removed from the air by the lungs during nasal breathing.

A key finding from Dallam's study was that after six months' training with only nasal breathing, the athletes achieved the same peak performance and oxygen consumption when nasal breathing as they did during oral breathing. They were pushing themselves to their limits yet still managed to breathe in an effective way. Breathing was also more economical. The 22% reduction in ventilation meant that breathing required less effort and the muscles of the respiratory system didn't have to work as hard. Achieving the same intensity with 22% less breathing represents a significantly greater economy. Dallam concluded that it is possible to maintain $VO_2$ max and peak performance after a period of training using only nasal breathing. The body naturally adapts to nasal breathing by increasing its tolerance to changes in $CO_2$, so air hunger decreases.

These findings are relevant for everyone, whatever your level of fitness. If a walk to the corner shop leaves you gasping for breath, nasal breathing will help you. To limit air hunger during physical exercise, work to achieve a higher BOLT score and breathe light, slow, and deep (LSD):

- **Light:** Only breathe the volume of air that you need (don't overbreathe).
- **Slow:** Reduce your respiratory rate.
- **Deep:** Breathe with greater amplitudes of diaphragm movement.

If you are healthy and exercising at the appropriate level to improve your aerobic fitness, you should be able to breathe only through the nose without needing any specific adaptations[66]. If the air hunger is so strong that you need to open your mouth, simply slow down and allow your breathing to calm. By breathing nasally throughout, you should finish your workout feeling relaxed and full of energy instead of exhausted and dehydrated.

### Recreational Athletes

Healthy people exercising at the lower levels necessary to improve aerobic fitness can breathe entirely through the nose,[66] without needing any specific adaptations. Recreational athletes should maintain nasal breathing at all times. If the air hunger is so strong that you need to open your mouth to breathe, simply slow down and allow your breathing to calm.

### Competitive Athletes

It is best for competitive athletes to alternate nasal breathing with mouth breathing. High-intensity training helps prevent muscle deconditioning and will require an athlete to periodically breathe through their mouth. For less-than-maximum intensity training, and at all other times, nasal breathing should be used. A competitive athlete may spend 50% of training with their mouth closed.

Research has shown that healthy adults are able to maintain nasal breathing to 85% of $VO_2$ max,[69] indicating that it is possible to breathe nasally at much higher intensities of exercise than we might choose.

- Use mouth breathing to maintain muscle condition when working at an all-out pace.
- During competition, there is no need to intentionally take bigger breaths. Instead, achieve a higher BOLT score and apply the OA precompetition preparation. (You can find this in Chapter Two.)
- Nasal breathing combined with breath-holding during your warm-up can be very advantageous. As can practicing light, slow and deep breathing during the warm-down. (You will find instructions for warm-up in Chapter Two.)

## SNIFFING OUT SUCCESS

One function of the nose we haven't yet discussed is the sense of smell via the olfactory nerve. In ancient yogic texts, while breath control is associated with a "pristine" state of mind, the condition of the olfactory nerve is seen as indicating the general state of health. Is this relevant to nasal breathing? Scientists say it could be.

In 2019, researchers at the Weizmann Institute in Israel suggested that nasal inhalation could be linked to cognition as part of an evolutionary survival mechanism.[70, 71] A sense of smell is, after all, equated with sniffing out danger. For our distant ancestors, this meant accurately assessing their surroundings to make life-or-death decisions. The Weizmann team theorized that this ancient sensory system might benefit from nasal inhalation and that, in modern life and competitive sports, nasal inhalation might automatically trigger conditions in the brain that optimize visuospatial focus. They demonstrated that nasal breathing synchronized electrical activity in the brain on a wavelength that helped maximize visuospatial (VS) awareness.

Visuospatial awareness is the way we relate visual information to the space around us. It helps us perform everyday tasks like walking through a door rather than bumping into the door frame, picking up a glass of water, catching a ball, reading a map, driving a car, and even parallel parking. Visuospatial skills can be defined as

> the ability to observe the visual world, to form mental representations of the visual objects, to mentally manipulate these representations, and to in turn reconstruct aspects of the visual experience.[72–74]

VS ability is made up of several cognitive processes, including the perception and understanding of spatial orientation, reproducing actions through fine motor movements, and integrating parts into a whole.[72, 75–77] These elements all place different demands on working memory.[73] Visuospatial tasks are "complex and engage various spatial processes", and involve numerous areas of the brain.[72]

The fact that nasal breathing helps synchronize the complex mental processes required for VS awareness has applications for sports, such as tennis, where a keen awareness of the external environment and its dimensions is key. In team ball games like football, soccer, basketball, and ice hockey, the player must be able to catch, carry, kick, or hit a ball at the same time as scanning the pitch for teammates to pass to—all this while running at full pelt.[78] During any sort of sporting activity (and during activities like music performance), it's necessary to absorb and process a great deal of information in a very short time. Athletes have to become highly proficient at perceiving changes in play caused by their opponents and team members.[78]

Athletes and musicians display better performance in VS tasks than people who are physically inactive.[79–81] Older people can improve their VS skills by improving their physical fitness.[82] Several studies have examined the influence of more general physical exercise on VS ability.[83–85]

The influence of breathing on VS ability also has implications for children's intellectual development. A 2015 study demonstrated that visuospatial perception is instrumental when a child learns to read, and that assessment of VS abilities could help with the early detection of "difficulties in neurodevelopmental disorders associated with low academic achievement."[86] Another paper from 2016 suggests that VS skills are even important in learning mathematics, especially for things like problem solving.[72]

# CHAPTER FOUR

# THE VAGUS NERVE AND THE HEART-BREATH-BRAIN CONNECTION

To really understand the powerful interconnections between the breath, heart, and brain, we must take a journey along the wandering *vagus nerve* and through the autonomic nervous system (ANS). This chapter will cover a lot of ground. If we seem to be heading away from the central issue of breathing, you will soon see how the vagus nerve connects with the breath in powerful, life-transforming ways.

The vagus nerve (the tenth cranial nerve or CN X) has multiple branches that diverge from two thick stems rooted in the cerebellum or "little brain" (the area at the lower back of the brain) and the brain stem.[1-3] It can be found behind the artery in your neck where you feel for your pulse. Vagus, *to wander* in Latin, comes from the same root as our words *vagabond*, *vagrant*, and *vague*. The name gives some clue to just how extensively this nerve travels. During its journey through the body, the vagus nerve supplies nerves to the heart, respiratory system, and gastrointestinal tract, reaching the lowest viscera of the abdomen. It is the most wide-ranging cranial nerve in the human body and is responsible for, among other things, many functions of the mouth, including speech, appetite control, and even vomiting. Ultimately, it conducts nerve impulses to every major organ in the body.[4]

The vagus nerve is made up of 80% to 90% *afferent* (body to brain) nerve fibers.[2] This means that most of the information it conveys travels from the body to the brain. Instead of orders flowing from the brain, affecting the various physiological systems and organs, the afferent fibers take information back from the body *to* the brain.[5] The heart, however, is innervated with *efferent* (brain to body) vagus fibers—a top-down line of communication.[6] The resulting two-way flow of data provides the building blocks for feedback loops in which information from the brain impacts the physical systems of the body and vice versa.

Many studies have shown the vagus nerve's positive potential to influence physical health, mental health, and cognition. This nerve can be stimulated to reduce anxiety, alleviate depression, and even inhibit inflammation to fight disease in the body by combating the cortisol-producing stress response we know as fight or flight.

To understand the vagus nerve's importance to the heart-breath-brain connection, we need to start our journey by looking at the two sides of the ANS, beginning with the fight-or-flight response.

## THE VAGUS NERVE AND AUTONOMIC BALANCE

The fight-or-flight response is the body's instinctive survival mechanism. From a simple evolutionary perspective, it allows mammals, including humans, to react to situations that may be life threatening. When humans lived in constantly unsafe environments, it was useful for fighting off enemies and hunting for food. While it still has a valuable role to play in keeping us safe in the modern world, problems arise when we have the same response to things that are probably not fatal. We might be fearful about giving a presentation, turning up for an interview, receiving an unexpected bill, or even being blocked on social media. When fight or flight is constantly in overdrive, the result is chronic stress, that all too common modern-day malady.

Fight or flight is controlled by the *sympathetic nervous system* (SNS), which is one-half of the overall ANS. The vagus nerve is the main driver of the other branch of the ANS, the *parasympathetic nervous system* (PNS)[1]. While the sympathetic nervous system triggers fight or flight, the vagus-led PNS is responsible for rest and digestion, the state in which the body perceives no threat, the mind is relaxed, and digestion is active. Crucially, as we will discover, it is through the ANS that the respiratory system, lung ventilation, and blood-gas exchange connects with the working of the heart rate and blood vessels. Ideally, the two responses of the ANS, fight/flight and rest/digest, work in balance.[7] The primary purpose of the ANS is to regulate the body's main functions.

The SNS (sympathetic nervous system) prepares the body for external challenges. It increases metabolic output, stimulates and prepares the muscles, and mobilizes existing energy reserves. It also constricts the blood vessels, increasing heart rate and blood pressure. In contrast, the PNS (parasympathetic nervous system) focuses inward, supporting growth, restoration, reproduction, relaxation, and conservation of energy. It maintains the balance of heart frequencies; notably, it reacts much faster to external and internal changes than the SNS, responding within just one second, in contrast to the five or more seconds it takes the SNS to kick in.[8]

These two opposing forces within the ANS are never static. The system continually fluctuates to maintain a stable internal environment that operates within healthy parameters. This constant balancing act to maintain *homeostasis* is key to keeping organs working properly. For example, if your body temperature is too high, the ANS adjusts to bring it back to the optimal temperature of 37° Celsius (98.6° Fahrenheit). This is not just a reactive system that waits passively to meet the next external crisis; it works incessantly to promote stability within the body.

While the two branches of the ANS may seem to function in opposition, they often operate in synergy to meet metabolic demands. For example, during exercise, PNS tone decreases while SNS activity increases. There are even unique situations when both PNS and SNS are either inhibited or activated.[9] For example, sexual arousal in adult humans is characterized by the excitement of both.

Homeostasis (balance or equilibrium) is a fundamental goal of all biological systems.[10] In humans, it operates at the level of the whole body, within tissues, and even in individual cells. Where homeostasis can be described as a healthy, dynamic feedback and regulation system, stress can be defined simply as any autonomic state that reflects a disturbance of that balance. Stress is a state where a psychological, environmental, or physical situation, whether a single event or a long-term issue, disrupts the body's ability to self-regulate. Modern life presents us with a world where it can be difficult to maintain that balance. Think about some of the terms used to describe an emotional upset: you are "out of whack," you feel "all over the place," or you are literally "off balance."

Stress can manifest itself in each of the three dimensions of dysfunctional breathing. It can show up biomechanically as imbalances in the respiratory muscles. This can lead to neck and back pain, upper chest breathing, and poor diaphragm control. Biochemically, chronic hyperventilation can impact the body's delicate pH balance. Psychologically, anxiety, depression, and anger can destroy your equilibrium.

Living in a constant state of fight or flight poses the danger of *cortisol* overload. Cortisol is the primary stress hormone.[11] When released into the bloodstream, it enhances the brain's use of glucose (blood sugar) and makes substances that repair tissues more available. In essence, it prepares the body to escape from the saber-toothed beast and not bleed too much if that doesn't work out. Aligned with that purpose, cortisol also curbs bodily functions that aren't immediately essential to the fight-or-flight situation. It alters immune system responses and suppresses digestive, reproductive, and growth processes. As you might expect, it communicates with the parts of the brain that control mood, motivation, and fear.

Ideally, the body's stress response is self-limiting. Hormones go back to normal levels after the perceived threat has passed, and the body returns to homeostasis. However, when stressors are constantly present or stress is chronic (which is like signing up for a long-term fight-or-flight subscription), a cortisol imbalance occurs. Considering how many of the body's processes cortisol can suppress, it is hardly surprising that people who suffer from high levels of stress display a plethora of physical and mental conditions, including anxiety, heart disease, weight gain, digestive problems, depression, headaches, sleep disorders, poor memory, and decreased ability to concentrate.

On the other (balancing) side of the ANS, we find the well-studied connection between the vagus nerve and the parasympathetic nervous system (PNS), the rest and digest side of the ANS. The vagus nerve, which sends impulses to all the major organs and is particularly connected to the heart and respiratory system, secretes a brilliantly useful substance called *acetylcholine* or ACh.

Acetylcholine (ACh), the first neurotransmitter ever to be identified,[12] was discovered in 1913 by English chemist Arthur Ewins.[12] Later, in 1921, the Nobel Prize winning physiologist Otto Loewi determined its functional significance. Loewi found that activating the vagus nerve reduced heart rate.[1] He did this by isolating the heart of a frog and stimulating the vagus nerve to release something he called "Vagusstuff." This substance, later identified as acetylcholine, caused the frog's heart to slow, replicating relaxation, the reaction to a nonthreatening environment—or the rest-and-digest state. The implications of this are huge. It means that stimulating the vagus nerve can activate the PNS, subduing or balancing out the fight-or-flight reaction of the SNS.

This "Vagusstuff" (ACh) released by the vagus nerve is a neurotransmitter—a chemical messenger released by nerve cells to send messages to other cells. This neurotransmitter is found in all motor neurons, where it stimulates smooth muscles to contract, slows the heart rate, and dilates the blood vessels. It is also present in many brain neurons where it has a role in vital mental processes such as cognition and memory. Severe depletion of acetylcholine has been associated with conditions such as Alzheimer's.[12]

## STRESS, INFLAMMATION, AND ILLNESS

From a health perspective, if we define stress as a disruption of homeostasis, inflammation often begins as the body's natural response to stress. What's more, chronic, low-grade inflammation has been proven to indicate an overactive fight-or-flight response.[10] It makes sense, therefore, to deduce that inhibiting the fight-or-flight reaction (as the ACh released by the vagus nerve does) could reduce inflammation.

Inflammation is a defense mechanism triggered by injury or infection. It is at the extreme end of the spectrum that ranges from homeostasis to stress response to inflammatory response.[10] It combines different immune mechanisms that work to neutralize invading pathogens such as bacteria and viruses, repair injured tissues, and heal wounds. However, when out of balance, inflammation plays a key role in the development and persistence of many diseases. It can be triggered by extreme internal imbalances or by external challenges that disturb homeostasis. After a stressor occurs, the inflammatory response kicks in.

While modern life has its benefits, including a much longer life span,[13] advanced technology, and home grocery deliveries, the nature of stress has changed dramatically. When stress is severe and prolonged, it causes the body to compensate, physiologically and behaviorally, to maintain homeostasis. Long term, this can put an unsustainable load on the body's systems.

There is increasing evidence that chronic stress increases the risk of both physical and mental health disorders. It can play a critical role in the onset and progress of stress-related illness, including diseases of the heart, digestive system, brain, and many forms of cancer. Chronic stressors are known to suppress immune function. In fact, while not yet fully understood, studies show that stress is a common risk factor in 75% to 90% of human diseases.[13] That's nearly all of them.

Scientists at Carnegie Mellon University discovered a direct relationship between chronic mental stress, the body's inability to regulate inflammation, and the progression of disease.[14] Their study, which used the common cold as a model, found that prolonged stress decreases the body's sensitivity to the stress hormone cortisol in such a way that the immune cells become insensitive to it. This negatively affects the ability of cortisol to regulate inflammation. Inflammation gets out of control, and disease sets in. The research demonstrated that the symptoms of a cold are not actually caused by the virus. They are a side effect of the body's inflammatory response, which is designed to fight infection. People who suffer most when they have a cold don't have "Man Flu"—they are actually experiencing a more extreme inflammatory reaction.

The study also confirmed that stress led to the immune cells being less able to respond to signals that normally regulate inflammation. Participants who were stressed were much more likely to develop colds when exposed to the virus than those who weren't stressed, and those people also produced more *cytokines*—the chemical messengers that trigger inflammation. Because inflammation is pivotal in so many illnesses, this offers a valuable window into the impact that psychological stress can have on health.

## VAGAL STIMULATION AND THE IMMUNE SYSTEM

A clear connection between the nervous system and the immune system was discovered by neurosurgeon Kevin Tracey in 1998. In an experiment on a rat, he investigated the idea that stimulating the vagus nerve could alleviate harmful inflammation.[4] He found that the nervous system could be used almost like a computer to trigger commands that stop a problem in its tracks. The results of his experiment were so unexpected that Tracey's colleagues were apparently in the corridor outside his lab, running bets against his theory even as he was in the middle of testing it![4] Further trials confirmed Tracey's findings. Using electronic implants to stimulate the vagus nerve in humans, he produced a dramatic reduction and even remission in rheumatoid arthritis, a condition with no known cure.[15] This helped illuminate the vagal system's close interrelationship with the inflammatory system.

The first steps of an inflammatory reaction involve the release of those pro-inflammatory chemicals called cytokines.[8] When the body produces too many cytokines, they can cause more damage than the invading pathogens. For example, in sepsis, the body's own immune reaction can cause tissue injury, dangerously low blood pressure, and even death. Chronic inflammation can also feature in many diseases where no infection or injury is present. In obesity, for example, an overload of storage in fat cells leads to a stress response that causes the release of inflammatory cytokines.[10]

The conversation between the immune system and the brain that moderates this inflammatory response relies, in part, on the vagus nerve, which, in turn, is important due to the anti-inflammatory role of Vagusstuff/ACh. Crucially, ACh, the neurotransmitter secreted by the vagus nerve, blocks the release of many of the pro-inflammatory cytokines. In studies of diseases characterized by an excessive immune reaction, including sepsis and pancreatitis, vagus nerve stimulation was found to be sufficient to block cytokine activity. When the vagus nerve is stimulated electronically, the body's level of inflammatory cytokines decreases.[16]

As it turns out, the breath also provides a (natural) gateway to influence the vagus nerve and the ANS—through the role of carbon dioxide ($CO_2$) levels in maintaining the body's acid-base balance.[17] One of the functions of breathing is to regulate the level of blood $CO_2$ to maintain the blood's acid balance (or pH). When levels of $CO_2$ in the blood are too high, over time, $CO_2$ diffuses into the red blood cells as carbonic acid, making the blood too acidic, a condition called *acidosis*. When $CO_2$ levels are too low, respiratory *alkalosis* occurs. Both acidosis and alkalosis are serious, potentially life-threatening in their acute forms and damaging to health if they persist long term. Therefore, the proper management of $CO_2$ through the breath is crucial.

When blood pH changes even subtly, respiration will automatically decrease or increase to compensate. One example of this is ketoacidosis, a serious complication which can occur in diabetes. Ketoacidosis increases acidity in the blood, stimulating corrective overbreathing. This fast, upper chest breathing is also commonly seen after the acidosis following prolonged diarrhea and as a response to increased progesterone levels in women. Conversely, alkalosis can be induced by vomiting or the use of steroids or diuretics. The respiratory drive is then suppressed as the body works to restore homeostasis.[17] Information about blood $CO_2$ is sent to the respiratory center so that breathing can adjust via pathways involving the vagus nerve.

Therefore, breathing exercises to increase $CO_2$ have a "vagotropic effect."[18] $CO_2$ directly influences the sensitivity of the vagus nerve's nuclei. This slows the pulse and improves the blood-filling of the heart.[19] Increased blood $CO_2$

is the most likely mechanism to enhance the vagus nerve's slowing effect on the heart during exhalation. Increased $CO_2$ (hypercapnia) and exhalation are both vital in stimulating the vagus nerve.[18]

What's particularly exciting is that the effects of vagus nerve stimulation don't stop when treatment is finished. They are ongoing. Over time, the vagus system develops and maintains much greater resilience to stressors. This long-term conditioning of the vagus nerve, its functionality, and ability to react to maintain homeostasis is known as *vagal tone*. This vagal tone is key not just to reducing inflammatory responses but also to a healthy and resilient functioning of the heart.

## VAGAL TONE AND HEART RATE VARIABILITY

While we often associate heartbeats with rhythm and may believe an absolutely regular heartbeat is a healthy one, heartbeats are not all the same.[9] In fact, they change constantly, and the more coherent the fluctuations are in speed and intensity, the healthier you are likely to be, both mentally and physically.[16] The heart is not a metronome. Its oscillations are complex and constantly changing. The cardiovascular system needs to adjust to external and internal stimuli to maintain homeostasis.

*Heart rate variability* (HRV) measures the difference between consecutive heartbeats. In clinical settings, readings are taken to the millisecond with the help of an ECG signal. With modern technology, you can now measure your own HRV using a smart watch or other wearable fitness tracker. Results are presented as time series data, a way of recording information collected over a period of time to show variations within that period. Daily high and low tide data is a familiar use of a data time series. Using HRV as an objective indicator of fitness and resilience has been gaining traction among fitness enthusiasts. While many people enjoy using gadgets and apps to measure their own HRV, remember that technology doesn't change HRV; it simply provides the information that allows you to assess it.

HRV is predominantly controlled by the ANS. Growing evidence associates an ANS imbalance with a higher prevalence of disease and death, which makes HRV a useful tool in predicting and assessing illness. When you are in a fight-or-flight state, HRV changes. As the system restores homeostasis, those changes settle down. However, if the body is under constant stress, the heart rate becomes less resilient and less flexible. The variation between oscillations decreases, and the body can't shift gears as easily. The potential impact is massive. Because lower HRV can be caused by stress, emotional distress and chronic stress directly impact wellness. Studies indicate, for example, that stress increases the risk of heart attack in people who have no prior heart disease and that emotions like anger, hostility, and aggressiveness can contribute to coronary artery disease.[10]

HRV declines significantly with poor health.[20, 21] People who are emotionally sick, older, or less physically fit often have a lower HRV.[16] High concentrations of cortisol are associated with low HRV,[8] and HRV is an established tool in diagnosing diabetic neuropathy, the nerve damage, often to the legs and feet, suffered by diabetics. Correlations have also been found between changes to HRV and many high-mortality conditions, including heart disease, cancer, stroke, Alzheimer's, diabetes, chronic lower respiratory diseases, and intentional self-harm.

Low HRV is related to a wide range of physical and mental illnesses and a lower life expectancy.[8] Even the stress caused by a single significant life event can have an impact. Scientists looking at the health of divorced people discovered that participants who had gone through a marriage breakdown had a lower resting HRV than those who were married.[22] The upset caused by divorce actually made those people less healthy.

While low HRV is associated with disease, people with high HRV are likely to be healthier, both physically and mentally. All of this explains why some people seem to be more resilient to stress, better able to field challenging situations and take difficulties in their stride, while others get thrown off balance. Scientists have so far failed to find satisfying answers about the genetics of the stress response,[23] but inherited conditions can certainly contribute to aspects of health that result in low HRV. For example, studies have shown that vagal tone is passed on from mother to child.[24] Mothers who are depressed, anxious, and angry during their pregnancy have lower vagal activity. Once the baby is born, he or she also displays a low vagal tone.

The good news is that it is possible to build better vagal tone. Just one note of caution: it is not always better to increase vagal tone.[25] For instance, parasympathetic hyperactivity can occur in athletes who overtrain. Several studies indicate that symptoms of overreaching may be related to down-regulation of the SNS and/or changes in the balance between vagal and sympathetic tone. This can cause fatigue and adversely affect performance during periods of regular competition.[26] The key is to *optimize* HRV, not just blindly augment it. Slow breathing at 4.5 to 6.5 breaths per minute has been found to optimize sympathovagal balance, creating an ideal balance between the two branches of the autonomic nervous system.[27]

Because it is closely connected with the working of the ANS, especially the parasympathetic branch (PNS), HRV is considered a reliable measure of how well the vagus nerve is working, that is, of vagal tone. Scientists believe that vagal tone in the heart forms one of the connections between breathing and emotion.[28] It is influenced by the breath and is essential to the stimulation of the vagus nerve, which is closely tied to aspects of human connection such as emotional regulation, reactivity, expression, empathy, and attachment. At the other end of the emotional spectrum, dysfunction of the ANS is common to people suffering from anxiety, depression, PTSD, panic disorder, and other stress-related mental and physical conditions. Parallels have even been found between vagal tone and cognitive functions such as visual recognition memory and alertness. HRV, used as a measure of vagal tone, provides doctors with a way to physically quantify stress and vulnerability to stress. That means that stress can be defined by its effect on the function of systems like the heart, rather than just on the way a challenging life event makes you feel.

## RSA: THE HEART-BREATH CONNECTION

The activity of the vagus nerve can be accurately measured using HRV and the way the heart interacts with the breath. When vagal tone is healthy, there are small differences in heart rate during the in-breath (when it speeds up) and out-breath (when it slows down). Inhaling, an increase in heart rate is caused by a rhythmic partial withdrawal of vagal tone. Exhaling, a release of acetylcholine causes the heart to slow, just as it did in Loewi's frog. This phenomenon is called *respiratory sinus arrhythmia* (RSA). It's a good indicator of how well the nervous system is functioning. In simple terms, HRV measures rhythmic changes between heartbeats, whereas RSA is HRV in synchronicity with the breath.

For most of us, breathing frequency is around 9 to 24 breaths per minute.[16] Corresponding oscillations in heart rate that produce respiratory sinus arrhythmia can be regarded as the effects of breathing on the region of the heart that initiates the electrical impulses for it to contract. The oscillations of RSA can be affected by stress, alterations in breathing patterns, or sudden bouts of exercise. RSA controls the rate of gas exchange inside the alveoli, the tiny air sacs in the lungs.[16] The heart beats faster when the air in the lungs is richest with oxygen, whereas the impulse to exhale is triggered when $CO_2$ in the lungs is highest. Gas exchange is most efficient when the heart rate is synchronized with the breath such that the heartbeat begins to increase at the start of an inhalation and begins to decrease at the start of an exhalation.

RSA is controlled entirely by the vagus nerve. Mirroring the function of the ANS,[16] it reveals how well the parasympathetic (or rest and digest) branch is working.[29] Because the vagus nerve activates during the exhalation, many studies have explored whether longer exhalations and slower breathing would produce greater differences in RSA and HRV. HRV is linked to breathing frequency, and greater changes occur when the breath is controlled and slower. Reducing the rate of respiration, increasing the amount of air delivered to the lungs with each breath, and breathing from the diaphragm have all been shown to increase RSA significantly. The best results for HRV, RSA, baroreflex sensitivity (more on this later), *and* optimal gas exchange are achieved with a breathing rate of 5.5 or 6 breaths per minute.[27] It has also been suggested that RSA has a central role in the resting state of the cardiorespiratory system. RSA maximizes during sleep, relaxation, and slow, deep breathing but is reduced in states of anxiety.[27] Energy expenditure is naturally minimized with improved pulmonary gas exchange.

## HRV BIOFEEDBACK

In the 1990s, clinician and research psychologist Paul Lehrer and his colleagues began to experiment with heart rate variability biofeedback (HRVB). The central focus of the technique is on slowing the breath to obtain beat-by-beat heart rate data so the participant can maximize RSA and match it to heart rate patterns. The participant uses feedback or a breath-pacing device to produce a heartbeat more rhythmically "in tune" with the breath. This synchronization provides the best conditions for gas exchange in the lungs.

Significant evidence supports the benefits of HRVB for a variety of common disorders,[16] as well as for enhancing athletic performance. While controlled studies are still needed for many specific conditions, scientists believe that training to optimize the rhythms of the breath and heart has potential applications for illnesses as varied as asthma, irritable bowel syndrome, COPD, cyclic vomiting, recurrent abdominal pain, fibromyalgia, cardiac rehabilitation, hypertension, chronic muscle pain, pregnancy-induced hypertension, depression, anxiety, PTSD, and insomnia. The improved gas exchange achievable with HRVB training may help people with respiratory diseases and stress-induced hyperventilation.[16] HRVB has been proven to restore the balance of the nervous system to combat inflammation.[30] It may also have advantages as a diagnostic tool for cardiovascular system dysfunction and its resulting illnesses.[31]

While most research in the field focuses on helping people who are sick, HRVB can also be used to reduce stress in otherwise healthy individuals. A study of young athletes who were taking their university exams found that the breath training resulted in long-term improved resistance to stressful situations (i.e., better vagal tone).[32] Another small study of women suffering from fibromyalgia concluded that actively participating in HRVB treatment restored a level of control to the patient, improving self-esteem and feelings of empowerment.[33]

## RSA, THE BAROREFLEX, AND BLOOD PRESSURE

Respiratory sinus arrhythmia (RSA) is also significantly connected to blood pressure. Remember, RSA describes changes in the heart rate during the respiratory cycle. Its functioning is highly dependent on the flexibility of the vagus nerve, or the heart's vagal tone, as measured using HRV.

One of the most important mechanisms of RSA is the *baroreflex*, a homeostatic function that helps maintain blood pressure at healthy, near-constant levels. The baroreflex is a reflex mediated by blood pressure sensors in the aorta (the largest artery in the body) and carotid arteries (the ones that supply blood to the brain, neck, and face).[34] Even during rest, blood pressure constantly fluctuates as breathing causes the pressure in the chest cavity to change. Scientists consider the strengthening of homeostasis in the baroreceptors to be the most obvious mechanism at play during HRVB training.[16]

All major blood vessels contain pressure receptors. These detect the stretching of the arteries as blood pressure increases. When blood pressure rises, the baroreflex immediately causes the blood vessels to dilate and the heart rate to drop. Conversely, when blood pressure falls, the baroreflex ensures that the blood vessels constrict and heart rate increases.[16] Under stress, the baroreflex reduces sympathetic outflow and increases vagal tone to protect the heart against unhealthy arrhythmias.[34]

The baroreflex is optimized when the relationship between breathing and heart rate is at its most efficient with regard to blood gas exchange. This means that breathing is a natural way to provide the external stimulation to increase HRV. At the same time, each breath stimulates the baroreflex. Heart rate and blood pressure are linked to the amount of air we breathe and to the exchange of oxygen between the lungs and the blood. During HRV biofeedback, the baroreflex works more effectively. This is associated with better mental and physical health, because as with higher oscillations in RSA and HRV, the body is more adaptable.

The sensitivity of the baroreceptors is also a good indicator of the body's response to a buildup of $CO_2$.[35] The respiratory system reacts to $CO_2$ buildup with involuntary contractions of the breathing muscles after an exhalation, triggering an inhalation. The stronger the reaction to blood $CO_2$, the harder it is to hold your breath after exhaling and the sooner you need to breathe in. The baroreceptors are most functional when the body is less sensitive to $CO_2$. Imagine being able to wait much longer before needing to breathe in. A high BOLT score, indicating comfort with slower breathing, signifies a reduced sensitivity to $CO_2$ in the blood. A healthy baroreflex with less sensitivity to $CO_2$ results in more frequent reflexes, slower heart rate, and increased vagal tone.

The cardiovascular and respiratory systems are tightly interconnected by the ANS which controls major functions of the body without conscious direction.[8, 36] Blood pressure receptors are triggered by the workings of RSA, which can be measured through HRV, providing strong indicators of mental and physical health. The fight-or-flight reaction (SNS) causes blood vessels to constrict, increasing heart rate and blood pressure, while ACh, the neurotransmitter released by the PNS-controlled vagus nerve, slows heart rate, dilates blood vessels, and suppresses the inflammatory response.

The baroreflex system is more than just a control mechanism involving heart rate and blood pressure. The activity of the baroreflex affects vascular tone—the sensitivity with which blood vessels expand and contract.[31] HRV also changes when there is inflammation. There is a clear relationship between various pro-inflammatory cytokines and lower HRV. The impact of the immune system on HRV, and the implications of that for health and disease, is probably underestimated.[8]

The common denominator in all these systems is the breath, especially slow breathing. Reducing the number of breaths per minute improves vagal tone, reduces stress, and supports health and cognition. The practices of slow breathing and relaxation benefit the heart and respiratory system in many ways. The baroreceptors become more responsive to changes in blood pressure, the heart rate becomes more lively and elastic, the vagus nerve more reactive, and the ANS shifts away from fight and flight toward less stress—which supports social interaction and enables the body to thrive.

## BETTER BRAIN FUNCTION: SLOW VAGAL BREATHING

It may seem obvious that it is easier to think when we are less stressed, and that when we concentrate on a breathing exercise, there is less room for the brain to worry. However, there is also evidence that slow breathing exercises have a *direct* impact on the way the brain works.

In one Belgian study, scientists discovered that vagus nerve stimulation (VNS) in rats clearly produced a memory-enhancing effect.[37] The rats performed a gambling task in which they could learn to use reasoning to maximize their food reward. Those that were treated with VNS developed better decision-making. Further trials, from another Belgian lab, found that vagal breathing could be used as a possible intervention against stress and its negative effects on decision-making in humans.[38] Other experiments have shown a connection between the vagus nerve and enhanced working memory.[39] Patients given inhalant anesthetics experience an increase in vagal tone as they regain consciousness[9]. Diaphragmatic breathing can directly lower cortisol levels,[28] reducing the negative physiological responses to stress and improving cognitive function.

Research into the connection between the breath and the brain in nasal breathing found that the breath directly affects neural activity in the brain.[40]

Breath actively promotes oscillatory synchronicity, which produces the conditions for optimal gas exchange and information processing in areas of the brain that mediate goal-directed behaviors. Nasal breathing offers an entry point to areas of the limbic brain that modulate cognitive function, which has interesting implications for mental agility given that the structures in the limbic system are involved in motivation, emotion, learning, and memory.[41] For example, experiments demonstrated that breathing influenced a participant's ability to identify fearful emotions in other people and their memory of visual objects. Passive inhalation of air through the nose enhanced reaction time to scary stimuli.

While there is a need for more research into the applications of VNS, slow breathing, and activation of the PNS on cognition, these correlations have been studied to some extent in other fields. For example, investigations into the impact of yogic breathing exercises have produced interesting insights into the connection between breath and brain. A study looking at *Nadi Shodhana*, yogic alternate nostril breathing, used EEG measurements (from scalp electrodes) to assess the balance between the two halves of the brain. It found that the practice generated more beta and alpha brain waves.[42] Beta waves are characteristic of a strongly engaged mind. A person who is in active conversation or focused on their work is in beta. Alpha represents nonarousal. It is associated with down time and relaxation. This suggests that the breathing practice allows participants to become more mentally active while remaining calm and clear headed. Another study looked at the way a combined practice of breathing and meditation improved memory and influenced academic performance.[43]

We will look in more detail at the correlation between these contemplative practices and the science of slow breathing, but it's worth noting that even meditation that doesn't focus on the breath can have the effect of reducing the respiratory rate. Scientists have concluded that regular yogic practices might improve cognitive functions, largely because they tilt the autonomic balance in favor of the PNS. Further experiments reported that EEG readings showed increased beta brainwaves under all conditions in advanced meditators, that long-term meditation practice improves gray matter atrophy, that attention and working memory improve, and that these techniques improve brain function in multiple pathways and may even offset age-related cognitive decline.[43]

Perhaps even more important, severe depletion of ACh, the neurotransmitter secreted by the vagus nerve when it is stimulated, has been associated with Alzheimer's. Parallels have been found between the working of the PNS and visual recognition memory and alertness. It has also been observed that both stress and inflammation can factor in the development of Alzheimer's[13] and Parkinson's disease. Breathing dysfunction can be related to impairments of attention or vigilance in patients with dementia.[28]

## VAGUS NERVE STIMULATION: THE SECRET TO BETTER HEALTH

Many clinical applications of vagus stimulation, including those approved to treat mental conditions like depression, bipolar disorder, and anxiety, involve a small surgical implant that electronically activates the nerve.[44] However, there are less-invasive, readily accessible options available. Countless studies, including those into HRVB, have shown that the power of the vagus nerve can be accessed *indirectly* to relieve imbalances in the nervous system.[25] This is particularly helpful with stress. When the vagus nerve is activated, the messages received by the brain become calmer. This begins a top-down feedback loop where the brain reports back to the body that it is safe, perpetuating a feeling of relaxation. Techniques to stimulate the vagus nerve include humming, laughing, and any sort of conscious breathing practice, including holding the breath, diaphragm breathing, nose breathing, and slow, relaxed exhalations.[45]

To recap quickly, fibers from the vagus nerve innervate systems that include the heart and lungs. When you breathe in, the sympathetic nervous system (SNS) facilitates a brief acceleration in heart rate.[46] On the out breath, the vagus nerve secretes Vagusstuff/ACh. ACh slows down the heart rate via the PNS. In other words, exhalation is under the direct control of the vagus nerve,[47] while vagal activity is suppressed during inhalation.[48, 49] By increasing the duration of the out breath, it may be possible to access the vagus nerve's connection with the rest and digest state, stimulate the on-demand release of ACh to calm the nerves, and shift the system out of its primal fight-or-flight response by signaling a state of relaxation.

The concept of slow breathing to restore and enhance health is not new.[27] A variety of breathing techniques have long been central to contemplative practices such as yoga, martial arts, Tai Chi Chuan, and meditation. The essential idea, encapsulated by the yogic practice of *Pranayama*, is that the mind and the breath are inextricably linked. The Sanskrit word *Prana* means the body's vital energy, and *yama* is control or mastery of that. Some practices that don't consciously focus on breath can also have an impact. For example, in deep transcendental meditation, the breath can gradually become so faint that it even stops for a while.[50] What most of these practices have in common is breathing through the nose.

Numerous scientific studies back up the centuries of tradition and experience. Research into the effects of slow breathing on the body shows significant impacts on the ANS and on the functions of the cardiovascular and respiratory systems, including baroreflex sensitivity, HRV, blood flow dynamics, RSA, and the balancing of the two branches of the ANS. Controlled slow breathing and breath holding can be used to optimize the very physical functions associated with health and longevity and which may provide greater resilience against disease.

Studies looking at the physical mechanisms of breathing indicate a connection between breath, cognition, and emotion, which involves the ANS.[28] Breathing well contributes to emotional balance and social adaptation. A 2017 review in the *Journal of Yoga and Physiotherapy* explains that, since exhalation is the relaxation phase, holding the breath after exhaling activates the PNS, increasing relaxation.[18] The paper suggests that to experience long-term benefits from breath-hold exercises, we need to spend time daily in parasympathetic dominance. The best way to do this is to develop a habit of controlling the breath most of the time in an easy, spontaneous way. Another study found that yogic breathing exercises altered autonomic responses to breath holding by increasing vagal tone and decreasing sympathetic activity.[51]

## COLD WATER RESILIENCE AND EXPRESSIVE FACES

While direct stimulation of the vagus nerve is only possible using an implanted device, diaphragm breathing, meditation, and singing can all be used to increase vagal tone. The popular breathwork guru, Wim Hof, uses a combination of breathing techniques and cold water immersion to activate the vagus nerve.

Scientists have proven that immersing the face in cold water or splashing cold water on the back of the neck increases parasympathetic activity.[52, 53] In fact, one study recommends the practice to moderate sympathetic activation after exercise to relieve stress on the heart.[52] However, full body cold water immersion can cause potentially fatal cardiac arrhythmia due to autonomic conflict, where both parasympathetic and sympathetic inputs to the heart are activated simultaneously.[54] This is because rapid submersion in water less than 59° Fahrenheit (15° Celsius) with simultaneous breath-holding activates two powerful autonomic responses: the cold shock response and the diving response.

At the same time, empirical evidence indicates that stronger vagal tone can make the body more resilient to cold. Magnus Appelberg has taught Ashtanga Yoga for nearly 20 years in Helsinki. He also enjoys ice swimming—an activity popular in Finland, in which bathers dive into holes in the ice, the hard-core among them staying in the water for several minutes. About four years ago, Appelberg met the long-time yoga exponent, physiotherapist, and research scientist Simon Borg-Olivier. Olivier's message boiled down to the simple principle: breathe less, stretch less (while getting more flexible), eat less, and move from the core. He taught Appelberg about the Bohr effect, the dilation of blood vessels, and the body's response to $CO_2$. In particular, Olivier explained how to balance the ANS using the breath, stimulating the parasympathetic, vagal branch with the exhalation.

Appelberg decided to change his breathing practice to include a simple prolonged exhale and breath holding after exhalation. He had been a winter swimmer for 20 years and his ability to adapt to the cold had never been particularly great. That winter, having adjusted his breathing, ice swimming was a little easier. The following year, he tried applying the slow exhalation in the water and discovered he could swim for 200 meters in freezing water— four times farther than the previous winter. Still, this wasn't completely out of the ordinary. In February 2019, he became a social media phenomenon with videos that showed him dropping into the ice hole directly from a yoga pose. He was interviewed on TV and radio, and this propelled him to experiment further.

Appelberg started using very long exhalations and breath holds, practicing these for 15 minutes before entering the water. Remarkably, this practice, using the breath to augment levels of $CO_2$ in his blood, increased the time he was able to stay in the cold water without pain or hypothermia from 5 minutes to 30 minutes—within 2 months. Appelberg found he could maintain his core temperature better by practicing breath holds in the water. He experienced none of the pain in his toes or fingers that would indicate the usual constriction of blood vessels, and the controlled breath kept him present in his body. In a June 2020 email to me, he wrote,

> The greatest help has been my almost 20 years of Vipassana meditation, after all cold is only a sensation . . . . Right now, I'm trying to find sources that could actually explain what is going on in the body. This adaptation is a fact and I've found the circumstances that are necessary for that: the stimulation of the parasympathetic nervous system and the higher levels of carbon dioxide to counteract the vasoconstriction. The effect on life in general has been amazing.

Few people have Appelberg's curiosity, resilience, and ability to push the boundaries.

It is important to emphasize that the practice of breath holds in the water is not recommended unless you are working under the supervision of a qualified breathing coach. For the rest of us mere mortals, the good news is that you can gain considerable benefits by practicing the breathing exercises on dry land.

Interestingly, research that demonstrates that immersing the face in cold water stimulates the vagus nerve is echoed in the work of behavioral neuroscientist and psychiatry professor, Steven Porges. Porges put forward a theory suggesting that the vagus nerve comprises three neural circuits, the most primitive of which is related to evolutionary behaviors like the "freeze" response of extreme stress, while the newest is linked to social communication and self-soothing. Porges says that one way that breathing exercises produce vagal stimulation is via sensory and motor nerves that regulate facial muscles.[55] This is in line with studies that show babies with more expressive faces have higher HRV[56] and with Wim Hof's assertion that it is possible to stimulate the vagus nerve by activating the parts of the body it innervates. The vagus nerve is responsible for speech, the gag reflex, and many movements of the mouth.[57] In fact, according to Porges, the very process of using the muscles in the face and head to actively interact changes our physiological state by increasing vagal influences on the heart and calming the sympathetic nervous system's fight-or-flight response. Conversely, the cosmetic treatment Botox, which is used to smooth away signs of aging by effectively paralyzing the face, actually works by inhibiting the release of ACh.

## THE DIAPHRAGM

The diaphragm is the main muscle for the physical act of breathing. It, too, is innervated by the vagus nerve.[58] It should therefore come as no surprise that diaphragmatic or deep breathing is one of the most common and ancient methods for body-mind training and holistic treatment of stress and psychosomatic conditions.[28] Inhaling and exhaling from the diaphragm slows the breath and maximizes the exchange of blood gases.[28] In a study, healthy participants who were trained in diaphragm breathing had slower rates of respiration and were more likely to achieve the goal of three to seven breaths per minute than those who breathed normally.[27]

Studies of the function and movement of the diaphragm muscle show that optimal breathing requires active diaphragm control. Ideally, during the inhalation, the lower ribs stay low, expanding only laterally, with the abdomen expanding instead of the chest. The amount of movement in the diaphragm correlates with changes in lung volume. The more the diaphragm moves between the in and out breaths, the greater the tidal volume (the amount of air breathed in with each normal breath).

Inhalations and exhalations are driven by a group of muscles collectively referred to as the respiratory pump, the largest of which is the diaphragm. During the in breath, the diaphragm contracts and flattens.[27] It pushes on the abdomen, and the lower ribs move upward and outward. Coordinated contraction of various muscles expands the rib cage, and the chest opens outward. The resulting changes in pressure trigger ventilation and gas exchange in the lungs. The out breath is more passive. The diaphragm returns to its dome-shaped resting position, the lungs deflate, and air is expelled.

Importantly, it is possible to support optimum gas exchange with controlled slow respiration *as long as it is paired with an increase in tidal volume*. Diaphragmatic breathing at a rate of six breaths per minute reduces the chemoreflex response to both *hypercapnia* (where $CO_2$

levels are too high) and *hypoxia* (where oxygen levels are too low).[59–61] Conversely, increasing the speed of the breath to a faster-than-normal rate does nothing to improve its efficiency: less of the air reaches the alveoli due to increased "dead space." As we saw in Chapter Three, slower breathing is simply more efficient. Air reaches and distends more of the alveoli in the lungs, so more oxygen enters the bloodstream. In a study comparing oxygen levels in the arteries during normal breathing and at 15, 6, and 3 breaths per minute, the rate of 6 breaths per minute was found to be the best for reducing dead space in the airways, increasing oxygen uptake, and for ease of sustainability.

A paper published in *Frontiers in Psychology* found that diaphragmatic breathing, which itself naturally results in a slower respiration rate, has the potential to reduce the impact of stress and improve cognitive performance in otherwise healthy adults.[28] The results suggested that this may be because HRV increases during diaphragmatic breathing, indicating a better balance of activity between the SNS and PNS. Scientists inferred that deep breathing might impact cognitive performance by influencing the ANS, and that breathing may link the mind and body together to regulate the information processing necessary to maintain attention.

A review of the possible pain-relieving effect of deep breathing further underlines the mind-body-breath connection. Scientists found that the perception of pain was reduced when participants held their breath after a deep inhalation, a position where the diaphragm is lowered. Notably, this appeared to involve the intervention of the baroreceptors.[58] The study suggested that the pain response is not simply a neural process but that a close relationship exists between the breath, the emotions, and the working of the baroreceptors. Stress can lead to anxiety and depression, which can adversely affect the way the diaphragm works. Equally, changes in emotional state can cause a greater perception of pain. The study concluded that the diaphragm influences the working of the baroreceptors and the perception of pain, and vice versa. This may be because the movement of the diaphragm changes the pressure within the body, and the resulting flow of blood in the body determines the baroreceptor response, but there is not yet clear research to confirm this.[58]

## SIX BREATHS PER MINUTE

To recap what we have already learned, slow breathing causes the oscillations in blood pressure to synchronize with the rhythm of the heart, creating the conditions for optimum blood gas exchange. Remember, there's a significant connection between RSA, HRV, baroreceptors, and the ANS. Scientists have shown that slow breathing at a rate of six breaths a minute, with increased tidal volume (achieved by activating the diaphragm), rather than suppressing the fight-or-flight activity of the sympathetic nervous system, appears to optimize the balance between the sympathetic and parasympathetic branches of the ANS and to enhance autonomic reactivity to both physical and mental stress.[27]

Breathing at six breaths per minute has a powerful effect on many body systems. In the respiratory system, it increases air in the lungs, enhances the function of the diaphragm, improves ventilation efficiency, pulls more oxygen into the blood, and is thought to increase blood flow back to the heart (venous return). This has been demonstrated in studies of athletes at high altitude. Athletes climbing to the peaks of Everest and K2 without oxygen supplies were able to achieve similar oxygenation with slower breathing rates after two weeks of acclimatization in lower atmospheric oxygen levels. It was concluded that efficiency of breathing is more important than quantity.[62]

In the cardiovascular system, breathing at six breaths per minute increases the filling of the right heart and the amount of blood pumped by the heart per minute.[27] It causes blood pressure oscillations to synchronize with the rhythm of the heartbeat, increases HRV, and potentially decreases mean blood pressure. In the cardiorespiratory system, it increases baroreflex sensitivity and HRV. In the ANS, it increases vagal tone, promotes a shift toward PNS dominance, and improves the responsiveness of the ANS toward physical movement. The rate of six breaths per minute optimizes the release and metabolism of acetylcholine, maximizing RSA.[27] It is also the threshold for triggering the baroreflex and is the respiration rate with the highest increase of HRV.

For centuries, people have practiced techniques like meditation and yoga for their positive effects on physical and mental health and cognition. What all these activities have in common is that breathing is attentively guided or regulated. Even simple awareness of the breath can influence the rate of respiration. This, in turn, explains the health benefits of such practices through their impact on the balance of the ANS. The physical functions underlying these breathing techniques have been studied to explain the impact of respiratory vagal nerve stimulation on inflammation, the working of the heart, general physical and mental health, stress relief, and enhanced brain power, including a better working memory and greater creativity.

There has also been research into the way the body interprets the top-down (brain to body) and bottom-up (body to brain) signals and into the possibility of training the autonomic responses.[25] It has been confirmed that respiratory vagus nerve stimulation (rVNS) reduces stress and inflammation long-term. While rVNS produces an immediate shift in PNS activity during and after practice, it also results in a shift in autonomic balance, increasing vagal dominance both in resting states and in those active states requiring behavioral and cognitive flexibility.

Evidence shows that breathing exercises with a low respiration rate can stimulate the vagus nerve. Though how this occurs is not proven, scientists believe the baroreflex mechanism causes this stimulation. The health benefits felt by people practicing slow and controlled breathing are due to a prolonged increase in vagal tone. Dominance of the PNS depends on the consistent ability of the body's systems to relax. This provides a release from chronic stress and prevents stress-related illness.

## LONG EXHALATIONS

Practicing breath holds, in particular, provides a tool to control the ANS. Breath holding also helps the body adapt to higher blood $CO_2$ (hypercapnia) and provides a direct way to hack the body's stress response. As one paper puts it, by practicing breath holds, you will eventually be able to "maintain self-control in most stressful settings."[18] Short term, the benefits include stress reduction, better regulation of blood pressure, and more focused attention. Prolonged practice improves cognitive function and enhances autonomic balance, improving your ability to come back to baseline and respond to external and internal challenges from a balanced physical and psychological perspective.[18]

Studies into the different systems, such as the PNS, respiratory ventilation, and HRV, have settled on a rate of six breaths per minute as optimal.

However, given that the vagus nerve is activated purely during the out breath, why isn't there more exploration into inhalation/exhalation ratios? Does the vagus nerve work even better when exhalations are longer than inhalations?

One study carried out by scientists in Taiwan looked at this idea in detail by examining healthy college students to discover the differences in breathing with longer exhalations compared to breathing with equal in/out ratios in the effect on subjective feelings of anxiety and physiologically on HRV.[63] Specifically, they explored two very similar breathing rates—6 breaths per minute and 5.5 breaths per minute—each with inhalation to exhalation ratios of 5:5 (equal) and 4:6 (longer exhalation).

They expected slow breathing with longer exhalations to create more intense feelings of relaxation and higher HRV than an equal ratio pattern. Previous studies showing the beneficial effects of 6 breaths per minute for heart and lung functions had already confirmed that inhaling quickly and exhaling slowly (2:8 respectively) was more effective in reducing mental and physical arousal in threatening or stressful situations than inhaling slowly and exhaling quickly.[63] There are also various breathing exercises, for example in yoga, where techniques such as 2:1 breathing, during which exhalations are twice the length of inhalations, are recognized as beneficial.[64] However, contrary to expectations, the Taiwan study revealed that a respiration rate of 5.5 breaths per minute with equal length in/out breaths (5:5) significantly increased HRV.[63] What's more, it increased vagal nerve/PNS activation and baroreflex function more than the other breathing patterns, meaning it has the potential to help patients with conditions where low HRV is a feature.

Several papers point out that slow breathing can be uncomfortable. This might explain why people are attracted to activities like yoga and meditation where the focus is on the breath, but the practice is guided to make breathing effortless. To comfortably breathe at a rate of 5.5 breaths per minute with an equal inhalation and exhalation ratio, a BOLT score of at least 15 seconds is required. There are programs in Chapter Two designed to improve the BOLT score to 15 seconds, making slow breathing practice more attainable.

It is certainly worth your time and effort, given the indications that this breathing pattern increases PNS and baroreflex function and simultaneously enhances relaxation.

## SYNCHRONIZED BREATHING—MANTRAS AND MUSIC

The age-old breathing practices cultivated in Eastern traditions have significant scientific basis in terms of physical and mental influence.[65] However, various other customs and activities have also been found to synchronize cardiovascular rhythms by reducing breathing to the optimum rate. Recitation of both the yoga mantra *"om-mani-padme-hum"* and the rosary prayer in Latin, with one person reciting the priest's part: *"Ave Maria, gratia plena, Dominus tecum, benedicta tui mulieribus et benedictus fructus ventris tui Jesus,"* and the other the response: *"Sancta Maria, Mater Dei, ora pro nobis peccatoribus, nunc et in hora mortis nostrae, Amen,"* has been found to lower the respiratory rate to, you guessed it, around six breaths per minute.[65]

This is no coincidence. Mantras, which are usually repeated in sequences of more than 100, similar to the rosary, which is recited 150 times, may have evolved as a device to slow respiration, induce relaxation and enhance concentration.[66] The length of time required to perform over 100 mantras or to get through 150 recitations of the rosary is significant, suggesting that one of the aims might be to induce physical changes as well as altering mental state.

Given that many of the physical aspects at play here are rhythmical, it is also worth looking at the connection between music and the PNS. Humans interact with music at behavioral, emotional, and physiological levels, both consciously and unconsciously.[67] Over 100 years ago, it was suggested that the ANS forms a sort of "sounding board" that reverberates to changes in consciousness.[67] Many centuries earlier, classical Greek philosophers believed music and sports to be the two fundamental aspects of well-being. Contemporary experiments have explored how elements of music such as beat, tempo, and pitch trigger emotional and behavioral responses, as well as reactions in the physical and nervous systems.

Singing has been found to reduce tension, increase energy, and improve mood. It directly activates the vocal cords and the muscles at the back of the throat—which are connected to the vagus nerve.[68] Regular singing can even increase vagal tone. However, the impact of singing on HRV was found to be dependent on whether the singer experienced the task as stressful or not. A greater heart rate variable was found in professional singers after a singing lesson, while amateurs showed lower HRV. Heart rate increased after solo singing but decreased after choral singing, indicating that when a person is performing music, rather than just listening to it, the perception of the task as safe or scary influences the resultant physical reaction. It has also been found that trained musicians have a lower baseline breathing rate than nonmusicians.[69]

One study into the physiological responses to music found that even a short listening session could bring about measurable cardiovascular and respiratory effects.[69] The level of arousal or focused attention was largely determined by the tempo (speed) of the music. Regardless of taste in music or whether the listener was previously familiar with the piece, slow music from a variety of genres reduced cardiorespiratory response. A pause or period of silence in the music produced a higher level of relaxation than the music itself, suggesting that music may give pleasure and potential health benefits as a result of the controlled alternation of arousal and relaxation. It was concluded that music can be used to induce relaxation and reduce SNS activity and that it may be useful in the management of cardiovascular disease.

In a therapeutic setting, music has been used to enhance parasympathetic activity and decrease congestive heart failure by reducing levels of inflammatory cytokines.[70] Patients undergoing a 14-day music therapy course exhibited changes in HRV patterns that indicated enhanced activity of the cardiovascular system.[71] One experiment into the impact of music on the autonomic response compared healthy participants with patients in a vegetative state or with unresponsive wakefulness syndrome. Those participants with disorders of consciousness showed replicable changes in the balance between the SNS and the vagal system after passive listening to symphonic music.[72]

## USING HRV IN THE REAL WORLD

As part of the training that I run for our Oxygen Advantage instructors, I was fortunate enough to organize an online coaching webinar in August 2020 with Dr. Jay T. Wiles, a clinical health physiologist. Dr. Wiles specializes in sports performance and holistic and integrative health, and he is board certified in biofeedback and HRVB.

Dr. Wiles came to HRV through his clinical practice, working with patients with clinical stress, PTSD, and anxiety. As he learned about HRV, he became fascinated by its implications not only for peak performance and sporting excellence but also for its potential applications in a clinical setting. He became determined to present information about HRV in a way that is easy to access and practical in day-to-day life.

The way you use HVR depends on your starting point and your goals. This is also true for the breathing exercises in this book. It's helpful to avoid preconceptions about what is "good" or "bad." For instance, it may surprise you to know that elite athletes often have very poor vagal tone because they have taxed their nervous systems through years of overtraining and over-reaching. These athletes often come to HRVB to find out what is impeding their performance.

If you want to understand how well your nervous system is functioning, HRV provides the best inexpensive, noninvasive way to do this. It has a wide-ranging and diverse clinical utility, but as it increases in popularity among fitness enthusiasts, its purpose and application are frequently misunderstood. In many cases, the readings that people get from their consumer-based devices are useless because they lack the contextual framework to understand or improve them.

Dr. Wiles originally became interested in HRV through his work with trauma patients. He wanted something that would allow him to objectively quantify the stress response. In clinic, he found that most information came from his patients in the form of subjective, qualitative data about how they were feeling. While this was valuable, HRV offered quantitative data that helped him build a clearer picture of what was going on with those patients so he could help them better. He began using HRVB with the chronic pain population, with patients who often had a variety of conditions including pain, depression, stress, and anxiety, all existing comorbidly. He began to see improvements in all these symptoms and syndromes as a direct result of HRVB.

Dr. Wiles explained to me that we have trillions of processes going on in the body in any given second. As we go about our day, the heart has to adjust to everything we encounter in our environment, and to all of the processes in the body. For this reason, higher HRV, which signifies greater adaptability, is normally preferable.

The widely held belief that the processes of the ANS are entirely involuntary is incorrect. We can control HRV very easily, but we lose control due to stress. Dr. Wiles believes that, because HRV is data driven, research-supported, and quantifiable, it is incredibly valuable in breathwork. In a sense, it strengthens the scientific basis for the work because results can be so clearly and accurately measured.

As we already discovered, HRV is measured in time domains (the time difference between each heartbeat). It is also measured in frequency domains (the frequency or the individual components of each heartbeat). These two elements, time and frequency, are the two main aspects of HRV. While the time domain data gives an important baseline for our HRV at rest, the frequency domain data gives us insight into our overall stress response. If you have high vagal tone and good HRV, you will see an increase in high frequencies and a decrease in low frequencies. This is because the high frequencies receive predominantly PNS contributions.

Another common belief that confounds HRVB training is that "higher is normally better" in terms of HRV measurements. As we touched on earlier, this is not always the case. For this reason, a self-comparison strategy is always more valuable than a comparison against some imagined "norm." HRV may become too high because you are too much in a parasympathetic state. The aim is not to be in a parasympathetic state all of the time; rather to modulate the ANS and to learn to control HRV.

There is no "good" or "bad" in terms of short-term readings, and the "normal" measurement range changes as we age, so the idea of an ideal or goal HRV is somewhat irrelevant. It's important to remember that HRVB devices measure two different things: time (RSMMD) and frequency (SDNN). Be careful not to confuse the two. In frequency readings over 24 hours, 100 is considered a healthy reading, between 50 and 100 is "compromised," and, if your reading is below 50, you may be at risk of a heart attack. However, even if your reading is just 20, don't worry. The focus should always be on self-comparison, your ability to modulate HRV, and progress in an upward direction.

Dr. Wiles stressed that the purpose of HRVB is not necessarily to raise your baseline reading. "The primary thing," he said, "is to be able to modulate HRV in acute situations, to get you out of the stress state and help you perform at your highest level."

One useful side effect of HRVB is that you will start to become more aware of your own stress response, both physically and mentally, thereby increasing your ability to self-regulate. The human brain doesn't distinguish stress caused by physical danger from the stress caused by less life-threatening situations, such as relationship problems or financial worries. That is why it is so easy to become conditioned to being in a state of permanently high SNS activation. HRVB gives you the tools to take back control, to change gear when you need to. One of the techniques used for this is breathwork.

Dr. Wiles explained that while the HRVB studies discussed earlier got many things right (focusing on low, slow breathing, the mind-body connection, data tracking, and replication), they overlooked some things. For instance, they failed to focus on biochemistry, the depth of breath, light and quiet breathing rather than heavy loud breathing, nose breathing instead of mouth breathing, and the importance of hypercapnia (high blood $CO_2$) for vagal tone.

You can influence HRV by engaging:

- Nasal breathing
- Light breathing
- Slow breathing
- Deep breathing

In fact, even without biofeedback, by using the exercises in this book, you are already training your HRV. Biofeedback tools come in useful when you want to see exactly what is happening from a physiological standpoint.

Nasal breathing can have a significant impact on HRV due to the influence of the baroreflex system and increased vasodilation. According to Dr. Wiles, this vasodilatory response sends a cascade of biochemical messages through the baroreflex to stimulate the vagus nerve. Simply switching to nasal breathing will influence HRV, whether or not you engage in diaphragm breathing or work to slow the cadence of your breath. To illustrate this, Dr. Wiles described how free divers need to be able to activate both branches of the ANS. These divers will generally breathe nasally, but just before a dive they inhale through the mouth. This increases blood pressure, so that the diver's blood pressure levels out as he or she dives, rather than dropping below normal.

Nasal breathing also promotes increased HRV due to hypercapnia (high blood $CO_2$). Be aware that when you practice breath holds or light breathing with air hunger, HRV may dip initially. This is because the body perceives stress and responds accordingly. As you practice, the body will adapt. Interestingly, what often happens after the practice is that, even when HRV has dipped, when you resume normal breathing, it becomes significantly higher.

According to research, changes in $CO_2$ that accompany conscious manipulation of breathing patterns independently influence autonomic control
of the heart and modulate HRV. Increased $CO_2$ in people who are awake
enhances high and low frequency power, indicating better vagal tone[73]. The
connection between $CO_2$, HRV, and vagal tone is the reason you feel relaxed
when you engage in light, slow breathing. From a biochemical perspective,
light, slow breathing, and hypercapnia also result in a flood of hormones,
an increase in acetylcholine, an influx of dopamine, and a reduction in
adrenaline and inflammation.

It is much easier to use HRV than it is to explain it in a simple way. It
provides a really good way to not only subjectively feel better, but to objectively see the change in the nervous system. This can be very motivating. If
you have the opportunity to do so, it can be immensely valuable to work with
a professional breathing instructor who can demonstrate how HRV changes
as you alter the biochemistry, biomechanics, and cadence of your breath.

You can also buy your own HRV measurement tools. However, Dr. Wiles
cautions that they are "not all created equal." Devices in the $300 range,
such as the Lief Therapeutics wearable ECG, Oura Ring, WHOOP Strap,
BioStrap, HeartMath Inner Balance™ or emWave2®, and the Polar H10 Chest
Strap with the Elite HRV app, are all reliable.

## SOME TIPS FOR TRAINING

If you have a serious health condition or suffer with anxiety and panic
symptoms, the same principle applies as for the breathing exercises—begin
any practice or training gently. Some people find the air hunger produced
by the *Breathe Light* exercise (found in Chapter Two) can cause an intense
stress reaction. Adjust your training accordingly and work your way up from
just a few minutes' practice. If you do experience a stress response, this is
not necessarily a bad thing or something to be concerned about. However,
too strong an activation of the SNS can put you off trying the exercises
altogether. Be reassured that as you get into the rhythm of HRVB training,
your nervous system response will begin to modulate.

If, after exercise, your HRV drops by more than 20%, you have over-
trained; your nervous system has had enough. In sports performance, HRV

is one of the greatest predictors of future injury. Dr. Wiles uses overnight readings with his clients. The differences between these readings dictate how hard the athlete trains the following day. He explained, "You have a much greater chance of a successful workout if your HRV has not dropped too much."

> One thing I like to mention is my 20% and 40% rule. If your over-night HRV reading is 20% lower than your normal baseline, this should indicate "caution." This does not mean you should not train, but you should be aware of a suppressed nervous system. When this happens, I tell athletes to do a lighter training day. When your HRV drops below 40%, this should be a day off where the athlete should utilize "strong caution" as they will be much more susceptible to injury and overtraining.

Dr. Wiles told me that teaching these athletes how to modulate HRV to get themselves back into flow is vital. They need enough stress that they can perform but not so much that it impairs performance. This is fundamentally true for anyone who needs to perform, whether in a sporting, Arts, or corporate setting. And this is where HRVB training can be truly valuable.

Mouth breathing during sleep (discussed in Chapter Seven) is also a big "no." Many of the Oxygen Advantage instructors report that their HRV improves just from nasal breathing during sleep. According to Dr. Wiles, this is a "non-negotiable" for athletes in his care. He described the case of an ATP top level tennis player in his early thirties who had very low HRV when he first attended the clinic for training. After working on light, slow, deep breathing and taping his mouth at night, the player's HRV measurement increased markedly. His performance on the court improved, and his risk of injury decreased.

One more tip: if you engage in public speaking, big presentations, or performance of any kind, when you are midperformance, your focus should be on what you are doing, not on your HRV. The trick is to condition your response before the event and then trust that you'll experience a significant change during the event. Focus on the task at hand and rely on your body to kick into high gear because your ANS is in a better state. This is the power of HRV.

# CHAPTER FIVE

# FUNCTIONAL BREATHING, THE SECRET OF FUNCTIONAL MOVEMENT

From birth, breathing is our first and most basic motor pattern.[1] As toddlers, we learn to stand up against gravity and control posture with the support of the diaphragm. As we grow, breathing is central to both posture and functional movement. Throughout our lives, breathing and posture sustain each other. But if breathing pattern disorders are present, this relationship becomes dysfunctional. The result is poor core muscle function and the onset of disabling conditions, such as lower back pain. If you want a simple reason to correct poor breathing patterns, it's this: when your breathing is less than optimal, it will adversely affect your freedom of movement, eventually causing chronic pain.

In 2017, researchers at Evansville University, Indiana, demonstrated that dysfunctional breathing (DB) directly and adversely affects the musculoskeletal system.[2] The musculoskeletal system includes the bones of the skeleton, muscles, joints, tendons, cartilage, ligaments, and other connective tissue. If the function of this system is compromised, it becomes impossible for the core muscles to support the spine and pelvis properly. Research has linked DB to a host of conditions that limit movement and cause pain, including lower back and neck problems, and it is now acknowledged that core muscle dysfunction plays a role in a variety of musculoskeletal disorders and an overall increased risk of injury.

Dysfunctional breathing can be at the root of recurrent and chronic symptoms including lumbopelvic, chest and neck pain, fatigue, anxiety, an irritable bowel or bladder, "brain-fog," paresthesia, and cold hands, fingers, feet, or toes.[3] However, there is a gap between research and practice. Core muscle exercises—such as pelvic tilts and exercises using a stability ball and hip bridge (a strengthening posture that involves lying on the back and lifting the hips off the floor while the shoulder blades and feet remain lengthened into the ground)—are often prescribed during physical rehabilitation,[4] but breathwork is not. Despite the recognized links between breathing function and postural support and the known prevalence of breathing pattern disorders, the connection is rarely made in therapy. In fact, breathing is usually overlooked.[2]

However, underlying breathing pattern disorders are common enough to warrant more attention. In the United States, as many as 10% of patients in general internal medicine practices have hyperventilation syndrome as their main diagnosis.[5] Dysfunctional breathing is even more widespread.[6] Everyday physical symptoms, such as headache, back pain, chest pain, and abdominal pain, which account for half of all primary care visits in the United States,[7] can potentially be made worse by dysfunctional breathing.[8] The good news is that dysfunctional breathing can usually be resolved by practicing simple exercises like the ones in this book.

While dysfunctional breathing often indicates poor health and goes hand-in-hand with dysfunctional movement, it is not necessarily related to cardio-vascular fitness. It is surprisingly common to be incredibly fit and still have symptoms of dysfunctional breathing. In fact, many of the clients I work with to restore functional breathing are top-level athletes. Even when high levels of fitness are achieved and maintained, DB can indicate problems elsewhere in the body. Ultimately, poor breathing patterns will have a significant and long-term impact on both mental and physical well-being. Breathing is one of the body's critical functions. When its fundamental processes break down, the body will compensate, calling on structures such as the core muscles to help maintain respiration. If breathing is not efficient in a normal restful waking state, it is never going to be optimal during physical exercise. It will also be dysfunctional during sleep, when the body needs to restore, repair, and revitalize its systems.

## BREATHING, CORE STABILITY, AND BALANCE

Your core connects and supports the movement of your upper and lower body. Whether you are kicking a ball, rowing, cycling, or vacuuming the floor, the action originates in or moves through the core. Weak or unstable core muscles will affect the functioning of the legs and arms and cause poor balance and stability. This can lead to falls, injuries in sport, or ongoing pain and discomfort.

A stable core is the foundation of functional movement. It underpins basic activities such as bending to put your socks on or pick up your child, sitting or standing, and the many day-to-day things we barely notice doing until they become painful. Core strength isn't just needed for manual work. Even sedentary desk jobs require core muscle strength so that the muscles of the back don't become strained.

The common narrative is that back pain and poor core stability can be prevented by exercises that balance and strengthen the core muscles, specifically the abdominal muscles. However, this conception of "core strength" misses the true foundation of core stability: the breath. According to a 2013 review by physiotherapist Josephine Key, breathing is a root mechanism for core control. Breathing is integral to postural stability and vice versa. Functional breathing supports posture and functional movement via the diaphragm muscle. However, if the spine and pelvis are not stable, there will never be optimum space for the diaphragm to descend during inhalation. Key remarks that "If the posture is 'good' so too is the breathing pattern and conversely, if the breathing pattern is healthy, so is the posture."[1] However, according to Key, the concepts of core strength and function are often misunderstood. She quotes the spine biomechanics specialist, Stuart McGill, who said, "There's so much mythology out there about the core. The idea has reached trainers and through them the public that the core means only the abs. There's no science behind that."[9]

Certainly, many people still understand the core to mean only the transversus abdominis muscle. There's a widely held idea that this muscle alone supports and stabilizes the spine and pelvis, but this is simply not the case. The core can be described anatomically as a box, with the diaphragm on the top, the abdominals at the front, the gluteal and spinal muscles at the back, and the pelvic floor and hip muscles at the base.[10] Notice that the mechanisms of core stability include *both* breathing and postural control.

Core stability, breathing, and posture are inextricably linked by the pressure generated in the abdominal cavity by the movement of the diaphragm. This is called intra-abdominal pressure (IAP). Intra-abdominal pressure fluctuates through the breathing cycle. When you breathe in, your diaphragm moves downward, producing positive pressure in the abdominal cavity. This pressure works a bit like an inflating balloon. It has a stabilizing effect, supporting the spine and pelvis. When breathing is fully functional, the diaphragm is better able to generate optimal IAP—and better spinal stability.

This affects balance, as well as posture and movement. One small 2017 study explored the connection between diaphragm breathing training and static and dynamic balance. Thirteen participants practiced breathing exercises over eight weeks. Balance and breathing were assessed every week. Researchers found that each week, as breathing scores improved, participants showed fewer errors in single-leg balancing.[11] This suggests that diaphragm breathing may help improve balance.

The stability of the trunk and pelvis is essential for athletic performance and injury prevention,[12] but it is also important for anyone who wants to enjoy a good quality of life, pain free. Instability around the pelvis can cause excess movement in other joints. That is why an athlete with poor gluteal control may experience knee and foot pain. Instability in the lumbar spine can cause stiffness in the thoracic spine, leading to compensating movements in the shoulder and pain or tears in the rotator cuff tendon[12]. Likewise, people with back pain tend to brace the superficial muscles of the abdomen and diaphragm. This, combined with poor core muscle activation, inhibits normal functioning of the diaphragm and encourages upper chest breathing.[13, 14] These problems are not confined to sports. Between 50% and 80% of adults suffer lower back pain at some point in their lives, and it is the most common cause of disability among working age people worldwide.[15]

A stable spine supports the body during movement. You may have seen weightlifters breathe in before a lift and hold their breath during the lift. The breath hold on the inhalation is intended to generate high levels of intra-abdominal pressure and "stiffen the spine." Instead, Josephine Key argues that if the weightlifter maintained a regular breathing pattern when lifting, IAP levels would actually be better and the risk of spinal compression less. In other words, a weightlifter with functional breathing would be better able to generate adequate levels of IAP during a lift. Instead of the lift relying on a breath hold, the weightlifter could actually generate greater IAP as the diaphragm moves downward.

It has been known for some time that IAP increases during many tasks that load the spine—for example, static and dynamic tasks such as walking, lifting, and jumping. However, it had been argued that the pressure generated during these basic movements isn't enough to significantly increase spinal stability. Studies failed to identify whether mechanical support of the spine was provided by IAP or by the abdominal muscles. However, one 2005 paper *did* find that IAP increases stiffness of the lumbar spine *without any concurrent activity* from the abs and back extensor muscles.[16]

When breathing is shallow and confined to the upper chest, it is difficult to build up IAP. Instead, the body must rely on the back and neck muscles for support. Proper movement of the diaphragm prevents upper chest breathing. When the diaphragm moves freely, the lower rib cage expands laterally. The diaphragm must be unrestricted, because this expansion, with the lower rib cage opening out to the front, back, and sides, only occurs if the movement of the diaphragm creates sufficient pressure to push the ribs outward[1]. This outward movement provides enough space between the thorax and pelvis for the diaphragm to descend, and this helps keep the posture balanced. (You will find an exercise to develop this lateral expansion of the ribs in Chapter Two.)

According to a 2018 study, the diaphragm plays another role in the stability of the trunk. When the diaphragm contracts, it minimizes the displacement of the abdominal contents, such as the digestive organs, into the chest, maintaining the hoop-like shape of the abdominal muscles.[17] This increases spinal stability through tension in the connective tissue or fascia that covers the thoracic spine and the deep muscles under the back. The thoracic spine is the longest part of the spine, from the lower neck to the abdomen, and is the part connected to the rib cage. The study found that the two functions of the diaphragm—breathing and postural stabilization—operate independently of whether we are breathing in or out. This observation led researchers to conclude that the diaphragm's response may be regulated by the central nervous system[17]. This would make sense since the diaphragm is also responsible for the pain threshold and plays a role in the perception of pain.[17]

The focus of that 2018 study was to determine whether a relationship existed between the health of the diaphragm muscle and maintaining static balance. Scientists found that balance was better, both with eyes open or closed, when the diaphragm was thicker and moved more freely during quiet and deep breathing. The diaphragm is a striated muscle—the same type that moves the joints.[18] A thicker diaphragm indicates better respiratory muscle strength,[19] which goes hand in hand with functional breathing. A diaphragm ultrasound (an easy-to-perform, easily reproducible, noninvasive diagnostic tool) can determine the thickness and excursion of the diaphragm. An ultrasound is a good supplement to (but not a replacement for) respiratory muscle strength testing.

In the 2018 static balance study, the same results were demonstrated in patients diagnosed with lung cancer, those undergoing lung resection, and healthy people. It also showed that deterioration in diaphragm function after chest surgery closely correlated with worsening balance. Problems with the diaphragm, such as atrophy, paralysis, and reduced muscle thickness, were clearly linked to the development of static balance disorders. It confirmed that stable balance depends on the diaphragm's ability to generate optimal IAP. The study concluded that balance is "inextricably linked to breathing."[17]

In an article in the 2017 *Journal of Yoga and Physical Therapy* (exploring the subject of reduced blood carbon dioxide and vagus nerve stimulation), U. P. Singh talks about the connection between the body and breath and its importance to properly aligned posture and a well-balanced outlook. Describing the concept of "grounding" as a sure sense of reality and self, with an openness and responsiveness to new ideas and input, he argues that this "sense of self" is achieved by restoring appropriate patterns of posture and breathing.[20]

This concept is integral to contemplative practices the world over. Even the word *yoga*, from the Sanskrit root "yuj (युज्)," means union—between body and breath and, in spiritual terms, between the self and the higher consciousness or divine. At the heart of this body-breath connection is the ability to perform a full, relaxed exhalation, allowing the diaphragm to achieve a natural domed position, in contact with the internal rib cage. Singh points out that, when it comes to functional movement, "We are always under the influence of gravity." Holding the breath after exhaling is an excellent exercise to rehabilitate and strengthen the core muscles. Once this skill is perfected, "it becomes a natural self-care; an invisible, but vital skill."[20]

Athletes also need to consider the role of normal breathing mechanics in posture and spinal stabilization. Studies have shown that breathing pattern disorders can lead to increased pain and contribute to problems with motor control, causing or contributing to dysfunctional patterns of movement.[21] The diaphragm performs the dual functions of respiration and postural support, but when all the body's systems are challenged, breathing always takes precedence and wins.[22]

## BREATHING AND EXERCISE: FUNCTIONAL MOVEMENT AND INJURY

When athletes are physically active, dysfunctional breathing can manifest as premature breathlessness or muscle fatigue, inevitably resulting in suboptimal performance[23]. A combination of upper chest breathing and overbreathing can cause significant changes in respiratory chemistry. In particular, dysfunctional breathing can decrease carbon dioxide ($CO_2$) levels in the blood. When $CO_2$ is depleted, blood pH increases, triggering respiratory alkalosis—the blood becomes too alkaline. Respiratory alkalosis can trigger changes in the nervous system and in physical and mental states that can have a detrimental effect on the musculoskeletal system[21] as well as on general levels of health and performance.

Respiratory alkalosis produces an array of symptoms, such as exhaustion, headaches, dizziness, light sensitivity, trouble sleeping, chest pain, cramps, and feelings of breathlessness. The common maxim, "no pain, no gain," implies that stressing the body to let it recover is a helpful strategy, when in fact, forcing yourself past the point of discomfort can affect mind-body coordination[24] and create a negative experience that does little to boost health and fitness.

Studies by Dr. John Douillard into an exercise technique that uses 5,000-year-old Vedic concepts of integrating mind, body, and environment to achieve flow and requires the athlete to practice a form of deep nasal breathing called *ujjayi* (the same form of breathing used in yoga practices like Ashtanga), found that the technique produced less feelings of exertion and greater comfort during high-intensity training than did normal aerobic exercise.[24] This breathing practice contributes to a feeling of deep calm during exercise and to increased respiratory sinus arrhythmia, helping promote fitness, endurance, strength, and better mind-body coordination with less effort, strain, and fatigue.[24]

Exercise increases demands on the respiratory, cardiovascular, and muscular systems and requires the body to adapt to biomechanical, biochemical, and psychological changes through the breath. Even top-level athletes can succumb to injury if their breathing is dysfunctional. Rates of musculoskeletal injury are relatively high among physically active people. One review in the *Journal of Athletic Training* cites an average of 13.79 injuries per 1,000 athletic "exposures" during competition.[25] Outside of sport, across a variety of professions, the breath may be at the root of repetitive strain injury (RSI).[26]

Since breathing pattern disorders are common in the general population—one study states that "normal patterns of breathing are the exception rather than the rule"[27]—prevalence will be similar in the athletic population. However, the effects of dysfunctional breathing may be amplified due to the extra physiological and biomechanical demands of exercise. Whatever the task, if the body is not able to recruit the appropriate muscles, the result will be compensatory patterns of movement.

In 2014, sport scientists Helen Bradley and Dr. Joseph Esformes studied the relationship between breathing pattern disorders and functional movement. Functional movement was defined as the "ability to produce and maintain sufficient mobility and stability along the kinetic chain while accurately and efficiently completing fundamental movement patterns." More simply, that just means all systems work in harmony to ensure healthy movement of the limbs. Thirty-four healthy men and women participated. The results showed that the most sensitive measures of breathing pattern disorders were resting *end-tidal carbon dioxide* (ETCO$_2$) and resting respiratory rate. In total, 70% of subjects were identified as having disordered breathing.[21]

In addition to end-tidal CO$_2$, they used the *Nijmegen Questionnaire* (NQ) and the *Functional Movement Screening*™ test (both also used in Kiesel's study discussed later in this chapter). Participants with poor breathing patterns scored lower on the FMS test, while 87.5% of those who passed were classified as diaphragmatic breathers. Functional breathing and functional movement were found to go hand in hand. The FMS test was also shown to accurately predict injury in people with suboptimal patterns of movement.

Participants who returned a higher NQ score had a higher respiratory rate and a lower ETCO$_2$ during the FMS test. In other words, those with a fast breathing rate had lower ETCO$_2$. In contrast, ETCO$_2$ readings at rest were significantly higher in diaphragm breathers than they were in chest breathers. The research also revealed a clear link between a high ETCO$_2$ and a better FMS score. These results unequivocally demonstrated the importance of functional breathing patterns for functional movement.[21]

| | Mean | Min | Max |
|---|---|---|---|
| Resting ETCO$_2$ (mmHg) | 33.70 ± 2.74 | 27.70 | 39.33 |
| Resting RR (breaths/min) | 18.39 ± 3.41 | 12.25 | 25.2 |
| Active RR (breaths/min) | 24.30 ± 3.06 | 17.65 | 30.64 |
| Breath-Hold Time (sec) | 19.22 ± 5.05 | 10.57 | 34.13 |
| Nijmegen Questionnaire | 9.24 | 0.00 | 27.00 |

(Bradley & Esformes, 2014)

According to a 2016 paper published in the *International Journal of Sports Physical Therapy*, it is possible to correct or reeducate disordered breathing.[23] Fresh neural connections can restore the central nervous system's normal motor control patterns. The paper suggests that breathing pattern disorders should be the starting point for all orthopedic investigations, stating, "If breathing is not normalized, no other movement pattern can be."

The adequate oxygenation of muscles during exercise is also worth looking at. Exercise, by its nature, is associated with a variety of corresponding cardiovascular and respiratory responses.[28] These generate the effort necessary for the orderly recruitment of motor units that cause the muscles to contract. A motor unit is the motor neuron (or messenger cell) and the muscle fibers activated by that neuron. The muscles of most mammals, including humans, store very little oxygen. In contrast, diving mammals like whales, seals, and otters have an oxygen-binding protein called myoglobin in their muscles.[29]

In Chapter One, we discussed how the extra resistance created by nasal breathing significantly increases the oxygenation of the blood. Oxygen gets from the air to the exercising muscles via the cardiovascular system. At rest, a young, healthy person weighing between 50 and 100 kilograms consumes between 0.15 and 0.4 liters of oxygen per minute. Around 80% of this oxygen is used by the brain, heart, liver, and kidneys.[28] Skeletal muscle does not generally use much oxygen unless those muscles are contracting.

During exercise, a young, untrained person can consume 10 or 15 times as much oxygen. In elite endurance athletes, it can be 20 times more, provided that they train with sufficient duration and intensity. According to a 2015 paper, this maximal oxygen uptake, or $VO_2$ max (first observed in the 1930s in Donald Lash, the first man to break nine minutes for two miles), is similar to that estimated for male hunter-gatherers and sheep or cattle farmers in nonmechanized societies. Values for women are around 10% or 15% lower due to lesser muscle mass, hematocrit, and hemoglobin.[28] Hematocrit is the volume percentage of red blood cells in the blood. Hemoglobin is the protein in the red blood cells that carries oxygen to the body's organs and tissues and transports $CO_2$ back to the lungs to be expelled during exhalation.

Oxygen consumption is driven by cardiac output, which increases from four to eight times during exercise, due to the faster heart rate and greater stroke volume. Cardiac output is the amount of blood the heart pumps through the circulatory system in one minute. Stroke volume is the amount of blood pumped from the left ventricle of the heart per beat. In elite athletes, stroke volume is enhanced by structural changes in the left ventricle.[28]

Exercise also prompts a two- or threefold increase in whole-body oxygen extraction. This is caused by differences in oxygen levels within the arteries and blood vessels, and by reduced blood flow to the less active skeletal muscles, kidneys, gastrointestinal tract, liver, spleen, and pancreas. The ability of exercising muscles to extract oxygen is also improved by increased capillary density. The muscles of trained athletes actually grow more blood vessels in response to regular exercise, which contributes to the rise in $VO_2$ max with training.[28] It has been known as far back as the late 1700s that "blood goes to where it is needed." This simple statement, made by the Scottish surgeon Hunter, underlines the fundamental idea that under most circumstances, metabolic demand (how much oxygen the muscles need) and the blood flow to the contracting muscles are well matched.[28]

It's also interesting to look at what happens when muscles become injured. When an injury occurs, the rupture of blood vessels results in ischemia (reduced blood flow) and *hypoxia* (lack of oxygen) at the site of the injury. One 2015 study explored the differing impacts of transient and prolonged oxygen deficiency on the regeneration of muscle tissue. Researchers found that short-term hypoxia stimulates "productive proliferation and differentiation" of satellite cells.[30] Satellite cells are muscle stem cells that can form new muscle fibers and differentiate and fuse to existing muscle.[31] These cells are involved in the normal growth of muscle and its regeneration after injury or disease.

The study demonstrated that while transient hypoxia is essential for the formation of muscle tissue and the stimulation of muscle stem cells, and is beneficial to recovery,[30] prolonged hypoxia is detrimental to muscle repair, inhibiting the ability of the satellite cells to differentiate. Differentiation is the important process by which cells change to perform a specific function.

Muscle injury is a difficult subject to study because, while injuries of this type are common, they are not reproducible in either severity or location in a trial situation, especially as they always, by nature, occur by accident. However, while the injuries of elite athletes may receive a high proportion of attention from a rehabilitative standpoint, muscle and tendon problems can affect anyone.

That study leaves open the question as to whether intermittent hypoxia achieved by breath holding could have therapeutic applications in muscle repair. Research is limited, but one master's study examined the curative use of intermittent hypoxia to repair induced muscle injuries in rats. It concluded that there was "absolutely no doubt" that the treatment would be beneficial to athletes.[32]

During breath holding following normal breathing patterns, levels of oxygen drop and $CO_2$ increase. This causes acidosis in humans through increased blood $CO_2$, decreased blood pH, and a reduced affinity for oxygen—which facilitates oxygen delivery to the tissues—known as the *Bohr effect*. The higher level of $CO_2$ causes the bond between hemoglobin and oxygen to weaken. This makes more oxygen available to the tissues. Therefore, it may be possible that breath holding could improve recovery of injured or fatigued skeletal muscles.

The increased oxygenation of the tissues seen after $CO_2$ therapy operates on the same principle. In 2011, scientists in Japan investigated whether absorption of $CO_2$ and the Bohr effect could be induced in humans by applying pure $CO_2$ directly to the skin. They found that 10 minutes after the gas was applied, the pH in the cells of the subject's calf muscle had decreased significantly. Four minutes after $CO_2$ was applied, there was a marked drop in oxy-hemoglobin concentrations, indicating better delivery of oxygen. The researchers concluded that $CO_2$, when applied directly to the skin, facilitates the absorption of $CO_2$ in humans and causes greater oxygenation of the tissues. This proved that the Bohr effect can be produced artificially in the laboratory. This has potential benefits for people with injuries or other disorders that can be treated with high levels of localized oxygen in the tissues.[33]

In 2017, scientists tested 27 rats to find out whether transcutaneous $CO_2$ ($CO_2$ applied directly to the skin) could speed up muscle repair. Each of the rats had an injury inflicted on a leg muscle—the equivalent muscle runs down the front of the human shin—and each rat was assigned to one of two groups. One group of rats was treated with transcutaneous $CO_2$, while the other group was untreated. In the rats treated with $CO_2$, the muscle injury had completely healed by the sixth week. In the untreated group, the injury was only partially repaired after six weeks.[34]

Endurance exercise produces $CO_2$ in the body through the aerobic metabolic processes. However, the full role of $CO_2$ is not yet clear. It has been established that external application of $CO_2$ to the skin promotes changes in the muscles and that these changes are linked to better endurance and greater power in the skeletal muscles. The 2017 study concluded that these changes also allow the muscles to heal more quickly. Scientists observed an increase in the number of small blood vessels in the muscles of the $CO_2$ group. This further confirms that $CO_2$ is beneficial for muscle development and performance in endurance sports and indicates that it may enhance oxygenation of the skeletal muscles and recovery from muscle fatigue.

## IMPROVING RESPIRATORY MUSCLE STRENGTH

Breathing patterns will change during intense physical exercise. When the system is under strain, respiration becomes the body's main concern. If push comes to shove, the system needs oxygen to survive, and so respiration will always be given priority over postural control. This is the underlying reason that while athletes might train to improve sports performance and while regular aerobic training improves cardiovascular and skeletal muscle function, physical training does not strengthen the breathing muscles. According to Alison McConnell's book, *Breathe Strong, Perform Better,* the lungs do not respond to physical training.[35] Research confirms that lung volume and function, including the ability of the lungs to transfer oxygen to the blood, is not improved by training.[35-38]

During intense physical exercise, the breathing rate can increase to between 40 and 50 breaths per minute. Since the volume of each breath is around 3 liters of air, this equates to a breathing volume of as much as 120 to 150 liters per minute. For Olympic-level male endurance athletes, the tidal volume (volume of air per breath) can be as high as 5 liters. This results in a minute ventilation of 200 to 250 liters.[35] Bear in mind that normal resting minute ventilation is between 5 and 8 liters, increasing to 40 to 60 liters during moderate exercise.

## WHEN THE BREATHING MUSCLES TIRE

Because breathing increases substantially in this way during physical exercise, the extra work of inhaling and exhaling places much greater demands on the breathing muscles. Unsurprisingly, this often causes fatigue in those muscles. According to the *Lore of Running*, by exercise physiologist Tim Noakes, there is strong evidence that the diaphragm (which is our main breathing muscle) and other respiratory muscles may become exhausted during both short-term high-intensity exercise, such as MMA or boxing, and extended activities like marathon running.[39]

The ventilatory response to $CO_2$ influences the work of the breathing muscles during physical exercise. If you have a low BOLT score, you will need to breathe harder. Effortful breathing like this requires significant increases in respiratory muscle work, both on the inhalation and on the exhalation.[40] As the breathing muscles tire, blood flow is diverted from the legs to help support respiration. The decrease in blood flow to the working muscles causes the legs to become fatigued, and you will be forced to slow down or stop. As the breathing muscles overexert, metabolic by-products, such as lactic acid, accumulate in the blood. Too high a concentration of these metabolites further reduces blood circulation, hampering blood flow to the limbs. Research into breathing techniques has shown that, when the effort of inhalation is reduced, blood flow to the legs increases by up to 7%.

Evidence suggests that the diaphragm is the most important breathing muscle to target during respiratory muscle training. For instance, one 2016 study demonstrates that over 50% of healthy athletes with varying levels of fitness will develop diaphragmatic fatigue after bouts of high-intensity exercise.[41]

## EXERCISING THE BREATHING MUSCLES

It is widely accepted that to stimulate any muscle to adapt, that muscle must be worked harder than usual. But since aerobic physical exercise is practiced

within the comfort limits of the breathing muscles, it cannot provide sufficient stimulus to cause the breathing muscles to adapt. In fact, it is impossible
for most people to sustain high-intensity exercise for long enough to provide
a load sufficient to improve the strength of the respiratory muscles. However,
the Oxygen Advantage exercises (see Chapter Two) provide a meaningful
strategy to improve respiratory muscle strength, as that extra load can be
added to the breathing muscles in a nonstressful and controlled environment.

In terms of function, respiratory muscles are divided into the inspiratory
muscles, used during inhalation, and expiratory muscles, used during exhalation. Exhaling requires less effort than inhaling, as the natural elasticity of
the breathing muscles helps push out the air. Therefore, it is the inspiratory
muscles that are most prone to fatigue. That is why the practice of breathing
against resistance, or inspiratory muscle training, specifically targets the
inspiratory muscles.

This resistance can be provided by a SportsMask, a training support that
makes the breathing muscles work harder. The SportsMask has an adjust-
able valve opening, making it possible to vary the level of resistance during
inhalation. This resistance conditions the breathing muscles in a manner
similar to the progressive muscle training achieved in weight lifting. The
technique of restricting airflow with a specialist device is called inspiratory
flow resistive loading (IFRL). Studies show that it can improve respiratory
muscle strength between 20% and 50%.

Breath holding, done properly, can also provide a workout for the respiratory muscles. Holding the breath after a passive exhalation creates a strong
air hunger and disturbs the blood's acid-base balance. When the breath is
held, excess $CO_2$ cannot leave the blood through the lungs, and the cells
continue to extract oxygen. This alters blood gas concentrations, increasing
$CO_2$ (hypercapnia) and decreasing oxygen saturation (hypoxia). Because
$CO_2$ levels are the primary stimulus to breathe, the excess $CO_2$ will cause
the breathing muscles to respond. To restore blood gas levels to normal, the
respiratory center begins to send messages to the breathing muscles to resume
breathing. As the breath hold continues, these impulses increase in intensity,
causing repeated contractions of the diaphragm. This is sometimes called
the "struggle phase." As the diaphragm continues to contract through the
breath hold, it essentially receives a workout. According to a 2013 study of
maximal breath hold in free divers, the relative intensity of diaphragmatic

and inspiratory rib-cage muscle contractions increases by around 5 and 15 times respectively, from the beginning to the end of the struggle phase, approaching potentially fatiguing levels by the time breathing is resumed.[42]

In 2016, scientists at the University of Zagreb, Croatia, ran a study to determine the effects of hypercapnic-hypoxic training on respiratory muscle strength among elite swimmers. Those swimmers who were subjected to a hypercapnic-hypoxic regimen significantly improved the strength of their inspiratory muscles when compared to swimmers who breathed normally. Participants who reduced their breathing improved their inspiratory muscle strength by 14.9% and expiratory muscle strength by 1.9%. The researchers noted that voluntary breath holding might have resulted in involuntary contractions of the breathing muscles, increasing diaphragm thickness.[43] The thickness of the diaphragm plays an important role in sporting performance and endurance.

The precise mechanisms by which respiratory muscle training improves exercise performance have not been fully determined. The positive effects on endurance may be due to the direct impact on fatigue in the respiratory muscles. Indirectly, the improved blood flow to working muscles that comes from more efficient breathing and better oxygenation is also beneficial. It is also likely that the increased resistance to breathing during respiratory muscle training may simply make normal physical exercise feel easier.[44]

When the breathing muscles are stronger, they are better able to cope with more intensive training. This means that more intense exercise is possible before the metaboreflex reduces blood flow to the legs. This ultimately improves performance as well as endurance. The effects of respiratory muscle training have been shown across a variety of sports, including rowing,[45] sustained heavy-endurance exercise,[46] and cycling.[47]

## A SIMPLE MEASURE OF DYSFUNCTIONAL BREATHING

As we've seen, breathing pattern disorders are multidimensional, comprised of a series of biochemical, biomechanical, and psychological components. So, it can be difficult to achieve a definitive diagnosis with any single test. Also, many methods to assess dysfunctional breathing rely too much on subjective information. As with any dysfunction, the body and mind can adapt to a certain degree until the problem becomes normalized, and so personal experience rarely provides clear information. This is perhaps part of the reason why breathing pattern disorders are so often overlooked in physical therapy.

In 2017, the lack of effective screening was addressed by a research team led by Dr. Kyle Kiesel, a professor and chair of physical therapy, who has done extensive research in areas including motor control of the core and functional movement.[2] The result was a simple screening procedure to enable fitness and healthcare providers to accurately identify disordered breathing in their patients.[2] Kiesel's study examined 51 subjects, 27 females and 24 males, with an average age of 27 years and a BMI of 23.3. Breathing was assessed in terms of biochemical, biomechanical, and psychological function.

The **biochemical** dimension of breathing was evaluated by monitoring $ETCO_2$. $ETCO_2$ is the average amount of $CO_2$ in exhaled air. This is measured using capnography, which measures the pressure of blood $CO_2$, because normally the pressure of $CO_2$ in the lungs determines the pressure of $CO_2$ in the blood. The normal range of $ETCO_2$ is between 35 mmHg and 40 mmHg. Less than 35 mmHg suggests the presence of dysfunctional breathing.[21]

The **biomechanical** dimension was assessed using a test called the *Hi-Lo*. This is a visual evaluation during which abdominal expansion and perceived displacement and functional movement of the upper and lower rib cage are recorded. The patient lies face up and breathes normally, with one hand on the chest and the other on the abdomen. How much the tummy and ribs move during a normal breathing cycle is measured.

For the **psychophysiological** dimension of the experiment, participants answered questions from the *Self-Evaluation of Breathing Symptoms Questionnaire* (SEBQ) and *Nijmegen Questionnaire* (NQ). The NQ has been a popular screening tool for the diagnosis of hyperventilation for over 30 years. It gives a broad view of symptoms associated with dysfunctional breathing and asks 16 questions about breathing discomfort. The patient responds using a numbered scale ranging from "never" (0 points) to "very often" (4 points). A score of 23 points or more is considered to indicate the presence of hyperventilation syndrome.[48]

I am not a fan of the *Nijmegen Questionnaire*. Its questions neglect some of the most common signs of breathing pattern disorders. It does not include frequent sighing or yawning, nasal congestion, fatigue, or wheezing. While it could be argued that these are omitted because they are all caused by organic conditions, people with these symptoms generally do have breathing pattern disorders. On the other hand, the NQ does include symptoms such as confusion, tingling and stiffness in the fingers, stiffness in the arms, and tightness around the mouth. In almost 20 years of teaching exercises to address chronic hyperventilation, I've only seen a handful of people present with those symptoms.

Kiesel's team failed to find any strong correlation between the 3 measures of disordered breathing.[2] This goes some way to explaining why these common methods of diagnosis are so continually unreliable. Of the participants, 5 were deemed to have normal breathing, 14 failed at least 1 measure, 20 failed at least 2 of the measures, and 12 failed all 3. Only 10% of participants who passed all three dimensions of breathing actually had normal breathing.

While the capnometer, *Hi-Lo* test, and self-evaluation questionnaires were found wanting, Kiesel discovered that a simple screening test could accurately assess the presence of dysfunctional breathing. The proposed test consisted of just four questions from the *Functional Movement Screen* (FMS) and a breath-hold time of 25 seconds.

FMS identifies physical weakness and imbalance. To assess movement patterns crucial to normal mobility, it uses a straightforward ranking and grading system of seven functional movements. These are deep squat, in-line lunge, hurdle step, active straight leg raise, shoulder mobility, trunk stability push up, and rotary stability. It pinpoints any functional limitations and asymmetries that may inhibit the ability to move correctly or train without injury. The four questions Kiesel found effective to diagnose dysfunctional breathing ask whether the patient feels tense, has cold hands or feet, yawns frequently, or mouth breathes at night. These symptoms are all common among people with breathing pattern disorders.

To accurately measure breath-hold time, each participant was directed to hold the breath at the end of a standard exhalation. The breath-hold was measured until the tester noted the subject's first involuntary contraction of the diaphragm or throat muscles.[2] This technique exactly replicates the BOLT measurement that we use in the Oxygen Advantage.

Kiesel's team concluded that, if an individual passed the screening composed of the four questions plus the breath-hold test, there was an 89% chance that their breathing was *not* dysfunctional. The test, therefore, provides an easy way for clinicians to accurately detect DB in their patients.[2] In the same way, the BOLT provides an accurate measure of functional breathing. By checking your BOLT score and observing what's going on in your body, you can assess your own breathing without the need for fancy equipment. This puts you in a strong position to tackle the problem.

## WHAT DO FUNCTIONAL MOVEMENT SCORES MEAN FOR PERFORMANCE?

Dr. Paul Sly is an Oxygen Advantage Master Instructor in Canada. He has more than 25 years' experience as a practicing chiropractor and is an acupuncture provider, certified in Functional Movement Systems. He sent me this explanation of functional movement screening and its implications for functional breathing and performance:

> In Functional Movement Systems, there is the Functional Movement Screen (FMS) and the Selective Functional Movement Assessment (SFMA). The FMS is a performance enhancement tool, while the SFMA is the clinical arm, designed to arrive at a diagnosis. I use both, but as a clinician I use the SFMA a lot. In particular, "breakouts" of the movement patterns determine whether a specific dysfunction is a Tissue Extensibility Dysfunction (TED) or a Stability or Motor Control Dysfunction (SMCD).
>
> Take the classic standing toe touch. If an individual can't do that, there are two possibilities. Either something (typically the hamstrings) along the posterior chain is too tight (TED) or the patient can't stabilize their core well enough to allow the hips to shift back and the spine to flex (SMCD).
>
> We are finally coming around to the idea that functional breathing, recruiting a strong diaphragm with appropriate timing, is a big part of core stabilization. When breathing is dysfunctional, it can create a SMCD. What also happens, however, is that TEDs will cause an individual to change their breathing patterns. For instance, people often hold their breath in order to try to overcome the dysfunction. A TED can therefore cause a breathing pattern disorder, which in turn can cause or exacerbate a SMCD. So, breathing can

be, and often is, central to both types of dysfunction. If you can't breathe functionally through a particular movement or posture, then you don't "own" that movement or posture.

This has significant implications for professional athletes. It also contributes to the huge rise in incidence and cost of repetitive strain injury in many occupations and workplaces.

The other overlooked and interesting application of functional breathing is for cognition in sport, especially team sport. I always tell the hockey players I work with that, while the mistakes you see players make, especially toward the end of a game, are often attributed to "pressure," they are also, at least in part, due to the continual hyperventilation you see on the bench during recovery. During recovery, players breathe through an open mouth, resulting in a decrease in cerebral blood flow that impacts their ability to think clearly. Nasal, functional breathing during recovery from an acute anaerobic bout, makes a difference to cognitive ability which is vital for performance. I'm not aware of any study backing this up, and I'm not sure how such a study could be designed, but I have seen it in action, and it makes sense.

*—Paul Sly*

## FUNCTIONAL BREATHING *IS* FUNCTIONAL STRENGTH

Tim Anderson is cofounder of Original Strength and has been a personal trainer for more than two decades. He is a well-known author and a sought-after speaker. He has written and cowritten books on this subject, including *The Becoming Bulletproof Project*. As I was preparing the final manuscript for this book, Tim wrote to me with the following practical explanation of the science we have covered in this chapter:

Strength starts with breath. Proper breathing literally strengthens the body from the center out. The diaphragm is the chief spinal stabilizer of the inner core muscles. When it is functioning properly, when it is being used to fill the lungs from the bottom to the top, it rhythmically dances with the pelvic floor. This dance, which also involves the transverse abdominus and the multifidi, stabilizes the spine and pelvis. When the diaphragm is functioning properly, the pelvic floor and the other spinal stabilizers are getting the stimulation they need to function properly. This is the foundation for a strong, powerful and efficient moving body.

A body that has a properly functioning diaphragm, a nasal breather who keeps their tongue on the roof of their mouth and fills their lungs up from the bottom to the top, has a nervous system that feels safe to express itself without restriction. Not only does this result in better performance in speed, strength, power and efficiency, it results in a more resilient and durable body, a body that is less prone to injury.

Trying to express strength and power while mouth breathing not only throws the nervous system into the sympathetic mode, it causes the body to recruit prime movers to stabilize the spine because the inner core unit's chief stabilizer (the diaphragm) is not functioning optimally. This compensation can lead to poor performance and even injury.

It may help to think of the body as an "X"? Functional breathing creates a body with a solid center, a reflexively strong inner core unit. When the body has a strong center, the forces it creates and encounters can easily and efficiently travel from one side of the body to the other, through that solid center. The result is a body that can move with grace, ease, and power.

Dysfunctional breathing creates instability of the spine because the inner core muscles are not able to properly do their job. This means when the body creates or encounters force, those forces cannot efficiently travel through the center of the body. Instead, they may end up in regions of the body they shouldn't causing movement issues, pain, or injury. Typically, the body of a dysfunctional breather, does not express optimal, fluid posture, or ease of movement. It lacks a poetry of movement because the body cannot express its full movement potential.

I like to tell people that breathing properly, nasal breathing with your tongue on the roof of your mouth, filling your lungs up from the bottom to the top, gives you a center of strength. It makes the body and mind strong and resilient. Improper breathing, mouth breathing, filling the lungs up from the top, rarely filling the bottom of the lungs; gives the body a soft or hollow center. It leaves the body and mind weak and fragile.

In other words, mouth breathing can create fragility while nasal breathing can create resiliency.

*—Tim Anderson*

# CHAPTER SIX
# WHEN BREATHING MAKES YOU HURT

---

## PAIN IS A SIGN OF DYSFUNCTION

As we have been discussing, the diaphragm, the primary respiratory muscle, is essential for stabilizing the core, spine, and posture. Dysfunctional breathing can compromise the body's fundamental stability. Poor breathing patterns can also cause pain in sometimes unexpected places. Over time, poor breathing patterns create faulty movement patterns that lead to pain and injury in the muscles, tendons, and joints. For instance, if you breathe into the upper chest, alterations occur in the position of your lower ribs, which need to move up to allow enough air into the lungs. The result is likely to be pain or dysfunction in part of the spine.

If you continually neglect the primary muscles that hold your body upright, such as the core and the diaphragm, the body will compensate by overusing smaller muscles that aren't really designed for the job. This is why muscular adaptations caused by breathing pattern disorders can contribute to all sorts of pain conditions that you might not intuitively associate with breathing. For example, paradoxical breathing, a dysfunctional breathing pattern in which the abdomen contracts on inhalation and expands on exhalation, often coexists with muscle imbalances and pain in the cervical spine. Weakness in the pelvic floor muscles can show up as injuries in areas as varied as the knee,[1, 2] ankle, anterior cruciate ligament,[2] and lower back.[3] Problems in the hands can be caused by tension in the shoulders and neck stemming from dysfunctional breathing.[4] Poor blood flow to the brain caused by chronic hyperventilation can result in excruciating headaches.[5]

Imbalances in the autonomic nervous system, which can be influenced by breathing, can also lead to pain. For the body to move, the nervous system and muscles must work together. If problems exist in either system, the other will adapt to compensate. This is why autonomic dysfunction caused by psychological stress can display as physical symptoms.

Stress has been clearly identified as both a contributing and a risk factor in musculoskeletal injuries and chronic pain. In one 2012 study, researchers observed patients with ongoing shoulder and neck pain and found that sympathetic activation was dominant and the parasympathetic system was suppressed, suggesting an imbalance in the autonomic nervous system.[6] When the nervous system is in a state of heightened arousal, the body is likely to adjust breathing patterns to restore homeostasis. This alters the recruitment of respiratory muscles, impacts motor control, and leads to chronic or acute musculoskeletal pain.

Another valuable window into how well the body's systems are functioning is provided by *myofascial trigger points*. These are tender areas in the muscles that often cause referred pain, a phenomenon where pain originating in one place shows up elsewhere in the body. Trigger points manifest as muscle stiffness, weakness, dizziness, nausea, and postural distortions.[7] Left untreated, they can result in ongoing disruption of movement patterns. Trigger points can be activated by psychological stress. In 1994, researchers observed what happened to a trigger point under different conditions, including mental stress induced by an arithmetic task. The results showed that the trigger point was stimulated during stress, suggesting that physical pain is directly influenced by the emotions.[8] A new paper from 2020 suggests that the stronger stimulation of the baroreflex that occurs during guided slow, deep breathing may offer a "cheap-and-easy way to 'behaviorally' stimulate the afferent vagus and reduce pain," but still, not much is known about this pathway. The stimulation and function of the baroreceptors have not been well studied in research examining the impact of slow, diaphragm breathing on pain, but it is known that the pain-blocking effects of baroreceptor stimulation are lessened during mental stress.[9]

A 2016 study explored the assessment and treatment of breathing pattern disorders in three patients whose musculoskeletal pain complaints were related to trigger points, motor control adaptations, and muscle imbalances.[10] The participants were treated using breathing exercises and manual trigger point therapy. Breathing reeducation focused on a physical exercise called the "clamshell exercise," which is designed to alter intra-abdominal pressure and prompt the patient's breathing reflex. Pain decreased in all three participants, although it was unknown whether this was due to improvement in diaphragm function and core stability, lessening of tender trigger points, or the restoration of functional movement.[10] According to researchers, breathing therapy is not typically considered to be as effective as physical therapy in the treatment of pain conditions, yet there is clear evidence that it is possible to achieve similar improvements in pain, function, and physical and emotional factors with both techniques.[11]

While we have so far focused on the diaphragm, both in terms of its importance for functional breathing and its role in spinal stability, it's also helpful to acknowledge other respiratory muscles. The diaphragm is responsible for around 70% to 80% of the work of respiration under quiet breathing conditions. The other 30% is performed by the scalene, external intercostals, sternocleidomastoids, and parasternal intercostal muscles.[12]

The scalene muscles are a group of three pairs of muscles in the sides of the neck. They are called secondary breathing muscles but are considered by some scientists to be primary to respiration as they lift and expand the rib cage during inhalation and are active at a low level even during light breathing.[13] It's easier to see these muscles at work during exercise, when ventilatory demand is high.[13] Trigger point pain in the scalene muscles is often associated with pain radiating to the arm, which is commonly misdiagnosed as disc herniation or prolapse, neck pain, or carpal tunnel syndrome. This type of misdiagnosis leads to mismanagement of the condition which can perpetuate the existing problem.[14]

## BREATHING AND THE PERCEPTION OF PAIN

How we breathe directly affects how badly something hurts. Beyond factors such as postural control and muscle tension, breathing pattern disorders can play a role in the amplification of pain.[15] For instance, respiratory alkalosis caused by overbreathing can induce muscle spasm and heighten the body's response to stress hormones including adrenaline. These factors combine to create inadequate blood flow and poor oxygenation of the tissues and organs.

One 2006 study used functional magnetic resonance imaging (fMRI) to explore the way that hyperventilation influences pain mechanisms.[16] Researchers found that low blood $CO_2$ may affect the processing of motor tasks and pain input. They discovered changes in the relative levels of oxygenated and deoxygenated blood, which they believed indicated widespread constriction of blood vessels in the gray matter of the brain. This was thought to represent an acute reaction to reduced blood $CO_2$.

Constriction of the blood vessels due to overbreathing stops the blood from flowing freely to the brain and limits oxygenation of the tissues.[17] This has implications for the excitability of nerve cells in the brain and can potentially impact both motor control and pain perception. Respiratory alkalosis, caused by low levels of blood $CO_2$, increases the sensitivity of the peripheral nerves. The peripheral nerves send messages from the brain and spinal cord to the rest of the body, allowing us, for example, to sense whether our feet are cold and to move our muscles to walk.[18] This increased sensitivity is what causes the muscular tension, spinal reflexes, muscle spasm, and a much greater perception of pain, light, and sound, which are all typical of alkalosis. Alkalosis can also cause mood swings, panic attacks, anxiety, and phobic behavior,[19] all of which can result in a negative feedback loop of poor breathing and deepening psychological distress.

The impact of hyperventilation on the excitability of the neurons was explored in a 1991 paper in *Brain*. Researchers looked at the effects of low blood $CO_2$ on two conditions that impact movement, *paresthesia* and *tetany*.[20] Paresthesia is an abnormal tingling or prickly sensation, like pins and needles, which is caused by pressure on or damage to peripheral nerves. Tetany is a condition characterized by spasms of the hands, feet, and voice box; cramps; and overactive neurological reflexes. Tetany, which is generally caused by very low blood calcium levels, can also be the result of severe alkalosis.

Scientists monitored the excitability of nerve fibers in six healthy subjects. Participants were asked to hyperventilate until paresthesia occurred in the hands, face, and trunk. This occurred when the pressure of alveolar $CO_2$ had decreased by, on average, 20 mmHg. Spontaneous EMG activity—muscle activity in response to stimulation by the nerves—developed when $CO_2$ had dropped by a further 4 mmHg. Neuronal excitability increased progressively in all participants as $CO_2$ levels dropped, producing a "statistically significant inverse correlation." When neurons or nerve cells are "excitable," it means they are generating electrical impulses that transmit information throughout the nervous system. The changes in the neurons happened before any sensation of paresthesia or tetany developed. Two of the subjects also perceived spontaneous bursts of neuronal activity to be pins and needles. The study concluded that the physical symptoms of paresthesia and tetany induced by hyperventilation were entirely the result of changes in neuronal excitability.[20] This is best described as hyperventilation causing an imbalance in the electrical equilibrium of the brain due to constriction of blood vessels in the brain, and this causes the physical symptoms.

## BACK PAIN

When researchers looked for links between health, pain histories, and faulty breathing, they found a much higher prevalence of dysfunctional breathing than expected. Their 2003 paper published in the *Journal of Bodywork and Movement Therapies* examined 111 patients attending a clinic for chiropractic pain. To their surprise, more than half of the study participants demonstrated faulty breathing on relaxed inhalation, and three-quarters breathed in a dysfunctional way when taking a deep breath. Nearly 90% of the subjects had experienced some kind of musculoskeletal pain in the head, neck, back, buttocks, leg, or arm. Based on their findings, the report's authors comment that clinicians can expect three in every four new patients to have faulty breathing patterns.[19]

As we already know, in a healthy body, the diaphragm dynamically stabilizes the lumbar spine, lowering on inhalation. Together with the expansion of the lower ribs, this creates sufficient intra-abdominal pressure for postural stability. In people with chronic lumbar problems, the diaphragm remains higher and flatter, moving less. During inhalation, the ribs do not move, and the diaphragm does not lower to its usual fixed point. Consequently, the body becomes less able to regulate IAP, and the lumbar and sacroiliac regions become unstable.

According to a 2016 study from the Osteopathic Centre for Research and Studies in Ancona, Italy, people who suffer from pain in their lower back and sacroiliac joint often have early fatigue of the diaphragm, otherwise described as poor diaphragmatic endurance, which can be caused by overexertion of the respiratory muscles.[21] Breathing too hard, a feature of chronic, effortful, inefficient overbreathing, can exhaust the breathing muscles.

A 2004 research paper by Dr. Leon Chaitow, a well-regarded osteopath and naturopath, explains that the core stability of the diaphragm and abs can be compromised if both poor breathing and a "load challenge" to the lower back are present.[3] A load challenge is anything that adds a "load" or weight to the task at hand, which, in this case, is movement. Chaitow uses the example of shoveling snow, but digging the garden, pushing a pram, using a vacuum cleaner, and many other day-to-day tasks have the same effect. Results showed that, after only 60 seconds with elevated blood $CO_2$, muscle function was reduced or lacking in postural muscles and in the muscles used for movement. This underlines the extent to which chronic dysfunctional breathing can interfere with the body's ability to move freely. Although more research is needed, Chaitow's results were clear: increased respiratory demand compromises postural control so that the likelihood of spinal injury is significantly higher. This is especially true during strenuous exercise when the load on the spine is greater.

In 2018, scientists at South Korea's Konyang University carried out a study to monitor the effectiveness of breathing exercises in patients with lumbar instability and dysfunctional breathing.[22] Instability in the lower spine causes pain even during simple activities like walking and sitting, and it creates imbalances in the motor system. Many studies have reported that the activation of muscles in the trunk is different in people with chronic lower back pain. For instance, pain and dysfunction in the lower spine affects the transversus abdominis muscles, leading to abnormal muscle recruitment patterns and excessive use of other supporting muscles to compensate.[22]

Twenty-seven adults aged between 20 and 40 years took part in the study. Each person was assigned to a breathing exercise group or to a trunk stabilization exercise group where they focused either on diaphragmatic breathing or on physical exercises for 15 sessions over five weeks. One focus of their breathing education was avoiding involuntary breath holding when an extra load is applied. At the end of the study, significant differences were observed in the lumbar area in the breathing exercise group. Diaphragmatic breathing exercises had improved the mobility of the sternum and ribs, allowing for thoracic extension, increasing intra-abdominal pressure (IAP), and stimulating the abdominal muscles.[22]

Back pain is incredibly common in the general population. It is also a significant factor in sports. Lower back pain is the primary reason for missed playing time among professional athletes.[23] Again, this is often due to compensatory muscle activation. For example, dysfunctional breathing correlates with an increased resting tone in the superficial abdominal muscles.[24] Studies show evidence of delayed activation of the transversus abdominis muscle and heightened activity of the superficial lumbo-pelvic muscles. If these muscles are overactive at rest, they can behave almost like a corset. That bracing of the trunk, often associated with overinflation of the lungs, may be the body's attempt to boost spinal stability with IAP. However, because the abdominal muscles are not working with the diaphragm, it ultimately reduces stability.

In treating back pain, it is important that clinicians and physical therapists consider the role of breathing and the respiratory muscles as well as the stability of the trunk. While there are many exercises for the muscles of the lumbar and pelvic regions, most fail to integrate breathing. Adopting a holistic, whole-body approach, in which respiratory patterns are incorporated into various postures, makes it possible to better address back pain. Just as important, correcting breathing pattern disorders can be preventive, providing optimal stability for the spine and functional movement, and better oxygenation of working muscles, meaning less risk of injury in the first place.

Dysfunctional breathing creates levels of anxiety that can be high enough to alter physical balance and motor control.[3] Changes in respiratory chemistry caused by dysfunctional breathing can have profound effects on the body's systems. A 2010 study of patients with back or neck pain found that all participants had low $ETCO_2$.[25] Remember, low $ETCO_2$ is considered a measure of breathing pattern disorders because it indicates a low level of blood $CO_2$, which is associated with hyperventilation. None of the patients had had any success using manual therapy and exercise to help with pain and mobility. However, when they practiced breathing pattern retraining, all experienced improvements in $ETCO_2$, pain and function, with 93% achieving clinically significant changes.[25]

When $CO_2$ levels are chronically low, the result is respiratory alkalosis. This causes symptoms such as decreased oxygenation of tissues and organs (including the brain), higher pain perception, constriction of blood vessels, and the onset of myofascial trigger points. Each of these, on their own, can change the normal motor control of skeletal muscles.

## NECK PAIN

It is easy to understand why poor diaphragm control might cause back trouble, but it may be less obvious why faulty breathing might frequently lead to neck pain.[19] Between 10% and 20% of the population suffer with neck pain every year.[26] But how could this be connected to the way they breathe?

The answer may lie in the biomechanics of dysfunctional breathing. One of the most common respiratory movement pattern faults involves lifting the thorax with small muscles, such as the scalene muscles (the pairs of accessory muscles at the sides of the neck), instead of allowing it to widen naturally by IAP. This interference or "overdoing" puts a strain on the upper spine and the muscles around the neck and can cause recurring pain.[27]

Like so many of the issues we've covered in this book, neck pain is both caused by and the cause of dysfunctional breathing. A 2014 study observed patients with chronic neck pain before and after a 30-minute breathing reeducation exercise. Researchers evaluated movement in muscles including the anterior scalene muscles during normal and deep breathing. They found that pain intensity and muscle activity were significantly reduced after breathing reeducation. The study concluded that breathing exercises can change breathing patterns and increase expansion of the chest, leading to an improvement in the range of motion in the neck.[28] This improvement could be attributed to better diaphragm function or to reduced compensatory activity in other breathing muscles.

A reduced ability of the abdominal muscles to maintain postural control is also believed to lead to increased tone in the diaphragm and cervical accessory muscles. In other words, when the core is not functioning well enough to support the body, the diaphragm muscles and the breathing muscles in the neck work harder to compensate. More muscle tone is not always a good thing. Instead of implying good health, it can indicate that a particular muscle is overactive or tense. Increased tone of the diaphragm and neck muscles has been observed in people with forward head posture, chronic sinus problems, and temporomandibular joint dysfunction,[12] a condition characterized by pain and dysfunction in the muscles that move the jaw and connect it to the skull.

A 2002 empirical study showed a link between work-related musculoskeletal disorders in the upper extremities and job stress. Previously, it had been unclear how psychosocial stress contributed to the development of muscle and joint pain.[15] Researchers explain that the respiratory alkalosis caused by excessive loss of $CO_2$ during hyperventilation triggers an unhealthy domino effect in the body, causing physiological reactions, including muscle tension and spasm.[15]

The shift from diaphragmatic to chest breathing typical in chronic over-breathing causes biomechanical stress on the neck and shoulders. When we breathe "big" into the upper chest, muscles in the neck and shoulders compensate for the lack of diaphragm function. A theory centering on hyperventilation provides a new way to understand how job stress factors into the physical processes leading to work-related musculoskeletal disorders. It also offers important insights into how employers might focus interventions and manage individual stress in their employees. Understanding work-related injury in terms of hyperventilation provides a unique opportunity to address job stress and associated musculoskeletal pain through breath reeducation, light exercise, and rest breaks.[15]

Forward head posture can be caused by many different things, not least being the habitual tension that comes from spending many hours in front of a computer screen.[29] When the head is pushed forward, the deep flexor muscles in the neck become inhibited, while the muscles at the base of the skull become overactive. Habitual forward head posture can be caused by hours in front of a screen, compounded by eyestrain and the effort of maintaining a healthy seated posture in a sedentary job.

It can also develop as the result of long-term ongoing breathlessness and nasal congestion. Some people develop a forward head posture in childhood due to untreated swollen adenoids and mouth breathing.[30, 31] This can lead to poor airway development, affecting breathing and posture into adulthood, and resulting in pain. (We'll learn more about this in Chapter Eight.) Others begin mouth breathing as the result of chronic respiratory conditions. When mouth breathing is caused by nasal obstruction, the head pushes forward as a way to increase airflow through the oral airway and ease feelings of air hunger.

It is likely that neck pain is directly related to chronic stress. Tension in the neck and shoulders can be a direct result of stress, even in the absence of a physical load.[32] The "startle" reflex, the normal response to a sudden, intense stimulus such as a loud noise, may also contribute. During the startle reflex, the shoulders lift and the head juts forward in a complex flexion pattern that begins in the head and travels down through the entire body.[33, 34] These reflexive movements are normal and designed to keep us safe, but when they become embedded in the nervous system so that the body defaults to this reaction under relaxed conditions or when the trigger is no longer present, they become problematic.

In a study where three-quarters of participants were found to have dysfunctional breathing, the relationship between chronic neck pain and chest breathing was found to be statistically significant.[19] Researchers noted that, while only 38% of the study's participants experienced neck pain (compared to 53% who suffered with headaches and 65% with lower back pain), 83% of those found to have faulty breathing had some experience of neck pain.[19]

## TEMPOROMANDIBULAR JOINT PAIN

Low blood $CO_2$ is common in people with chronic pain disorders.[16] It is known that stress and acute pain, or a combination of the two, can cause a hyperventilation-induced decrease in blood $CO_2$.

Growing evidence suggests that the onset of idiopathic pain disorders (with "pain of unknown origin"), such as temporomandibular joint disorder, peripheral neuropathy, and fibromyalgia, is linked to both physical and psychological triggers. From a physical point of view, joint or muscle trauma can contribute. Emotionally, stress responses may initiate pain amplification and mental distress. Idiopathic pain disorders are characterized by pain and a variety of abnormalities in motor function, autonomic balance, and sleep.

Temporomandibular joint disease (TMD) is the name given to several conditions of the chewing muscles and the joint connecting the jaw to the skull. It causes pain and can contribute to migraines and tension headaches[35]. Traditionally, it was thought that these symptoms were related to misalignment of the jaw, but scientists have failed to identify a link. More recently, the significance of psychosocial factors has been accepted.[35] The term *psychosocial* refers to both psychological and social or interpersonal aspects and can involve problems, including anxiety, fatigue, and sleep disorders.

While relaxation techniques and coping strategies are often used in therapy, the role of breathing reeducation in temporomandibular joint dysfunction is seldom mentioned. However, breathing pattern disorders could offer a biomechanical explanation as to how and why the physiological changes in the joints and muscles occur. A 2011 paper published in the *Journal of Bodywork and Movement Therapies* suggests that a forward head posture could lead to increased pressure in the temporomandibular joint. Researchers also suggest that health professionals can gain valuable insights into temporomandibular joint disorder and its treatment by paying attention to breathing and postural rehabilitation.[35]

While gaps in research are acknowledged, the connections between TMD, breathing, and posture are detailed in a 1997 study. It examines the influences of dysfunctional breathing and describes the effects of poor core strength and diaphragm function on temporomandibular disorders. Overuse and overdevelopment of accessory inspiratory muscles; forward head posture; altered proprioception; increased compression of the cervical, cranial, and mandibular joints; hypermobility or hyperactivity in the temporomandibular joint; and craniofacial pain all contribute to the development of TMD.[12]

TMD is also linked with *bruxism*, which is grinding or clenching of the teeth. Bruxism can occur during both wakefulness and sleep. It has been connected with the use of antidepressant medication, a fact that may offer a window into the connection to the psychological and biochemical dimensions of breathing. A letter in the *Journal of Neuropsychiatry* in 2007 described the case of an 81-year-old man who suffered with depression. He was treated with paroxetine, a selective serotonin reuptake inhibitor (SSRI). While his depression was controlled, once his dosage increased to 30 mg per day, he began to experience night and day jaw clenching and sore teeth and jaws.[36] Similarly, a paper from The Netherlands Pharmacovigilance Centre, Lareb, describes 10 reports of bruxism in which an SSRI was the suspected cause.[37] The report explains that bruxism often exists alongside a dopamine imbalance and can result from disturbances to neurotransmitters or neuronal excitability. It should be noted that both of those can be caused by hyperventilation and low levels of blood $CO_2$.[38]

Bruxism during sleep, also called parasomnia, is experienced by around 8% of the adult population.[39] It is characterized by rhythmic tooth grinding and is associated with tooth wear and temporomandibular joint problems. Scientists are still unclear exactly what causes it, but recent studies suggest that it is the result of transient arousals during sleep. Evidence suggests that tooth grinding occurs simultaneously with apnea or hypopnea in patients with *obstructive sleep apnea* (OSA).[39] An apnea is when breathing stops completely and a hypopnea is a reduction to the flow of breathing for 10 seconds or more due to partial collapse of the throat.

A 2014 study found correlations between the occurrence of sleep bruxism and microarousal apnea or hypopnea events.[40] Researchers concluded that patients with OSA had a high risk of bruxism, and that the phasic episodes of teeth grinding were directly related to apnea events. This suggests that an improvement in OSA may prevent the worsening of sleep bruxism.[40]

A 2016 study explored the link between TMD and breathing further in looking at the relationship between craniofacial pain and daytime sleepiness.[41] Daytime fatigue is an indicator of sleep-disordered breathing. Researchers studied 1,171 patients seeking treatment for chronic pain, sleep-disordered breathing, or both. Each subject attended one of 11 international treatment centers. The results showed a high instance of comorbidity, in which patients experienced both sleep-disordered breathing and craniofacial pain, including headaches. The study also demonstrated, for the first time, a link between craniofacial dysfunctions, such as a locking jaw, and poor sleep scores. (We will look at sleep-disordered breathing, including OSA, in much more detail in the next chapter.)

As with other conditions where chronic pain is a characterizing factor, there is considerable evidence that heightened pain sensitivity and psychological distress can contribute to the onset and persistence of TMD.[42] Further evidence suggests that imbalances in the autonomic nervous system factor in the development and persistence of the condition. TMD is associated with a stronger sympathetic response and lower baroreflex sensitivity. In one 2018 study, researchers found that patients with TMD had significantly lower heart rate variability (HRV), higher pain intensity, and increased cortisol levels when compared with a control group of people without TMD.[43] The study's findings indicate that people with TMD could benefit from interventions such as breathing retraining to restore autonomic function and stress balance.

Breathing pattern disorders are also common in people with fibromyalgia.[44] This fact is not widely recognized, and the clinical effectiveness of breathing retraining is often overlooked.[44] It is, however, necessary to practice breathing exercises daily for several weeks or even months to achieve results. According to a 2017 article by Leon Chaitow, when a chronic pain condition such as TMD or fibromyalgia exists, the "layers of pain and fatigue" that build up as a result of dysfunctional breathing can be helped by improving breathing habits.[44] In these pain conditions, he recommends that manual therapy be used alongside breathing exercises to help restore functional movement, explaining that "active trigger points . . . may need to be deactivated manually." He also suggests that relaxation techniques can be helpful and that sleep disturbances are likely to require "attention and advice."[44]

## PROPRIOCEPTION: BREATH AND MOVING IN SPACE

Research has identified a connection between breathing pattern disorders and *joint position sense error*. A 2019 paper in the *Journal of the Korean Society of Integrative Medicine* found that patients with chronic lower back pain and joint position error had low levels of blood $CO_2$, fast respiratory rates, and chest breathing—all symptoms of chronic hyperventilation[45]. Joint position error can be best described as your ability to accurately return your head to a predefined position after a neck movement.[46] It is used by doctors to evaluate *proprioception* because joint position sense error can result from faulty proprioception.

The term *proprioception* is used to describe our perception of movement. It encompasses things like spatial awareness and how the body positions itself in space, ensuring that the brain knows where the arms and legs are so that the body can coordinate movement. It is controlled by cells called proprioceptors that process sensory information when the body moves.[47] Proprioception makes it possible to bring a cup to your mouth with appropriate speed and force so that you don't pour the contents all over yourself or throw hot coffee in your own face. People with poor proprioception often appear to have weak muscles and difficulty balancing.[47]

The muscles in the neck are instrumental in proprioception, so they are particularly important to postural control. The small muscles in the head and neck contain a high number of something called *muscle spindles*. Muscle spindles are stretch receptors (mechanoreceptors) in the muscle fibers. When you move your head, these spindles send information to the nervous system about the length of the muscles.[48] The high concentration of muscle spindles in the soft tissue of the neck provides the nervous system with information about the positioning of the head in relation to the rest of the body.

People with joint position sense error have an increased incidence of neck pain.[46] Many studies have shown reduced postural control with neck pain[49] and following fatigue, anesthesia, or vibration of the neck muscles.[50] According to one 2019 study, the neck area is the only region with direct access to the senses of sight and balance.[45] While many different mechanisms and systems contribute to a healthy sense of proprioception, disturbance to the nerve signals in the neck is believed to be one possible cause of symptoms including unsteadiness, dizziness, chronic lower back pain, and dysfunctional postural stability.[45]

## SUBSYSTEMS OF POSTURAL STABILITY

Problems in the three dimensions of breathing can lead to a variety of painful postural adaptations. In 1992, Yale University Professor Emeritus Manohar Panjabi suggested another way to understand spinal stabilization and its impact on the body's system.[51] Panjabi suggested that the stability of the spine relies on three subsystems:

1. The passive subsystem—the vertebrae, discs, and ligaments
2. The active subsystem—all the muscles and tendons surrounding the spinal column that can apply forces to the spinal column
3. The neural subsystem—the nerves and central nervous system, which assesses what is needed for spinal stability by monitoring signals and directs the active subsystem to provide that stability[51]

Dysfunction in any of these three subsystems may lead to short-term compensation by the other subsystems, long-term adaptation, or injury[51]. When adaptation is only temporary, it is still possible for the system to maintain normal function, but when the problem persists, alterations develop in the systems that stabilize the spine. When injury occurs, dysfunction is introduced into the whole system. This manifests as symptoms including lower back pain. Conversely, when these subsystems function correctly, the body can adapt to accommodate extra loads or complex postures. In this instance, the neural subsystem works to alter recruitment of muscles to temporarily "supercharge" spinal stability.

Significant evidence indicates how altered breathing patterns can negatively influence these neurological and muscular systems, contributing to the onset or persistence of dysfunction in the lumbopelvic region. Let's look at this in terms of the three dimensions of treatment for breathing pattern disorders:

**Biochemical:** Hyperventilation decreases levels of blood $CO_2$ and causes a higher pH in tissues and body fluids. This triggers changes in the nervous system and the way it moderates input from the eyes and ears, and negatively impacts postural control.[52] Breathing exercises that normalize levels of blood $CO_2$ help bring these systems back into balance.

**Biomechanical**: Fatigue in the inspiratory muscles causes "a rigid proprioceptive postural control strategy," like that observed in patients with lower back pain. You know how stiffly you hold your muscles when your back hurts in an attempt to avoid pain? This actually inhibits postural stability and may explain why many people with lower back pain experience recurrence of their injury.[53]

When the breathing muscles become overworked and exhausted, proprioceptive input from the lower back also becomes less reliable. This disrupts the way the brain receives and processes information and can impact postural control. Remember, diaphragm function is a key aspect of spinal stability through the creation of IAP. The diaphragm is the primary muscle of the respiratory system and sustains posture and stability. When chronic over breathing occurs, the diaphragm cannot maintain support of both systems. Postural control will be compromised as the body always prioritizes its need for oxygen. By practicing diaphragm breathing through the nose, you will increase oxygenation and gain better postural support of the spine and pelvis.

**Cadence:** A paper from 2020 reported that paced diaphragm breathing at six breaths per minute can reduce pain. This effect was enhanced when the exhalation was longer than the inhalation.[54] This may be because autonomic imbalance can itself directly contribute to pain. Breathing at six breaths a minute activates the parasympathetic nervous system, inhibiting sympathetic stress activation.

There is a direct relationship between the level of diaphragm dysfunction and the intensity of pain experienced by people who suffer with lower back problems. One explanation is that, when chronic back pain is present, the sympathetic nervous system, which is responsible for the fight-or-flight response, becomes overstimulated. An overactive stress response makes the body more sensitive to touch and increases perception of pain.[55] Also, when breathing is predominantly into the upper chest, as it is when the diaphragm is not functioning properly, it tends to involve a large volume of air and decrease in blood $CO_2$. This creates a biochemical trigger for panic symptoms, which feeds back into the stress response, making anxiety worse.

When treating musculoskeletal pain, it is important to look at the problem holistically. Trigger points can be deactivated with manual therapy. Pain in the spine and joints can be viewed in terms of muscle tension or as the body compensating for muscle dysfunction by recruiting smaller muscles. Alongside this, it is important to acknowledge the role of lifestyle, psychological factors, and habits including sleep, posture, and breathing.[56] It turns out that if you want to address chronic pain, the breath, the most fundamental and sustaining of all movement patterns, is a very good place to start.

# CHAPTER SEVEN
# SLEEP-DISORDERED BREATHING

---

Sleep is a behavioral and neurological state in which homeostatic functions essential to health and well-being occur.[1] Modern science doesn't yet fully understand the purpose of sleep or its physiological relationship with the autonomic nervous system. However, significant research confirms the relationship between quality of sleep and breathing—and highlights the fact that sleep disorders and sleep-disordered breathing (SDB) are increasingly prevalent.

When you are asleep, you probably are not aware that your breathing is causing problems. Your partner may complain that you snore, but unless you know how to spot the signs, there's little obvious feedback as to whether you breathe through your mouth or nose, or how fast, slow, shallow, or deep your breathing is.[2, 3, 4] Regardless of your awareness, the body prioritizes respiration. How you breathe when you are asleep is very important. Just as your waking breathing patterns affect the functions of your brain and body, nighttime breathing affects the quality of your sleep and to a large extent, how each day subsequently unfolds.

In the introduction to this book, I recounted how exhausted I felt during my teens and early twenties due to poor breathing and sleeping habits. This all changed after I learned to decongest and breathe through my nose and to slow down my breathing. Two days after switching to nasal breathing during sleep, I experienced what it was like to wake up feeling refreshed and alert. I remember being amazed at the difference. Even if you don't feel like you are sleeping badly, if you suffer with nasal congestion due to allergies, asthma, or rhinitis, you are almost twice as likely to experience moderate to severe sleep-disordered breathing.[5]

The following symptoms occur in people with SBD:

- Insomnia
- Snoring
- Sleep apnea

- Disrupted sleep
- Nightmares
- Nighttime asthma symptoms (usually around 3 a.m. to 5 a.m.)
- Needing to use the bathroom during the night
- Bed-wetting in children
- Fatigue first thing in the morning
- Dry mouth
- Symptoms upon waking, such as wheezing, coughing, breathlessness, or a stuffy nose

If you or your child commonly experiences one or more of these, it is likely that you already know how disruptive insomnia, snoring, and sleep apnea can be to sleep. A low BOLT score corresponds with strenuous, upper chest breathing and will result in many of the symptoms listed above.

If you would like to sleep better and wake up feeling energized and refreshed, this is easily achievable if you commit to adopting good breathing habits and increasing your BOLT score. The light, calm, nasal breathing taught throughout this book reduces snoring and obstructive sleep apnea and activates the body's relaxation mode, leading to deeper and better-quality sleep. By improving your BOLT score, you will regain control of your breathing and alleviate many common problems.

## MOUTH BREATHING DURING SLEEP

To some extent, the knowledge I'm about to share with you has been around for a long time. Yet for some reason, it has failed to become part of the common consciousness. Way back at the end of the sixteenth century, the Dutch physician and author Levinus Lemnius noted that breathing through an open mouth results in poor sleep quality[6]. Around 200 years later in 1869, the American painter, author, and traveler George Catlin published a book called *Shut Your Mouth and Save Your Life*. Caitlin observed that Native Americans had a technique to ensure their babies maintained nasal breathing during sleep. He saw that each time a baby breathed through its mouth, the mother would gently press the child's lips together to restore nasal breathing. In contrast, he described European settlers gasping for breath through open mouths as they slept.

Mouth breathing in adults has attracted only limited research. This creates some difficulty when it comes to determining exactly how common the problem is. However, many of us spend at least part of the night breathing through an open mouth. It has been proven that the habit of mouth breathing during sleep is to some extent age-related. By the time you reach 40, you are around six times more likely to spend at least 50% of your sleep switching between nasal and oral breathing.[7]

It is generally agreed that mouth breathing develops because the ability to breathe nasally is impaired in some way.[8] If the incidence and impact of mouth breathing still attracts debate among experts, it is simply because total mouth breathing rarely occurs.

A paper published in the *American Journal of Orthodontics and Dentofacial Orthopedics* in 1988 assessed the relationship between nasal obstruction and nasal-oral breathing in 116 adults. Researchers aimed to determine the switching range from nasal to nasal-oral breathing and to quantify the term "mouth breathing." They found that breathing habits are affected by the size of the nose—97% of subjects with small noses were mouth breathers to some extent, while only about 12% of those with an adequate airway habitually mouth-breathed[8]. What is not fully understood is whether the small size of the nose causes mouth breathing or whether mouth breathing results in an underdeveloped nasal airway.

There is significant evidence that mouth breathing influences the way the face, jaws, and upper airways develop—which is one reason why research in this area is so heavily weighted toward children. Mouth breathing in childhood can result in poor development of the airways and contribute to habitual mouth breathing in later life.

## INSOMNIA

Insomnia is defined as difficulty falling or staying asleep, waking early, and experiencing interrupted or nonrestorative sleep.[9] "Tired but wired" is the phrase often used by my clients. Insomnia is one of the most common sleep disorders. According to 2007 research, it affects between 25% and 30% of the general population, with 10% of people presenting chronic complaints and seeking medical help.[9] It is frequently caused, at least in part, by psychological factors, such as anxiety, depression, periods of prolonged stress, an overactive mind, or a reaction to a traumatic event.

Anyone who has had trouble sleeping will relate to the frustration associated with insomnia, the sense of irritation or even desperation, frequently aggravated by persistent thoughts that simply won't go away. Even if you have never experienced insomnia, I am sure you have, at some time, found it difficult to fall asleep due to stress or worry. A niggling internal monologue traipses back and forth through your mind, and you spend the night twisting and turning instead of enjoying restful, deep sleep.

If you do suffer from this common sleep disorder, spend between 15 and 20 minutes before sleep slowing down your breathing to achieve a tolerable air hunger. This technique works for two key reasons. First, by paying attention to your breath, you take your focus away from the mind, thereby reducing thought activity. Second, reducing the breathing volume activates the parasympathetic relaxation response, making you more able to deal with the physiological aspects of stress.

One 2019 article by US scientists in Georgia, explores the relationship between insomnia and the therapeutic role of slow breathing.[1] Deep breathing is often used for relaxation in insomnia, but much less research has been done into the therapeutic benefits of slow breathing. This is despite the fact that autonomic dysfunction often plays a role in insomnia and slow breathing can increase vagal tone, promoting better quality sleep.[10]

The average adult needs at least seven hours sleep every night. People who consistently get too little sleep are more likely to be obese[11] and physically inactive, to smoke, or to suffer with heart disease,[12] depression, diabetes, asthma, and other disorders.[13] Sleep deprivation is considered a public health epidemic, with more than a third of American adults regularly getting by on too little sleep.[14] Due to a culture where lightbulbs, computer screens, and stressful schedules make it difficult to find a reason to switch off, the study claims that between 35% and 50% of adults worldwide show symptoms of insomnia.[15] Many cases of insomnia are thought to be the result of hyperarousal, a disorder that is present during both day and night.[16]

As well as the cost to health, there are practical concerns regarding this chronic sleep deprivation. Around 109,000 road traffic collisions resulting in injury and 6,400 fatal crashes occur every year in the United States because of a drowsy driver.[17] Sleep deprivation costs the US economy $411 billion annually due to poor productivity and sick leave.[18] Approximately 4% of Americans take prescribed hypnotic sleep aids,[19] drugs that, along with a wealth of unpleasant and unhealthy side effects, can be habit-forming and cause disturbed sleep patterns.[20]

The authors of the 2019 insomnia study suggest that slow breathing can be used along with sleep hygiene techniques to reverse disturbed sleep, and this may provide a more desirable and effective long-term solution than the over prescription of hypnotic drugs. To explain the effects of slow breathing on insomnia, the study investigates the origins of the disorder in the context of "evolutionary mismatch." This is a term to describe diseases that result from evolved characteristics that were beneficial to our ancestors but due to the pace of change in the human environment and lifestyle, are now maladaptive[1]. It has been suggested that insomnia is one such disorder. The study's authors propose that a significant proportion of insomnia cases may be due to a chronically overactive sympathetic nervous system (SNS) or a depressed parasympathetic nervous system (PNS). This autonomic hyper-arousal can be counteracted with slow, diaphragmatic breathing practice. As the slow-wave sleep state promotes parasympathetic tone,[21] a regular cycle of healthy sleep stabilizes the autonomic nervous system (ANS), bringing the body back into a calmer state.

Slow breathing also causes the body to produce melatonin.[22] This is an essential sleep-inducing hormone that has been proven to improve vagal tone and inhibit the activation of the SNS.[23] Melatonin levels are lower in people with insomnia and even further depleted in chronic insomnia, indicating that the longer the sleep disorder is present, the more severe it becomes.[24]

This can create a vicious cycle of worsening insomnia in which stress increases, perpetuating hyperarousal of the SNS. New research also suggests that slow breathing may help orchestrate oscillatory brain activity, providing a mechanism to alter brain waves. This has implications for the potential modulation of brain activity to promote sleep.[1]

The researchers behind this extensive study conclude that slow breathing to regulate the ANS may be a more effective way to combat insomnia than the prevailing "standard care" pharmaceutical interventions. There is still limited research into the use of slow, deep breathing, although significant evidence points to its efficacy in treating insomnia. The paper's authors express the hope that their work will inspire more investigation into the effectiveness of slow breathing in relieving hyperarousal and thus treating insomnia.

There is a strong connection between insomnia and mental health disorders, including depression. It is quite normal for people suffering from depression to experience constant fatigue. While there is no doubt that depression contributes to feelings of tiredness and exhaustion, the question arises: Could it also be that poor quality sleep arising from insomnia, snoring, or sleep apnea may contribute to both depression and fatigue? In answer to this, I cannot help but think of a young woman in her early thirties who attended my clinic seeking relief from depression. She looked totally washed out. When I asked her how she felt upon waking up, she told me that she was exhausted most mornings. I asked whether her doctor, or any doctor in the past, had ever referred her for a sleep study, and she answered, "No." It seems obvious to me that there may be many people in a similar situation. The bottom line is, if you are feeling constantly tired, it is likely that your sleep quality is poor.

Research has shown that obstructive sleep apnea (OSA) can contribute to the development of depression.[25, 26] Up to 67% of people with OSA also experience insomnia, and depression scores are higher in individuals presenting with both insomnia and OSA.[25, 26] This means that people with sleep apnea may be at higher risk of depression because of the comorbid insomnia symptoms. It makes sense, then, that some patients with a primary diagnosis of depression should also be considered for a sleep study.

The diagnostic criteria for insomnia disorder include daytime fatigue, irritability, and difficulty concentrating. These are often the symptoms that prompt patients to seek treatment for their mental health. They are also all well-known consequences of both depression and OSA.[25] When symptoms are similar across several conditions, a little more investigation is needed to determine the root cause.

There is a direct interplay between breathing, the emotions, and sleep:

- If your breathing patterns are poor, mood regulation, and sleep will be poor.
- If sleep quality is inadequate, the emotions are unbalanced, you feel tired and anxious, and breathing is dysfunctional.
- If the emotions are high, you may have difficulty falling asleep or suffer from insomnia, and breathing will be fast, in the upper chest and effortful.

Poor breathing is closely linked with stress and anxiety and increases the risk of SDB. This is one reason why people with asthma are also more likely to experience higher levels of anxiety and fatigue.

Another factor that contributes to insomnia is fast breathing during wakefulness.[27] This means that, if you breathe too fast, you are more likely to be aroused from sleep. In a 2017 paper published in *Science*, researchers identified a neural circuit within a brainstem region called the pre-Bötzinger complex, a part of the brain that may be responsible for generating respiratory rhythm in mammals.[28] They suggest that this neural circuit may have evolved as a defense mechanism, "mobilizing the animal in the face of rapid, irregular, or labored breathing." The researchers point to the fact that fast, irregular breathing increases alertness and can cause panic and anxiety in humans[27]. Similarly, increased activity in the area of the brain responsible for respiratory rhythms, hyperventilation, and sighing appears to trigger arousal during sleep.[27] This contrasts with the practice of slow, conscious, controlled breathing, which is known to promote relaxation via the PNS and is effective in treating stress disorders.[27]

This would seem to tie in with the theory that insomnia may be caused by hyperarousal during wakefulness, and that an overactive sympathetic nervous system may contribute to the problem. An earlier study from 1992 supports the theory that hyperventilation or "increasing ventilation" prompts arousal from sleep, regardless of the stimulus that causes the increase in breathing.[29] Insomnia is a widespread problem not adequately resolved by doctors and generally addressed with medication. Knowing that fast breathing and hyperventilation causes us to wake from sleep can be key for people with insomnia and sleep apnea.

Light, disturbed sleep leads to feelings of lethargy, decreased productivity, and heightened stress levels.[30] In terms of physical well-being, researchers have consistently reported a relationship between poor sleep and high blood pressure, a connection that may be explained by the physiological load that insufficient sleep adds to the nervous system[31]. Ultimately, poor sleep results in a reduced quality of life. The good news is that disturbed or inadequate sleep is frequently connected to the way you breathe at night, and that is something I can help you change.

## DOES COUNTING SHEEP HELP?

Insomnia can manifest in two different ways: difficulty falling asleep and waking suddenly after four or five hours' sleep.

If you struggle to get to sleep, practice *Breathe Light* exercises during the day. Exercise only with your mouth closed and improve your BOLT score to over 20 seconds. Just before you intend to sleep, practice *Breathe Light* to create a tolerable feeling of air hunger for 15 minutes. Use MyoTape to ensure nasal breathing during sleep.

If you wake after a few hours' sleep, this may be due to heavy snoring or sleep apnea. If your airways narrow sufficiently during sleep to create an increase of negative pressure and a buildup of carbon dioxide, you are likely to wake. The techniques in this book can be very helpful for snoring and sleep apnea and for preventing this type of insomnia.

Once you are awake, it can be very challenging to get back to sleep. The mind is sufficiently alert to wander, but too groggy to get you out of bed. You can end up lying there for hours, worrying about how tired you will be when you eventually have to get up in the morning.

In both types of insomnia, the practice of "counting sheep" has historically been considered helpful. The idea is to count one imaginary sheep after another as they jump across a fence in your mind's eye. There is an early reference to this technique in the context of an anxious landowner in an 1832 book *Illustrations of Political Economy* by Harriet Martineau.[32]

The idea of counting sheep may be somewhat of an old wives' tale, but interestingly, scientists have demonstrated that it works. A team at Oxford University explored the use of an imagery task in reducing presleep cognitive activity and found that "imagery distraction" took up sufficient brain power to prevent unwanted thoughts and worries. Researchers examined 41 people with insomnia who were given either an imagery distraction task, a general distraction task, or no instruction. The imagery group were told to imagine a situation they found interesting, engaging, pleasant, and relaxing.[33] They were asked to spend two minutes picturing this scene in as much detail as possible. It was found that this task helped people fall asleep more quickly.

If counting sheep works for you, great, but if you struggle with visual imagery, cognitive tasks such as complex mental arithmetic problems also improve sleep latency by preventing the brain from engaging with negative, unwelcome thoughts.[34] If neither of these methods work, it is also helpful to bring your attention away from your mind and into your body. Unless the mind is calm, sleep will continue to elude you. Try bringing your attention to a small part of your body, such as your hand or foot, and hold your attention there. If you find that easy, practice expanding your focus to include a larger area of the body, say, perhaps, your feet and legs. Some people find a body scan meditation helpful. When you bring your attention into your body, it helps to bring space between your thoughts, quiet the monkey mind, and allow you to fall asleep.

Another way to calm the mind is to focus on and gently slow your breathing. It is normal for the mind to wander. When it does, quietly bring your attention to your breath. This becomes easier with practice. As you go about your day, make it a habit to bring attention to your breathing for short periods. It is more important to do this regularly throughout the day, than it is to be able to sustain the attention for a long time.

## SNORING AND OBSTRUCTIVE SLEEP APNEA

Snoring occurs when a large volume of air passes through a narrow space, causing turbulence in the nose, mouth, or back of the throat. There are two reasons this might happen: either the snorer is breathing too hard during sleep, or the upper airway—the nose, mouth, and throat—is too narrow.

Traditional snoring treatments, such as nasal dilators or surgical procedures, are generally designed to increase space in the upper airway. These focus solely on the airway, ignoring the role of breathing. It is common for children and adults with asthma, anxiety, and faster breathing habits to snore. Fast, hard breathing during the day translates into fast, hard breathing during sleep. This is what creates the turbulence.

To get clear about the link between breathing and snoring, it is helpful to deliberately make the sound of a snore through your mouth. Open your mouth, tighten your throat, and draw air fast into your mouth. You will feel the turbulence at the back of your mouth where it meets your throat. Now, close your mouth. Try to snore through your mouth when your mouth is closed. It might sound obvious, but this will prove to you that mouth snoring stops completely when you breathe only through your nose.

Next, make the sound of a snore through your nose. Nose snoring is also created by fast breathing through a narrow space. At this point, it is worth slowing down the speed of your breathing. Take a soft breath in through your nose and allow a slow, relaxed breath out. As you continue to breathe slowly through your nose, try to make the sound of a snore. You will find that when you breathe slowly through your nose, you are much less likely to snore. Snoring is not solely due to narrow or collapsed airways. Fast, hard breathing also contributes.

To reduce nasal snoring, breathe only through your nose during the day, and practice *Breathe Light* to improve your BOLT score to at least 20 seconds. For many people, this is enough to stop nasal snoring. If you have a compromised nasal airway or small nose, your snoring may continue at a lower intensity.

If you wake up with a dry mouth in the morning, indicating that you have been breathing through an open mouth, a support such as MyoTape can be very effective for maintaining lip closure during sleep.

Snoring can also lead to sleep apnea, a more severe symptom of SBD, where the sleeper involuntarily stops breathing during sleep. *Obstructive sleep apnea* (OSA) is becoming increasingly widespread. Statistics suggest that the condition affects up to 9% of women and 26% of men between 30 and 49 years old, and up to 27% of women and 43% of men aged between 50 and 70[35]. OSA is characterized by breathing that stops during sleep. People with OSA tend to snore very loudly, and they experience frequent episodes of shallow breathing (*hypopnea*) and pauses in breathing (*apnea*) lasting 10 seconds or more.[36] Aside from the apneas themselves, symptoms that indicate OSA may include:

- Daytime tiredness
- Limited ability to concentrate
- Sudden awakening, sometimes with a racing heart or feeling of breathlessness
- Dry mouth on waking
- Night sweats and a frequent need to urinate
- Waking with a headache
- Impotence and erectile dysfunction in men[36, 37]

When we inhale, air is drawn into the lungs, producing negative suction pressure in the upper airways. During the day, our upper airways are held open by various dilator muscles, but when we sleep those muscles become "lazy" and the airway is more vulnerable to collapse.[38] Collapse occurs when negative suction pressure exceeds the ability of the upper airway dilator muscles to maintain an open airway. There are four possible places where the airway may collapse during sleep:

- The soft palate can fall against the back of the throat
- The tongue can fall back into the airway
- The walls of the throat can collapse
- The epiglottis may close the airway[39]

To really visualize how breathing stops during sleep, I find it helpful to use the analogy of a paper straw. If you place one end of a straw into your mouth and suck air forcefully through it, the walls of the straw will collapse. If you then continue trying to inhale through the straw once it has collapsed, it will be impossible to do so. However, when you suck air into the straw more gently, the straw will maintain its shape and air will pass through it. As soon as you increase the speed of airflow, the straw becomes unable to withstand the increase in negative suction pressure.

In essence, that is what happens during OSA. As the inhalation begins, the negative suction pressure created by the effort to pull air into the lungs causes the walls of the upper airways to collapse. As the interruption in breathing continues, the body no longer gets enough oxygen.[36] The respiratory center in the brain sends increasingly urgent messages to the diaphragm, prompting it to resume breathing. As the diaphragm contracts to draw air into the lungs, this further increase in negative pressure reinforces the inability to breathe. Eventually, the oxygen saturation of the blood becomes low enough to partially wake the brain, and the sleeper starts breathing again with a loud gasp, followed by a series of heavy and intense breaths. This can trigger another collapse of the airways, and so the cycle is repeated throughout the night, often preventing the sufferer from ever entering deep sleep.[36]

Most people with OSA go undiagnosed and untreated.[40-42] This may be partly due to a lack of confidence in existing treatment options, but, in some cases, patients avoid diagnosis out of concern for their lifestyle or livelihood. I recently took a ride with a cab driver in California. During our conversation, he told me that he suffers from OSA. He had visited the hospital to undergo a sleep study, but, when he arrived, it was made clear to him that the licensing authorities would be notified if he tested positive. He was essentially told that a diagnosis necessary for his overall well-being might lose him his driver's license and therefore his job. Upon hearing this, he naturally turned around and walked straight back out the door.

Bearing in mind the percentage of road traffic accidents that are related to driver fatigue, sleep studies should not be a deterrent to drivers getting help. The results of a 2020 study suggested that more than a quarter of drivers hospitalized after motor vehicle crashes were at high risk for OSA.[43] Researchers concluded that diagnosed or undiagnosed OSA is an established hazard for drivers and represents a significant public health concern. This is relevant to other professions too. There have, for example, been numerous accounts of pilots falling asleep while flying. In 2013, the British Airline Pilots' Association reported that more than half of pilots have fallen asleep when in charge of a plane, with 29% reporting that they had woken up to find their copilot asleep as well.[44]

Other risk factors are associated with OSA, not least being the danger of sudden death. A 2015 study found that patients with OSA are more likely to die during the night than people without the disorder. Scientists observed 112 adults over a period of 16 years. Sudden cardiac death (SCD), a condition in which the patient suffers a fatal loss of heart function, was recorded in 46% of OSA patients, compared with 21% of people without OSA.[45] OSA more than doubled the risk of SCD. The severity of sleep apnea was found to relate directly to the relative likelihood of SCD between midnight and 6 a.m. When the results were evaluated in terms of sleep-wake cycles, researchers found that 54% of OSA patients died while asleep, compared with only 24% of non-OSA sufferers.[45] In this study, the severity and duration of apneas was linked with an increased incidence of high blood pressure and abnormal heart rhythms[45]. While the factors leading to increased risk of sudden cardiac death in sleep apnea are unclear, the scientists concluded that,

> apnea, hypoxemia, and hypercapnia act synergistically to elicit sympathetic activation, which is thought to be a major mechanism

underlying elevated risk of adverse cardiovascular consequences and mortality.

Vagal responses to apnea are also critical in triggering cardiac arrhythmias.[45]

In a 2019 study published in the *American Journal of Respiratory and Critical Care Medicine,* researchers discovered an inverse relationship between the duration of apneic events and overall risk of mortality in sleep apnea.[46] That study indicated that the people who are most at risk are not those with severe sleep apnea or those who stop breathing for a minute or more. Instead, they are the light sleepers who awake easily by slight abnormalities in their breathing, when $CO_2$ levels rise or negative pressure in the airways increases.[46] The constant interruptions to sleep are quite literally killing those people. That paper shows the importance of good quality deep sleep with few if any awakenings.

In the case of prolonged apneas, research from 2007 demonstrates that the increased levels of $CO_2$ may actually contribute to improved oxygen uptake and delivery through mechanisms including vasodilation, actually protecting the brain against injury caused by lack of oxygen (hypoxia). This paper concludes that the hypercapnia (high blood $CO_2$), which occurs during apneas, might be the body's way of adapting to severe, chronic, intermittent sleep hypoxia.[47]

During snoring and sleep apnea, the sleeper may not even be conscious of the noise created by their breathing. It is usually their sleeping partner who lies awake, sometimes too fearful or exasperated to sleep. After some time, and often with a little persistence from their partner, the sufferer might attend a sleep clinic. Here, the doctor or nurse will normally begin the consultation by requesting the completion of a questionnaire called the *Epworth Sleepiness Scale.* If the scale is positive, a referral for a sleep study is likely.

While the *Epworth Sleepiness Scale* is a validated questionnaire used by many sleep centers, I have observed that it does not capture everyone presenting with OSA. The problem with a questionnaire such as this is that some people are unaware of just how exhausted they are. Not everyone who suffers from a sleep disorder experiences or recognizes symptoms of tiredness—25% of patients with moderate obstructive sleep apnea have neither subjective nor objective sleepiness.[39] Also, up to 50% of people with OSA are not obese. These people are falling between the cracks of sleep medicine.

The test for OSA is overnight polysomnography in a sleep center. Polysomnography involves monitoring both sleep and respiration, with the primary measure being the number of apneas and hypopneas per hour of sleep. An apnea is categorized as a total collapse of the upper airway, during which the patient completely ceases to breathe for 10 seconds or more. A hypopnea is a partial collapse of the upper airway that causes a reduction in the amount of air taken into the lungs lasting for 10 seconds, with a corresponding decrease in blood oxygen of 3% or more, or EEG arousal. The number of apneas and hypopneas during the sleep test are added up and divided by the number of hours spent sleeping. The severity of sleep apnea in adults is then defined by the following scale:

- Mild sleep apnea: 5 to 15 respiratory events per hour
- Moderate sleep apnea: 15 to 30 respiratory events per hour
- Severe sleep apnea: more than 30 respiratory events per hour

While the *apnea hypopnea index* (AHI) is the measurement of choice for most sleep clinics, it is not without its limitations and should, at best, be considered a crude and imprecise measure of OSA.[48] Apneas and hypopneas have fundamentally different effects on the individual, but the index does not differentiate between the two. It could be argued that an apnea, which involves complete collapse of the upper airway, is more severe in its physiological impact than a hypopnea, which involves only partial collapse.[48] Furthermore, a hypopnea with a 4% drop in blood oxygen saturation is less severe than one that causes an 8% to 10% drop, but the index does not take this into account either. Apneas and hypopneas can occur evenly throughout the night or cluster during one period of sleep. If the sufferer experiences several events in a short period of time, it might still be possible to also manage 4 or 5 hours of decent quality sleep. This is a very different experience than that of the individual who experiences symptoms throughout the night, resulting in few, if any, hours of quality sleep. Finally, the AHI correlates poorly with the key causes and consequences of the disease.[49, 50]

Traditional treatment of OSA normally focuses on the use of a CPAP machine (continuous positive airway pressure)—a device that splints the airway open at night. Newer procedures involve widening the airways, either with the use of oral appliances or by bringing the lower jaw forward with surgery—a procedure called mandibular advancement. More recently, hypoglossal nerve stimulation has been introduced as a further surgical option since the approval of the Inspire® hypoglossal nerve stimulator implant by the US Food and Drug Administration (FDA).[51] The implant, which triggers the tongue to contract, stopping it from falling back into the airway, has been found to be effective in reducing the symptoms of sleep apnea.[52] A study of 27 participants found that preoperative AHI fell from an average of 46 down to 4.6 after surgery.[53]

While these interventions are relatively successful, it is still important to address the breathing patterns that underlie the condition. Over the years, I have seen many individuals reduce their AHI to near normal levels simply by applying the breathing exercises in this book, practicing nasal breathing day and night, maintaining a correct resting tongue position, and addressing their ineffective breathing habits.

Research from 2006 demonstrated that mouth breathing is a strong determinant of OSA in people with no nasal obstruction.[54] People with sleep apnea spend more time breathing orally and oronasally than people who snore. A strong relationship exists between the AHI (which indicates the severity of sleep apnea) and time spent breathing fully or partially through an open mouth. This was confirmed in a 2020 paper published in *Laryngoscope* in which worse OSA and greater oxygen desaturation was associated with mouth breathing than with nasal or oronasal breathing.[55]

## SECRETS OF A HEALTHY AIRWAY

The habit of breathing continuously and solely through the nose during sleep comes with many positive consequences. These include maintaining a moist upper airway, harnessing nasal nitric oxide, creating more stable breathing patterns (see "Phenotypes of Sleep Apnea" in bonus Chapter 18 online at www.HumanixBooks.com/The Breathing Cure), using the diaphragm, and helping keep the tongue out of the throat. All of these benefits have the added effect of improving and preventing the symptoms of sleep apnea. Conversely, mouth breathing can be a trigger and perpetuating factor in OSA as it increases negative suction pressure and dries out the nose, mouth, and throat. The loss of moisture inherent in mouth breathing causes inflammation in the airways, which, in turn, causes nasal obstruction, encouraging mouth breathing, and so the cycle continues.

The gas nitric oxide (NO) is produced in significant quantities in the nose and in the paranasal sinuses.[56] (The importance of this was discussed in detail in Chapter Three.) NO acts as a bronchodilator and helps keep the lower airways open. In general, the role of NO in the regulation of sleep apnea, though likely significant, is still not completely understood.[56, 57] It appears to help reduce obstruction of the upper airways and acts as a transmitter between the nose, throat muscles, and lungs.

The lower and upper airways (the lungs and the nose and throat) are mechanically connected, thus nasal breathing leads to improved lung volume[58] due to greater activation of the diaphragm.[59] Increased lung volume results in tautening and opening of the throat, reducing the risk of the airway collapsing during sleep.[38]

Anatomically speaking, breathing through the mouth causes the jaw to hinge downward and the tongue to fall back into the throat. When this happens, the airway size is compromised, increasing the risk of collapse during sleep (imagine a narrower straw). According to airway orthodontist Dr. William Hang, the difference between a healthy and a poorly functioning airway can be described by comparing the diameter of a garden hose to that of a pen. Dr. Hang has been instrumental in advancing awareness of the airway in orthodontics for several decades, and patients (including myself) often travel great distances to visit his clinic in California. The airway can be adversely affected when teeth are removed or jaws retracted to create a "better" smile, so it is vital to research the implications of this when considering orthodontic treatment.

In his 2017 research paper, Dr. Hang explains that many approaches that result in a reduction of the airway are currently standard practice in dentistry and orthodontics. He states:

> In light of the current epidemic of OSA and OSA related morbidities, such reduction in airway cannot be justified. Instead of arguing about whether or not a proposed orthodontic treatment protocol involves extraction of teeth . . . , we must substitute the question about how it affects the airway.[60]

When it comes to the modern human airway, there is not much room for error. Any infringement on that already narrow space is likely to be detrimental to health.

Thankfully, there is a growing awareness of this issue, largely driven by the general public. Initiatives such as RightToGrow.org in Canada and the Prevent Crooked Teeth campaign in the United Kingdom are helping people to recognize the importance of retaining all 32 teeth and instilling good breathing habits to promote lifelong health. Methods sympathetic to airway health and function, such as expansion of the jaws to make room for existing teeth, ensure a beautiful-looking smile without any negative consequences for respiration, sleep, or overall well-being.

Conventionally, if a patient has a problem with their nose, a referral is made to the ear, nose and throat (ENT) department. Chronic lung problems such as recurrent chest infections, wheezing, or coughing necessitate a visit to the respiratory consultant or pulmonologist. However, researchers are now recognizing that the nose and lungs constitute the same airway. Since inflammatory mediators and infectious pathogens can be transported along the respiratory mucosa and through the airways[58], inflammation in the lungs, which is prevalent in asthma sufferers, can travel up to the nose. Equally, inflammation in the nose can reach the lungs. Given this, it's no surprise that children and adults with asthma are more likely to experience problems in the nose. Physiological, epidemiological, and clinical evidence now support a **unified airway model**.[58]

Asthmatics are likely to experience nasal congestion that causes them to breathe through an open mouth. This results in a faster respiratory rate and shallow, upper chest breathing. It is this very same breathing pattern that contributes to SDB. People with asthma are more likely to experience fatigue too,[61] especially when they are suffering from asthmatic symptoms such as chest tightness, wheezing, or coughing.

Obstructive sleep apnea and asthma are common respiratory disorders. They are also frequently comorbid,[62] meaning that they occur simultaneously but not necessarily as a result of each other. Undiagnosed or inadequately treated OSA may adversely affect control of asthma and vice versa.[63] In one study, researchers demonstrated that approximately 74% of those with asthma also experience nocturnal symptoms of airflow obstruction[64] and that when an asthmatic is experiencing asthma symptoms, they are more likely to also experience OSA.[63]

Much can be learned about breathing patterns in sleep apnea by looking in more depth at the breathing habits of people with asthma. The exercises in this book have been shown to improve asthma control. Given the relationship between asthma and sleep apnea, these techniques are also likely to be helpful in reducing OSA.

## HOW TO SLEEP BETTER

Gravity plays a role in both snoring and sleep apnea. When you lie on your back, there is no restriction to breathing, so breathing volume increases and snoring becomes more severe. Sleeping on your back also encourages the mouth to open, causing the lower jaw to hinge downward and the airway to narrow. OSA sufferers who sleep on their back experience a higher number of apneas per night and stop breathing for longer during those apneas. In one study of 574 patients with sleep apnea, participants had at least twice as many instances of apnea or hypopnea when sleeping on their back as they did when lying on their side. Researchers concluded that "Body position during sleep has a profound effect on the frequency and severity of breathing abnormalities in obstructive sleep apnea patients."[65]

A similar assessment of 2,077 OSA patients over a period of 10 years found that nearly 54% experienced at least twice as many breathing abnormalities when sleeping on their back than when sleeping on their side. The paper acknowledged that "Avoiding the supine posture during sleep may significantly improve the sleep quality and daytime alertness of many positional patients."[65]

The techniques that follow will help you achieve better quality sleep.

### BREATHE LIGHT AND SLOW

You can do this while watching some light television or relaxing in bed.

- Place one hand on your chest and one hand on your abdomen.
- Gently soften and slow down your breathing to create a slight hunger for air.
- Continue the practice for approximately 15 minutes.

This is an excellent way to help with SDB. It also promotes relaxation and enables you to fall asleep more easily.

## MOUTH TAPE FOR NASAL BREATHING

We've already described why it is vital to breathe through your nose during sleep, but how can you make sure it happens?

When you wake up in the morning, your mouth should be naturally moist. If you have been breathing through your mouth at night, you will wake up with a dry mouth. You may also find that you have smelly breath.[66] Mouth breathers have a higher incidence of gum disease, halitosis, and tooth decay than nasal breathers.

If you tend to mouth breathe during the night, you can try taping the mouth, following these guidelines.

Taping the mouth at night may seem like a scary prospect at first. However, the method has been used with great success by Oxygen Advantage trained instructors and in Buteyko Breathing Clinics around the world. It may be reassuring to know that it does not take long to get used to. If you struggle to keep your mouth closed at night, placing MyoTape around your mouth before you go to sleep is an excellent way to eliminate SDB and encourage full-time nasal breathing. The tape, which I designed especially for this purpose, is placed around the lips rather than across the mouth and is designed to act as a reminder, using elastic tension to prompt you to close your mouth if it falls open.

I have no doubt that the single best thing I ever did to improve my sleep was to tape my mouth at night. MyoTape can be easily purchased online at MyoTape.com. You may also like to try a Micropore paper tape, which you can pick up at any pharmacy, or Lip-Seal Strips, which can be bought online from Simply Breathe.

To overcome any initial anxiety about having your mouth taped, try wearing the tape for 20 minutes before you go to bed. Also be aware that if you are accustomed to breathing through your mouth, the tape is likely to fall off during the first couple of nights. This will resolve fairly quickly. Within a few days, your body will relearn its natural nasal breathing pattern and the tape will remain in place. You may then begin to experience the best sleep you have ever had.

If your nose is partially blocked before going to bed, use the nose unblocking exercise to clear it before taping your mouth. Rest assured, however, that if you are wearing the lip tape at night, your nose will never become completely blocked. This is because nasal breathing actually helps dilate the nasal passages.

If you breathe heavily during the night while wearing the tape, your nose may partially block. If this is the case, you may also find it helpful to wear a nasal dilator, which you can purchase online or from your chemist. This small plastic dilator is placed inside the nose to open the nasal passages and alleviate snoring. In time, if you follow the breathing exercises and techniques in this book and as your nasal congestion improves, you will be less likely to require a nasal dilator.

In a recent study that tested the application of lip tape to assess difficulties with nasal breathing, researchers found that 83.5% of habitual mouth breathers were able to breathe comfortably through the nose with the mouth taped. Remember, your nose will only ever become completely blocked if you revert to mouth breathing.[67]

If, during the night, you find it difficult to breathe while using the tape, gently reduce your breathing until you feel comfortable. Try to acclimatize to the tape rather than removing it. Without it, you are likely to revert to mouth breathing during sleep, and this will only make your symptoms worse.

**Important: This method is not suitable for children under four years old.** While MyoTape does not cover the mouth, meaning that it is still possible to communicate while wearing it, any child taping their mouth at night must be able to remove the tape if they feel the need to.

**Do NOT use MyoTape or any other lip tape at night if you are feeling nauseous or have been drinking alcohol. If your child has a tummy upset or is likely to vomit, you must NOT tape his or her mouth during sleep.**

### Check your BOLT Score

To find out whether you are overbreathing during the night, measure your BOLT score before you go to bed and again when you wake in the morning. If your BOLT score is lower upon waking than it was the night before, this means that you have been breathing too hard or mouth breathing during sleep.

## ENSURE BETTER CPAP COMPLIANCE

If you use a CPAP machine, mouth breathing during sleep compromises the effectiveness of your treatment.[68] If you commonly mouth breathe at night, you may also find it necessary to wear MyoTape with your CPAP device. Some people find it difficult to wear a mask all night, and the full-face mask is naturally more uncomfortable.

Acceptable CPAP adherence or compliance is defined as 4 hours use per night,[69] at least 70% of the time.[70] But studies show that different levels of compliance lead to better or worse results and that adherence of more than six hours a night is necessary to reduce the risk of cardiovascular mortality.[69] Given that we need between seven and eight hours sleep every night, four hours of compliance is obviously less than ideal. Also, if you drive or fly for a living, it's worth noting that you are required to share your CPAP compliance data with the relevant authorities[70] and that if your treatment compliance is inadequate, you may lose your job.

Throughout this book, we explore the connections between SDB and many different aspects of health. There are links with conditions including diabetes, sexual dysfunction, heart failure, and high blood pressure. Clinical interventions like CPAP can help prevent and, in some instances, reverse these problems, but only when the device is used effectively, which means all-night compliance.

To achieve that, it is necessary to address mouth breathing, which is the primary cause of CPAP noncompliance.[68] Mouth breathing allows air to leak out through the open mouth before reaching the airways. This often causes the user to wake, which contributes to sleep fragmentation. When you breathe nasally during sleep, the air supplied by the CPAP device makes it to the airway as intended. It's so simple but just by closing your mouth, you improve your chance of staying asleep.

There are various products such as chin straps on the market designed to keep the mouth closed at night. These can be problematic. They fit tightly around the head, fixing the jaw closed, and can cause side effects including temporomandibular joint pain. This is another instance in which taping the mouth during sleep is the best solution. Whether you choose MyoTape or an alternative product, mouth tape is a gentle way to ensure CPAP compliance. It easily prevents oral air leaks without causing jaw pain, interfering with your CPAP mask, or adding a level of discomfort that stops you from sleeping.

Another problem with CPAP is that air leakage can cause irritation to the eyes. This is especially true for people who have floppy eyelid syndrome—loose upper eyelids that easily fold back, leaving the eye unprotected.[71] Sleep apnea is known to be an independent risk factor for blindness due to glaucoma,[72] and although the reason for the relationship is unknown, studies have found associations between OSA and various eye diseases including floppy eyelid syndrome,[73] Using mouth tape to prevent oral air leaks, there is less chance of eye irritation.

## PREPARING FOR A SLEEP STUDY

When you have been practicing breathwork for a while, you may find that your symptoms lessen and it's time to discuss reducing your CPAP use with your doctor. The best way to determine whether your sleep apnea is under control is by attending a sleep study.

You should only ask to take part in a sleep study once your BOLT score has been greater than 20 seconds for at least 2 weeks. You should have been practicing light, slow, deep nasal breathing with your tongue in the correct resting position and your lips closed. For men, another indication of healthy breathing during sleep is that you begin to notice yourself waking up with an erection each morning. The reason for this is covered in much more detail in Chapter Eleven when we look at the link between breathing and sex, but for now it's just worth understanding that "morning wood" is indicative of good cardiovascular health.

On the night of the sleep study, before you go to sleep, practice slowing down your breathing for 15 to 20 minutes to create air hunger. Then tape your lips using MyoTape. Over the years, I have advised many of my students to wear lip tape during the sleep study. The technicians organizing the study are often curious but have never, to my knowledge, vetoed use of the tape. This is important, because during the sleep study, you want to determine the severity of sleep apnea when breathing is through the nose, slow and low.

## THE BASICS OF GOOD SLEEP HYGIENE

There are several best practices for going to sleep that are considered the basics of good sleep hygiene. You can start by avoiding eating a large meal or drinking alcohol late at night. Although alcohol can send you off to sleep more quickly, it is actually a stimulant, which results in poor quality sleep and waking in the middle of the night. Eating too close to bedtime creates similar problems as it leaves the body needing to expend considerable energy digesting food while in a state of semirelaxation.

Reserve the bedroom, where possible, for sleeping, relaxation, and making love. Your bedroom should not be a place to watch television, work on the laptop, or browse the Internet on your mobile phone. In fact, having as little technology as possible in the bedroom will help ensure good quality sleep. Technology is increasingly implicated in contributing to poor sleep. Even the age-old ritual of reading before falling asleep has been compromised as backlit tablets and phones replace traditional paper books. When our eyes are exposed to bright light, especially blue light, such as that produced by these devices, the brain stops secreting the relaxation hormone melatonin, which is responsible for creating feelings of sleepiness. The human body is designed to be awake during daylight and to sleep when it gets dark. According to a *Harvard Health Letter* entitled "Blue light has a dark side," it is advisable to refrain from using a laptop or electronic device for at least three hours before sleep.[74] If this is not possible for you, it is a good idea to invest in a pair of blue-light-blocking glasses to wear when using your computer or phone in the evening.

## CABIN PRESSURE: USING BREATHWORK IN A LOW OXYGEN ENVIRONMENT

An email I received from a client who is a professional pilot provides an interesting perspective on the subject of breathing and sleep. Remember the report from the British Airline Pilots' Association about pilots who fell asleep while in charge of a plane? According to my client, fatigue, disrupted circadian rhythms, jetlag, sleep disturbance, and body-clock disruption are all part of the job, along with a high level of pressure and responsibility. These are significant, unavoidable issues that must be managed and closely monitored if performance is to be maintained at the necessary levels throughout the flight. My client explained:

> At a major airline like mine, which is notorious for its diverse operating schedule and network, these issues are amplified even further. A quick look at my logbook reveals that on average, 40% of my flights are operated at night and back-of-the-clock hours. This

cannot be taken lightly. In one month, I can typically fly one ultra-long-haul, two or three medium-haul trips and multiple short-haul return flights.

In order to optimize my mental performance, I need to take a number of steps to ensure I am well-rested and able to operate at an adequate cognitive level. This is in addition to the stringent rules and regulations employed by the industry, which ensure that our rosters are compiled and managed safely.

Since discovering breathwork, and its convincing benefits in terms of sleep, energy, and wellbeing, I have used this to my advantage consistently. I have a daily breathwork routine that allows me to sleep better, recover between flights, and perform optimally during a flight.

It all starts with sleep. In my experience, this is the most important variable to manage, whether I'm at home, staying in a hotel around the airline's network, or during critical rest periods onboard ultra-long-haul flights.

I use the principles behind Pranayama breathing, and the scientifically backed exercises from *The Oxygen Advantage* to create a sleep-management routine which consists of the following:

- Taping my mouth at night to ensure nasal breathing and deeper more restful sleep.
- A sleep hygiene routine consisting of a dark room, eye shades, and ear plugs.
- Presleep breathing exercises or meditation, to relax and activate the parasympathetic response. These include long deep and slow diaphragmatic breaths that emphasize longer exhalations to relax my body.
- Keeping hydrated before bed.
- Trying to be as consistent as I can and staying on a fixed "home time-zone" as best as possible.

My real-time breathwork practices during flights include:

- Box breathing using small breath holds after inhalation and exhalation. (You will find this exercise in Chapter Two.)

- Long slow and deep cycles of breathing, using the diaphragm, which is pretty much a habit now anyway.
- Consistent nose breathing to ensure maximum oxygen uptake.
- These techniques are essential during flights because we operate in a low oxygen environment of poor quality recirculated air. The exercises have obvious benefits not only for the operating crew, but also for passengers who are not used to the environment. In effect, we are already at a disadvantage because of the low air oxygen levels and the altitude of approximately 6,000 feet. This is compounded by the fact that a high percentage of the population has dysfunctional breathing habits.

My postflight exercises include:

- Any breathwork I feel like doing that emphasizes nasal and diaphragmatic breathing. I especially like to practice this before bed.
- Focusing on parasympathetic recovery and lowering my arousal levels, which are usually quite high after flights due to lengthy periods of elevated concentration.

I'm very aware of how physical and mental stress affects the quality and speed of the breathing. I use the breath as a powerful tool to control my state of mind, arousal, and general self-awareness. It is a two-way street. The mind can control the breath, and the breath can control the mind. This works particularly well in high-pressure training situations. These simulations, which we practice every three months, are similar to real-time combat training in the military special forces and police tactical groups.

The benefits I receive from breathwork are powerful and effective. I can literally help my body and mind change and adapt as I need it to, using the breath.

# CHAPTER EIGHT
# DEVELOPING HEALTHY AIRWAYS IN CHILDREN

---

## WHAT CAUSES CHILDHOOD MOUTH BREATHING?

B ack in 1909, an article, "Habitual Mouth-Breathing and Consequent Malocclusion of the Teeth," was published in *The Dental Cosmos*. In it, DeLong described how mouth breathing can cause the sleeper to wake with a dry mouth and throat in the morning, often accompanied by headache:

> A restless sleep, [and] much tossing in bed and snoring will be observed. The face is usually elongated, the bones of the face are underdeveloped, as the air spaces do not have the proper circulation, the nostrils are small.[1]

DeLong goes on to list other detrimental effects of mouth breathing, including recession of the chin and a high narrow palate with crooked teeth. Children who breathe through their mouths are observed as looking dull and expressionless and may be accused by their teachers of being inattentive in class.[1] When I first discovered this article, over 100 years after it was written, I could not help but feel a sense of disappointment that mouth breathing is still not taken more seriously by the dental and medical professions.

Humans were never designed to mouth breathe. In fact, in the entire animal kingdom, there are only a few creatures for which mouth breathing is normal. Diving birds, such as penguins and pelicans, whose respiratory apparatus differs from that of humans and other mammals, will take in a gulp of air before descending below water to hunt. Even dogs, while they are often depicted with their mouths open and tongues lolling, only ever pant to regulate body temperature.

From birth, a tiny baby will instinctively breathe through the nose. You may notice that a baby's tummy moves easily up and down with each inhalation and exhalation as the diaphragm engages. However, at just a few months old, many children switch to mouth breathing. Unfortunately, this is a habit that sticks. Mouth breathing is classified as a pathological condition, yet it is one that more than 50% of children exhibit. It is present in 60% of boys and 40% of girls.[2]

Mouth breathing in children has a variety of causes, all falling into two basic categories; obstruction to the airway and behavior.[3] The two most common triggers are chronic allergies and enlarged tonsils and/or adenoids. The adenoids are glands located toward the back of the nasal cavity where the nose connects to the throat. They form part of the immune system and produce white blood cells to help fight infection. Enlarged adenoids are common among children aged between two and seven years, typically shrinking by adolescence.

Other genetic and environmental factors that lead to mouth breathing in children include a high narrow palate, tongue-tie, lip-tie, a small nose,[4] constricted upper airways, asthma, bottle feeding, insufficient breastfeeding in infancy, and an overheated home. Habits such as thumb sucking, excessive use of pacifiers, overeating or eating too much processed food, lack of physical exercise, and even wearing too many clothes also play a part. A child with a high narrow palate is nearly three times more likely to breathe through an open mouth.[5] Equally, something as simple as the use of a conventional pacifier can increase the probability of mouth breathing by 25% for each year of use.[5]

Of all these influences, swelling of the adenoids (adenoid hypertrophy) is the primary reason for mouth breathing in children. Untreated adenoid hypertrophy results in *adenoid facies* or long face syndrome, an alteration in facial development characterized by an elongated, open-mouthed appearance. I see children with faces like this all the time. Tragically, it can hold them back in their lives.

## HOW THE AIRWAYS DEVELOP

A 1991 study published in the *American Journal of Orthodontics and Dentofacial Orthopedics* compared the breathing of normal and long-faced adolescents.[6] The purpose of the research was to assess tidal volume and ratio of nasal breathing in 32 children between the ages of 11 and 17. Those with long faces (vertical dentofacial morphology) due to juvenile adenoid hypertrophy had a significantly different lower face form than those who had developed normally. While the results showed that both groups of adolescents had similar tidal volumes, the long-faced subjects were much less likely to breathe nasally. Children who develop adenoid facies have smaller nasal airways.[6] This is an irreversible, lifelong consequence of mouth breathing during early development.

I live in the small village of Moycullen on the west coast of Ireland. Every few months, I visit my local dentist. He is in his early thirties and was educated at Trinity College in Dublin. During one of our conversations, I asked him about the implications of mouth breathing during childhood for oral-facial development. I was surprised to discover he doesn't believe mouth breathing contributes to crooked teeth or any negative development of the face. Given that he is a recent graduate, I expected that, if there were a relationship between mouth breathing and crooked teeth, he would know about it. Apparently, despite the topic having been hotly debated in dentistry for over a century, this is not the case. Unfortunately, the well-being of millions of children and adults is being sacrificed due to the unwillingness of the dental and medical professions to reach agreement about the connection.

I am living proof of the effects of mouth breathing on the development of the face. I have the same features described in the *Dental Cosmos* article. My palate is very high, my jaws were set back, and my teeth were crooked. It could be a coincidence, but it may not be. It is indeed still difficult to reach conclusions on several points. It is unclear how much nasal obstruction is necessary to cause mouth breathing, and there is as yet no comprehensive evidence to show how long a child's mouth breathing must persist in order to cause a lifelong problem or at what age mouth breathing does the most damage. There is, however, relevant research we will look at later, regarding the rate of craniofacial development in children at different ages.

In my case, it could be that I was born with a narrow facial structure that resulted in my mouth breathing. Or my mouth breathing may have caused my face to develop poorly. Either way, what I do know is that I was a mouth-breather during childhood, as is evident in many family photos, and that my dentist could have spotted this early on and advised my parents about the importance of nose breathing. The problem of my small jaws could have been easily addressed within months by using functional appliances to widen my palate.

What pediatric health professionals must realize is that dentists are in an ideal position to help children with these same facial structures and mouth breathing habits. With this understanding, procedures could be put in place to gently widen the jaws, to help promote forward development of the face, and to shape the airway. I believe that, if this were done, each child would be better placed to reach his or her full potential.

## THE INFLUENCE OF DISORDERED BREATHING ON LEARNING POTENTIAL

A stuffy nose will adversely affect a child's sleep. After a night spent breathing heavily through the mouth, the child will wake up exhausted. This manifests as poor concentration and frustration in school. If this inability to focus continues for a length of time, a psychological evaluation and possible diagnosis of attention deficit disorder (ADD) or attention deficit hyperactivity disorder (ADHD) may follow. Notably, scientists have demonstrated that it is common for children with ADHD to experience nasal congestion and hay fever.[7] Also, 40% of children who experience sleep disorders, including snoring or sleep apnea, develop ADD, ADHD, or a learning disability.[8] In fact, researchers have found that, if a child is snoring by the age of 8 and the problem is left untreated, there is an 80% chance that the child will consequently develop a permanent 20% reduction in mental capacity.[9] A 2012 paper by pediatric sleep expert Karen Bonuck demonstrated that mouth breathing, snoring, and apnea at 6, 18, and 30 months of age significantly increases the risk of neurobehavioral and neurocognitive disorders at ages 4 and 7.[10]

A 2017 study by pediatric behavioral and sleep scientists described the case of a 5-year-old girl named Carly.[11] Carly was brought for an interdisciplinary evaluation because her behavior at home and school suggested ADHD. Carly demonstrated average verbal, visual-spatial, and fluid reasoning IQ scores during psychological testing, but her processing speed and working memory were below average. Executive function skills (processes that monitor behavior) returned mixed results, and her working memory was borderline. The ratings given by her parents implied worse symptoms of ADHD and executive function than her test results showed. While factors such as the separation of her parents and inconsistent disciplinary approaches were noted, the researchers felt that her nightly mouth breathing and snoring were most significant. Carly displayed enlarged tonsils and a high, arched palate. A sleep study indicated that she also had OSA.

Carly underwent an adenotonsillectomy, after which her ADHD symptoms noticeably improved. However, her behavioral problems recurred one year after surgery.[11] The paper does not record whether Carly also reverted to mouth breathing after the operation, but it could be reasonably assumed that a failure to restore nasal breathing resulted in the recurrence of OSA.[12]

Unfortunately, doctors treating ADD or ADHD rarely consider nasal obstruction as a possible cause and are unaware that the condition can be greatly helped without medication or psychological therapy.[9] When I speak to any parent who has a child diagnosed with ADD, my first suggestion is to check the child's sleep habits. Is your child breathing through the mouth, twisting and turning during the night and waking up with the bedclothes tangled in the morning? Do they snore or stop breathing during sleep? Is their breathing audible during sleep? To experience quality sleep, nasal breathing is of the utmost importance. Any adult understands the knock-on effect that a poor night's sleep has on mood, so how can a child be expected to face the day with boundless energy if their sleep is inadequate?

While no parent wants to see their child feeling constantly tired and frustrated, more serious consequences are at issue. Children who breathe through an open mouth have a strong tendency to experience cognitive disorders and problems with memory, concentration, attention, and learning ability.[9] Those with sleep problems are much more likely to have special educational needs (SEN). The Avon Longitudinal Study of Parents and Children, also known as *Children of the 90s*, is a detailed and ongoing birth cohort study of children born in the United Kingdom between April 1991 and December 1992. The Avon research has shown substantial correlations between sleep-disordered breathing (SDB) and cognitive impairment in children.[13] Parents enrolled in the study reported on their children's snoring, witnessed apnea, and mouth breathing at 6, 18, 30, 42, and 57 months. SDB symptom trajectories, or clusters, were derived from the resultant data. By the time the children reached 8 years old, parental reports for 11,049 children with SDB indicated that children with SDB were 40% more likely to have special educational needs.[13] These statistics are echoed by a 2013 study in which 48 children had complete ear, nose, and throat examinations. Results showed that children with enlarged adenoids experienced greater learning difficulties than those with normal adenoids.[14]

Likewise, a 2015 study from the faculties of dentistry at Havana and Aden Universities found that children with excessive daytime sleepiness were almost 10 times more likely to have learning difficulties.[3]

Another 2011 paper compared cognitive function in children with varying severities of SDB against a control group with no history of sleep problems. In total, 137 children between the ages of 7 and 12 took part. It was found that there was a lower general intellectual ability in all children with SDB. This was the case whether or not the problem was severe enough to manifest as snoring or sleep apnea—children should not be snoring or even breathing heavily during sleep.[15] Children with SDB also showed higher levels of impairment in both executive and academic functioning.

The first important study to look at the potential link between OSA and its damaging effects on cognitive ability was published in 1998. The paper examined 297 first-grade children whose academic performance was in the lowest 10th percentile of their class. These children were found to have significantly higher incidence of OSA than their higher-achieving peers. The academic results of those children who received treatment for OSA improved considerably in the following year, while children who had OSA but were not treated showed no improvement.[16]

Another point regarding the cognitive and behavioral effects of OSA is demonstrated by a 2011 paper that examined the methods used to evaluate SDB in children.[17] The study reported that many children who suffered OSA at a level that was not picked up by traditional testing were on various medications to alleviate symptoms, all of which could be explained by poor sleep. Some children were prescribed a sedative at night and a stimulant during the day. Others were on a range of medicines including antidepressants, antiheadache, antiallergic, antigastroesophageal reflux, and antihypertensives. After treatment for SDB, 43 out of 99 children had their drugs withdrawn by their physicians.

## NONSURGICAL INTERVENTIONS

The good news is that sleep specialists are becoming increasingly concerned about the impact of open mouth breathing during sleep, especially in children. Dr. Christian Guilleminault, who had discovered in the 1970s that blood pressure dramatically increased when patients stopped breathing during sleep[18] and made many further discoveries in the field of sleep medicine, states in one 2015 paper, "The case against mouth breathing is growing, and given its negative consequences, we feel that restoration of the nasal breathing route as early as possible is critical." The paper goes on to explain that "Restoration of nasal breathing during wake and sleep may be the only valid 'complete' correction of pediatric sleep-disordered breathing."[12] After his death in 2019, Dr. Guilleminault was recognized for his pioneering work on sleep apnea and his contributions to the understanding of the negative impacts of mouth breathing during childhood.[19]

As we've already seen, the causes of mouth breathing during childhood can vary and may be related to nasal congestion or enlarged adenoids. When my daughter Lauren was four, I noticed her having disturbed sleep. I quickly made an appointment with the ear, nose, and throat (ENT) department at the Bon Secours hospital in Galway, Ireland. On examination, it was found that her tonsils were enlarged and in all probability, so were her adenoids. A date was set for her to have her tonsils and adenoids removed and to have her tongue-tie and lip-tie released. The operation went as planned, but the procedure was traumatic for Lauren and for us as parents. In the following months, there was no postop followup, and at no point was there any mention that the procedure might bring only short-term benefits to Lauren's sleep unless nasal breathing was restored.[20]

Soon after this episode, I sent papers to the ENT surgeon regarding the importance of restoring nasal breathing post-tonsillectomy and adenoidectomy. I received a thank-you email in reply. In hindsight, I would not now follow the advice to have my daughter's tonsils and adenoids removed without first having pursued less-invasive techniques such as developing her jaws. Had I been armed, as I am now, with more knowledge about functional dentistry, I would have known that the better solution would have been to embark on the development of her airways. Genetically, my daughter has a similar facial profile to me, with the same narrow upper airways.

Postsurgery, I brought her to the functional dentist, Dr. Tony O'Connor, where she had her airways developed using an easy and noninvasive appliance known as the advanced lightwire functional appliance (ALF). Since then, I recommend to any parent presenting a child with enlarged adenoids to look at *maxillary expansion* (widening of the upper jaw) and forward development of the face first. Try that, along with continued nasal breathing and practicing the *Steps* exercise for children (in Chapter Two). In most cases, this approach will result in maxillary expansion, develop the airway, restore nasal breathing, and reduce inflammation of the adenoids and tonsils within three months. All of these methods are noninvasive, so there is little or no trauma involved. The airways are developed, and good breathing patterns are restored for the long term.

If your child's breathing problem persists for more than three months, then consider an adenotonsillectomy. However, children must still be taught to breathe nasally after surgery, or SDB is likely to recur within three years.[12]

One 2019 review examined the effects of nose-breathing exercises in mouth-breathing children. The report concluded that nasal breathing is better for the respiratory system.[21] The authors also cited results from a 2008 paper, which demonstrated that a protocol of respiratory muscle training and nasal breathing improved respiratory muscle strength and nasal inspiratory flow in children who had mouth breathed.[22] This study discusses the importance of nasal respiratory training for reestablishing lung volume and nostril elasticity in children.

For over a century, researchers have investigated the effect of rapid maxillary expansion on the functioning of the nose.[23–26] Maxillary expansion involves wearing a dental appliance positioned in the roof of the mouth. The device exerts gentle pressure over time to widen the jaws and airways. Numerous studies have shown how this procedure causes positive development in the top jaw and nasal cavity and that the resulting changes improve breathing throughout a child's life.

## THE VITAL ROLE OF THE DENTIST

Dr. William Hang, a Los Angeles–based airway-centric orthodontist, describes the dentist as the gatekeeper to the airways.[27] Researchers Peter Catalano and John Walker also state,

> The most likely person to diagnose a child with SDB is their family
> dentist or orthodontist. This is directly related to the fact that nasal
> breathing has a tremendous impact on craniofacial development,
> which in turn determines dental profile and occlusion (how the teeth

align). Over 90% of children with crooked teeth, teeth grinding, or malocclusion (misalignment of the teeth) have compromised nasal breathing.[9]

In the United States, thanks to a joint effort by American Academy of Pediatrics and American Academy of Pediatric Dentistry, children are ensured a "dental home" by the time they reach the age of 1 year. This means that pediatric dentists have a higher frequency of patient encounters than most other allied health professionals.[15] A 2017 study of 55 children, more than 65% of whom were mouth breathers, concluded that "Recognition of mouth breathing in young persons by orthodontists is poor."[28] But why is this the case? Why isn't SDB in children, its causes and treatment, primarily the domain of the pediatric dentist? And why is it so often not even picked up by dentists?

The connection between nasal breathing and dental issues was first observed in the 1970s by a Norwegian orthodontist, Dr. Egil Harvold. Harvold noticed that many patients who came to him with dental issues were also mouth breathers, and he decided to investigate further. In 1981, he published the results of his landmark study, "Primate experiments in oral respiration," in which he compared baby monkeys whose nostrils were blocked with silicone plugs with a control group.[29] For six months, as the monkeys grew, those animals whose noses had been plugged began to mouth breathe by default. This led to many changes in craniofacial development. The faces of the monkeys whose noses had been blocked looked very different from those who were able to breathe nasally. They developed long faces, misaligned teeth, and altered face and neck muscles as the body adapted to form an oral airway. Even after the nasal obstruction was removed, they continued to mouth breathe for as much as a year, while their altered facial features were retained.[29]

A 1998 paper by American orthodontist Katherine Vig questioned Harvold's results. Vig explains that, while Harvold fully blocked the noses of the monkeys, total nasal obstruction in humans is "extremely rare."[30] However, I believe that Dr. Vig is missing the point. The issue is not the extent of nasal obstruction, it is whether or not the child is mouth breathing. The studies by Harvold investigated if persistent mouth breathing in monkeys caused craniofacial abnormalities. The study results showed this to be the case. A new review published in 2018 reported that children with nasal obstruction were 5.55 times more likely to mouth breathe.[5]

A study in the *American Journal of Orthodontics* in 1997 also looked at the effects of nasal obstruction on craniofacial growth in young Japanese macaque monkeys.[31] Researchers studied 11 animals, of which 7 were subject to either light or heavy nasal obstruction, while 4 acted as a control group. Nasal breathing was assessed in terms of nasal airway resistance, and craniofacial development was measured. In the monkeys whose noses were blocked, the mandible (lower jaw) rotated downward and backward, the condyle (jaw joint) grew upward and backward, and the gonial angle of the jaw changed. The monkeys also developed anterior open bites and spaced dental arches. Notably, these changes in growth were significantly more apparent in the monkeys who had the heavy nasal obstruction. These results support the theory that a blocked nose in childhood, before and during puberty, may result in permanent deformities in the structures of the face and skull. More specifically, it may result in skeletal open bite, a condition where there is no contact between anterior and posterior teeth, one of the most challenging dentofacial deformities to treat.[31]

Another paper from 2011 looked at the effects of short-term forced oral breathing on baby rats. Results showed that even very short-term nasal obstruction created significant hormonal changes, including an increase of stress hormones of more than 1,000%. While the stress hormone level normalized by adulthood, other hormonal changes persisted long term, the development of the olfactory bulb was impaired, and alterations were seen in the development of the respiratory muscles.[32]

A 2019 assessment of preschool children in Italy examined the relationship between mouth breathing and severe malocclusions.[33] Researchers observed oral habits in 1,616 children aged between 3 and 6 years to determine the prevalence of dental problems and the statistical significance of their connection with mouth breathing and sucking habits. The results showed that 38% of the children needed orthodontic treatment, and 46% had signs of malocclusion that required monitoring and risk factors that needed to be removed so that the problem could correct itself as the child grew. Only 16% of the children were completely healthy. Common dental problems included tooth displacement, tooth decay, and early loss of primary teeth, overbite, overjet, crossbite, and open bite—all symptomatic of dental misalignment and poor oral hygiene. It was found that oral breathing increases as malocclusion gets worse.[33] Separate research has confirmed the link between oral breathing and poor dental health, tooth decay, and halitosis.[2]

The 2019 study concluded that mouth breathing is a risk factor for dental malocclusion and should be intercepted and corrected as early as possible to prevent the development or worsening of craniofacial problems. However, a 2017 cross-sectional study of patients aged between 10 and 25 years old had concluded that recognition of mouth breathing in young people by orthodontists is poor.[28] Orthodontists must aim to address these risk factors to promote correct dento-skeletal growth. This requires pediatricians, allergists, orthodontists, speech therapists, and ENT specialists to work closely together to promote early diagnosis and treatment.[33]

SDB in children is serious and potentially life threatening. Numerous sources underline the fact that dentists may be in the best position to recognize a potential airway-related sleep problem.[34] It is vital, then, that dentists enter the profession with a reasonable knowledge of sleep disorders and their assessment. Only with this understanding can they ensure that timely referrals and appropriate treatments are offered. Currently, limited diagnostic norms exist for both children and adults, and more research is desperately needed, particularly into childhood sleep disorders. The dentist is trained to look into the mouth. The medical doctor is not. To meet the best standards of patient welfare, it is clear that sleep medicine requires an overhaul. Medical doctors must form partnerships with their dental colleagues.

Studies have defined the risk factors of obstructive sleep apnea in children as a narrow palate, long face, enlarged tonsils and/or adenoids, and minor malocclusions (misaligned teeth), and *not*, as some might expect, obesity. It should therefore be clear why dentists must be involved in identifying SDB in children. Indeed, since obstructive SDB affects between 1% and 5% of the pediatric population[35] and has been found to be implicated in sudden infant death syndrome, this fact should be considered with some urgency.[35]

Since 2018, the American Dental Association has endorsed sleep and airway hygiene risk assessment as a primary responsibility of dentists who provide services for children.[36] It is encouraging to see that the definition of optimal pediatric health is changing and now includes the ability to breathe nasally during wakefulness and sleep. However, from a conversation with a friend of mine, who is a dentist with 40 years of experience, it is clear that there is still some way to go. He explained to me that when he talks to colleagues about breathing, they

> are consistently resistant to talking with their patients about the problems of mouth breathing and dental health. . . . They are waiting for a "new" dental specialty to evolve . . . I tell them this responsibility belongs in every general dental practice. If their patients . . . ask them . . . what to do about dry mouth, snoring, tongue thrusting, anxiety, teeth grinding or clenching, and sleep problems, they might be nudged to get involved and really care for their patients.

A UK orthodontist who developed a technique called orthotropics to correct the effects of childhood mouth breathing has been heavily criticized within dentistry. Dr. John Mew, who promotes the idea of preventive measures in younger children rather than surgery later in life, was dismissed as an "idiot" by a prominent American orthodontist in 2020 in the *New York Times*.[37] Mew fell foul of the General Dental Council in 2017 when, at the age of 89, he lost his license after publishing an advert slamming the orthodontic community. His son Dr Mike Mew still practices Orthotropics and increasing research now supports his ideas. Dr. Mew strongly believes that the teeth should not be pushed or pulled. He works on the principle (called the "Tropic" Premise) that if the tongue rests on the palate, with the lips sealed and the teeth in or near contact, the growth and position of the jaws will be ideal. In other words, the teeth and jaws know how to grow, they only need guiding into position with correct posture. Over the years, Dr. Mew found that the teeth often align themselves if the posture is right. In this fundamental he is copying the natural growth of most mammals.

I first reached out to Dr. Mew in 2010, when I was writing my book *Buteyko Meets Dr. Mew* to help teenagers with their breathing. I immediately felt a genuine welcome from both Dr. John and Mike Mew, and their passion for helping children develop correct facial growth was obvious. I was fortunate enough over the course of two years to attend Dr. Mew's practice and sit in the clinic room as he and his son worked. While John Mew worked with one child, Mike would work with another, and there was often a lively interaction as the two would share opinions and argue concepts. The parents looked on as the particulars of each child's treatment unfolded between the two dedicated orthodontists. I have seen for myself the positive changes to children's faces. I also spoke with parents to get their insight, and I cannot remember anyone having anything negative to say about the treatment. To this day, I am in touch with both John and Mike Mew, and before the COVID restrictions struck, I brought my daughter Lauren to their clinic. I admire their work and their tenacity.

I sometimes feel a sense of bewilderment about the fact the dental industry has ignored the impact of chronic mouth breathing and incorrect tongue resting posture on craniofacial development. The Mews' arguments may not be perfect. Sometimes in their drive to generate awareness of the importance of forward growth of the face to make room for the airway, they can be critical of traditional treatments, but there is room for both approaches. The unwillingness of the orthodontic industry to even conduct a clinical trial of Dr. Mew's work makes me wonder why there is such a vested interest in the status quo. Perhaps the German physicist Max Planck was correct when he suggested that advances in science take place only when their opponents die out.

For the sake of the patient, medicine, like other industries, should be about continued development. While it is obviously essential to question everything and to ensure that new treatments are thoroughly tested, it is important that progress is not held back by dinosaur thinking, personality, or ego. The airline industry, for instance, works with a policy of ongoing improvement and has made continuous upgrades to safety a top priority since the first commercial airline flight in 1914.[38] I don't see any reason why dentistry shouldn't do the same.

## THE IMPORTANCE OF EARLY INTERVENTION

It may be that the dental industry is not more active in its approach to mouth breathing because there are still "chicken or egg" questions about its cause. In practical terms, however, the question is somewhat irrelevant. Does a child mouth breathe because he or she has been born with a small nose and nasal cavity? Or does habitual mouth breathing create the small nose and restricted airway? Either way, the solution lies in developing the child's airways at an early age. Unfortunately, most orthodontists will wait until their patient is 11 or 12 years old before acting. By then, the face is already grown, and it is too late to fully intervene. A study of 24 male and 24 female children discovered that not only does the face develop most significantly in the first five years of life, growth changes to the facial bones are most rapid during the first six months, decreasing incrementally thereafter.[39]

A 2018 article published in the *American Journal of Otolaryngology and Head and Neck Surgery* reports that 60% of facial growth occurs before the age of 4 and 90% by age 12. The speed of growth during the early years will not be news to any parent who is constantly replacing clothes their child has outgrown, but it underlines the fact that the window of opportunity is fairly limited when it comes to restoring nasal breathing and treating compromised airways and sleep problems in children. This does not mean that things are hopeless for preteens, teenagers, and even adults. Catalano and Walker explain that it's never "too late" to treat a breathing pattern disorder.[40] As time passes, the problem simply becomes more challenging for dentists and surgeons to correct and more difficult and unpleasant for the patient.

Incredibly, this exact issue was already written about in 1922. The dental profession has been debating it for 100 years, while millions of children have suffered. In 1922, Samuel Adams Cohen, a New York doctor, described how the normal growth of the teeth and jaws goes hand in hand with sound teeth, proper chewing, correct breathing, well-formed jaws, normal brain development, and normal speech[41]. He explained that nasal breathing does not naturally follow the removal of adenoids unless the child is taught to breathe properly. Cohen cites the example of children seen at the Forsyth Dental Infirmary, 75% of whom still breathed orally 3 years after the removal of their adenoids and tonsils.

His paper precedes the work of Dr. Kevin Boyd, whose research we will get to soon, in stating that breastfeeding gives a baby an advantage in terms of developing the mouth and jaw when compared with an artificial nipple and that soft food does not enable the child to develop the facial muscles responsible for chewing.

According to Cohen, misalignment of the teeth and jaws always indicates abnormal functioning. If there is no space for the temporary "milk" teeth, there is unlikely to be enough room for the permanent adult teeth. He states, "The presence of perfectly close, regular teeth after five years of age is an indication for treatment." At three and a half years, the dental arch should measure at least 27 mm. If, by four years of age, it measures less than 28 mm, the child will not have a normal dental arch unless intervention takes place.[41] About two years before the adult teeth appear, their growth within the tissues causes the dental arches to begin widening. This means that the baby teeth appear to be widely spaced. There should be space between all of the teeth at this point.

Cohen insists that once malocclusion is diagnosed, treatment should begin immediately, as early as possible. He suggests "thirty months of age" as the ideal time. In early treatment, only a slight "force" is necessary. He also states that

> treating dental deformity before the sixth year insures not only good mouth functioning but also correct breathing, since the width of the maxillary arch determines whether or not there is room for normal nasal breathing.

Cohen says that the child's brain at six years old is "within 40 grams of its weight at 19 years."[41] For this reason, it is vital that any problems in the growth of the face and teeth should be corrected before age six. He argues that the child's doctors and dentists should check for normal arches in children between two and a half and six years. Cohen concludes that the dental "apparatus" is not an organ with a single function in the same way as the eyes and ears. Any impairment in the teeth and jaws also impacts chewing, voice production and sound, dental health, facial expression, and the "beauty" of the face.[41]

Attractive faces are always forward grown.[42] I often use photos of Kate Middleton and Prince William (the Duke and Duchess of Cambridge) to illustrate this. They have distinctly different jaw sizes. When you look at a photo of them both smiling, try counting the number of teeth you can see in each of their mouths as they smile. In Kate, you might see 10 teeth. She has a beautifully wide-shaped face, good jaws, and with that, a good airway. On the other hand, it's only possible to see about 7 teeth as Prince William smiles. There are dark triangles to either side of his jaw. This indicates that his jaw is not wide enough. I don't know Prince William's dental history, but I would speculate that he may have had teeth removed to give him a nicer smile. As a result, the width of his jaw has been reduced so there is not enough room for the tongue. This would cause airway limitations, resistance to breathing, and possibly sleep apnea. Personally, I would rather have an ample airway and a poorer smile. At least, a poorer smile is not going to kill me!

## SAFE SLEEP FOR YOUR BABY

A further and extremely concerning consequence of SDB in children is SIDS. Dentists are well positioned to address the risk for children born with deficient airways, but, as yet, it is very rare for babies to be checked for tongue-tie or a high, narrow palate. In 2012, Caroline Rambaud of the Hôpital Raymond-Poincaré in Paris, France, and Stanford University's Christian Guilleminault looked at correlations between airway obstruction and SIDS in seven infants[43]. The authors compared the post-mortem findings for the seven dead children with seven age and gender-matched living children with OSA. In all seven SIDS cases, medical histories indicated chronic signs of abnormal sleep, and a significant proportion of the babies had presented with acute, often mild, rhinitis just before death. Four of the children normally slept prone (on their tummies). All of them displayed enlarged upper airway soft tissues and features consistent with a small *nasomaxillary complex* (narrow upper airway), with or without *mandibular retroposition* (backward displacement of the lower jaw). They all died of hypoxia (oxygen deprivation) in their sleep. The living children with OSA had similar facial features and upper airway complaints.

The paper explains that the anatomical risk factors for a narrow upper airway can be identified early in life. SDB is most frequently related to a small upper airway. When abnormal resistance to nasal breathing is present, the child will switch to mouth breathing. This leads to greater respiratory exertion during sleep. These traits are often inherited, so family dentists should be able to identify or even predict which children may be at risk. While more research is needed into the role of upper airway infection and anatomically small airways in SIDS, dentists must pay close attention to any sleep-related complaints in children with features consistent with a small airway.[43]

In the study, death was associated with abnormal sleep in six out of seven cases. Symptoms such as rhinitis or infection in the upper airways in the days prior to death were not marked enough to cause concern when mentioned to the child's doctor, but in each instance, the child essentially suffocated during sleep. Although many of the deaths were preceded by an abnormal sleep history, and the children displayed the anatomical risk factors for SDB, none were recognized as having SDB, so they were left untreated. Rambaud and Guilleminault concluded that it is vital to recognize the risk factors leading to a narrow upper airway as early in life as possible and that educating dentists and pediatric doctors regarding the facial features symptomatic of SDB may be valuable.[43]

The work of Dr. Kevin Boyd, a pediatric dentist who specializes in anthropology, helps us understand the connection between facial structure and SDB. Dr. Boyd works with young children from the age of six months old, developing the maxilla and nasal cavity in those with anatomically small airways. He believes that many craniofacial traits can be altered during the early childhood stages of dentofacial growth and that these features are likely to be a significant factor in SDB and OSA.[15] In his anthropological work, Dr. Boyd explains that sleep-related breathing disorders were not even part of the human experience until very recently. He points to the fact that skeletal malocclusion wasn't found in humans until the mid-eighteenth century. While he attributes many of the dentofacial and physical risk factors for malocclusion to the considerable changes in diet and lifestyle since the Industrial Revolution, he is also clear that these factors increase the incidence of SDB and OSA.[15]

The shape of the human face is changing. According to Dr. Boyd, it is likely that feeding behaviors in infancy are partly to blame. As his paper indicates, "ancestral-type" breastfeeding and weaning are important for the development of the face and jaw. While we might equate dental decay with diet in adulthood, the highly processed baby foods, artificial baby milk formulas, and "commercial nipples" that are all so common in use today were simply not available before the Industrial Revolution.[15]

Dr. Boyd concludes that treatment, prevention, or reversal of malocclusion may help to address SDB. From an evolutionary standpoint, he argues that pediatric dentists are uniquely placed to identify those patients who are at risk of OSA and SDB, and that their practices should acknowledge aspects that impact long-term health, such as airway size. The fact is that set-back jaws increase the risk of sleep apnea for the rest of a child's life. Dr. Boyd proposes that pediatric sleep medicine centers should employ at least one dentist experienced in dentofacial issues related to sleep problems and OSA, and suggests rewriting the rulebook when it comes to cephalometric norms (the models used by dentists to measure "correct" proportions of the skull and face).[15] The current models are almost entirely based on twentieth-century skulls and fail to take the evolution of the human chewing apparatus into account. These considerations apply to traditional orthodontic techniques such as tooth extraction and retraction of the jaw for aesthetic alignment.

In his paper on airway-centric dentistry, Dr. William Hang explains that it has been recognized for more than 30 years that the upper jaw rarely protrudes and is more commonly set back, yet treatment is still often directed to correcting protrusion of the upper teeth. Dr. Hang argues that extraction of bicuspid (premolar) teeth and retraction of the incisors and canine teeth negatively affects airway size and that dentists must consider how these procedures impact the airway, concluding, "Clearly, extraction/retraction must stop."[27]

## TREATMENT OPTIONS

Obstructive sleep apnea (OSA) is the most severe form of SDB. It is caused by a series of anatomical factors that reduce the size of the space at the back of the nose, mouth, and throat, and problems that make the upper airway more likely to collapse. This explains why children with craniofacial syndromes and conditions including cerebral palsy, allergic rhinitis, asthma, and obesity are more at risk. Anatomically, children with OSA have a soft palate that is on average 30% larger than normal.[44] This causes extra restriction to the airway. Further contributing features include a buildup of fluid in the eardrum and inflamed sinuses, perhaps indicating that a more general disorder affects the airway as a whole.[44] The simplest explanation is that most children with OSA have difficulty breathing through the nose.

Not all children with enlarged adenoids and tonsils suffer from OSA—craniofacial structure, genetic, and neuromuscular functions can also play a part—but the severity of OSA is related to the size of those tissues. One 2002 study confirms that the top two-thirds of the upper airway is around 50% smaller in children with OSA than in other children.[45] While further research is needed, it is thought that this narrow point is where airway obstruction occurs in OSA. For this reason, the most common treatment for OSA in nonobese children is surgical removal of the tonsils and/or adenoids.[15] However, adenotonsillectomy can leave a child with residual SDB.[43] Despite its popularity, the overall effectiveness of the operation as a treatment for OSA was unknown until the following 2010 study. It was acknowledged that success rates were likely to be lower than estimated, and factors that leave the child with unresolved OSA after treatment were still undefined.

In 2010, scientists from the University of Chicago's Department of Pediatrics carried out a multicenter review of otherwise healthy children undergoing adenotonsillectomy as a treatment for OSA.[46] The study looked at 578 children who were treated in pediatric sleep centers in the United States and Europe. Around 50% of the children were obese. Data included results from all preoperative and postoperative nocturnal polysomnograms—a polysomnogram is a test that records brain waves, blood oxygen levels, heart rate, respiratory rate, and eye and leg movements during sleep. Removing the adenoids and tonsils significantly reduced the number of apneas and hypopneas per hour of sleep (AHI), but OSA was only completely resolved in 27% of the children. While this was considered a significant improvement, symptoms persisted after treatment for a large number of subjects, particularly those who were obese, having asthma and older than 7 years.[46] The fact that nearly three-quarters of the children continued to have sleep apnea post-tonsillectomy and adenoidectomy points to causative factors aside from enlarged adenoids and tonsils. It is logical to argue that a child with underdeveloped airways and/or a habit of mouth/faster breathing is more likely to experience resistance to breathing during sleep and therefore suffer SDB.

There is growing evidence that medications including intranasal steroids may be helpful in mild OSA.[44] The very fact that nasal decongestants can help with minor instances of the condition points to nasal stuffiness as a problem. That means that exercises to unblock the nose can be used successfully in place of medication. Widening the upper jaw (maxillary expansion), known to be a useful treatment for SDB, can also be considered in cases of childhood OSA. According to an article published in the *American Journal of Orthodontics and Dentofacial Orthopedics* in 1987, the procedure may be warranted on the basis of airway size alone.[47]

## TONGUE-TIE AND BOTTLE FEEDING

Distinct from the adult condition, the onset of OSA in children can be caused by abnormal activity of the tongue.[48] This may be down to genetic and anatomical factors such as tongue-tie, though it is more commonly the result of bottlefeeding and habits including pacifier use, digit sucking, or sucking the lip, arm, or a blanket. In adults, OSA is affected by poor tongue resting position and tongue size.

In a healthy child, the tongue rests high in the palate.[49] This is the resting position conducive to nasal breathing. Correctly placed, the tongue shapes the upper jaw into a wide U, forming the basis for an attractive, well-proportioned face and jaws that are big enough to house all of the adult teeth without crowding. The activity of the tongue—sucking, swallowing, and chewing—stimulates oral-facial development, a process that continues until the child is around 13 to 15 years old. However, narrow jaws or constrictions of the tissues can make it difficult for a baby to suckle or hold his or her tongue in the correct place. When the mouth hangs open, the tongue cannot rest easily in the roof of the mouth, and poor breathing habits form.

A tongue-tie, or short lingual frenulum, occurs when the tissue that attaches the tongue to the floor of the mouth is too tight.[49] Babies with this condition may find breastfeeding difficult because they are unable to lift their tongue sufficiently to extract milk from the breast. This may cause frustration or fussy feeding in the baby, and the mother may experience nipple soreness, blocked ducts, or mastitis. When breastfeeding is problematic because of tongue-tie, the answer is usually to introduce bottle-feeding, while the underlying cause goes undiagnosed.

Tongue-tie is a relatively common condition in newborns, but it does have an impact on development if left untreated.[50] Without the freedom to suckle correctly, the child can develop a tongue thrust that leads to misalignment of the jaws, and infants with a tongue-tie are more likely to be exclusively bottle fed by one week of age. Lip-tie has not received the same attention in studies as tongue-tie, but it is also known to cause difficulty in breastfeeding.[51]

In older children, an untreated tongue-tie has been shown to create speech difficulties and contribute to SDB. The modified tongue position leads to mouth breathing, the development of an anterior and posterior crossbite, and imbalanced, disproportionate growth of both the upper and lower jaw. All these anatomical changes affect the size of the upper airway.

An article by Brian G. Palmer published in *Sleep Review* in 2003 explains that a high palate can also affect breathing and the alignment of the teeth.[52] Palmer writes, "Since the roof of the mouth is also the floor of the nose, any increase in the height of the palate decreases the volume size of the nasal chamber." This reduced size increases nasal air resistance. A high palate can cause the opening at the back of the nose to narrow, which means the soft-tissue region of the airway is smaller and more likely to collapse. Palmer points out that skulls from eras where children were universally breastfed rarely have small nasal apertures and conjectures that OSA may not have existed prior to the invention of artificial nipples. While the breast tissue is soft and shapes itself to the baby's mouth, bottle teats and pacifiers are firmer and require the mouth to adjust. Equally, the effort required for an infant to express milk from the breast gives the muscles of the face a workout, promoting the development of good muscle tone and ensuring nasal breathing. This cannot be replicated by an artificial teat.[52]

Tongue-tie may also contribute to the enlargement of the tonsils that is so prevalent in OSA.[53] The restrictive tissues can lead to mouth breathing, which increases upper airway resistance and causes inflammation to the back of the throat. Swollen adenoids and tonsils further obstruct the air-flow, exacerbate the need to breathe through the mouth, and contribute to abnormal oral-facial growth. Tongue-tie, left untreated, can therefore lead to SDB and OSA.

A tongue-tie in a newborn should be clipped to facilitate the necessary movement of the tongue during breastfeeding. I remember hearing a speaker at a sleep conference explain that sixteenth-century French midwives grew one fingernail extra long so they could use it to cut the tongue-ties of new-born babies. By today's standards, this may sound grotesque, but at a time when formula feeding was not an option, it may have saved the lives of those children.

*If you suspect that your child has a short lingual frenulum, seek advice from a healthcare professional or myofunctional therapist trained in identifying tongue-tie. You can find a specialist in your area by visiting AomtInfo.org.*

## DEVELOPMENT OF POSTURE, SPEECH, AND LANGUAGE

Mouth breathing in children also has impacts on speech, auditory process-ing, and postural development. In a 2011 study of the effect of chronic nasal obstruction on speech in children aged between 4 and 12 years, it was found that 76.6% of children with nasal blockages suffered dysphonia—problems speaking due to anatomical disorders in the throat, mouth, tongue, or vocal cords.[54] More than 68% of the children with blocked noses demonstrated vocal abuse, a behavioral condition that causes strain to the vocal cords.

A 2013 paper that explored the correlation between oral breathing and speech disorders in children found that mouth breathing could affect socialization, academic performance, and the development of speech.[55] Researchers underlined that early detection of mouth breathing is essential to reduce or prevent its harmful effects on development. Changes in posture, mobility, and muscle tone of the lips, cheeks, and tongue, when a child habitually mouth breathes, lead to a loss of efficiency in basic functions like swallowing, chewing, and speaking. This can encourage the development of flaccid jaw muscles, poor head posture, and speech disorders, including lisps and the inability to pronounce specific sounds. Children who mouth breathe may also have underdeveloped auditory processing.

In 2014, scientists undertook a first-of-its-kind study looking at speech difficulties in children who had swollen adenoids and found a connection between adenoid hypertrophy and articulation errors during speech.[56] The study compared 19 children with adenoid hypertrophy to a control group of 33 children with functional articulation disorders but no physical symptoms. The mean age of the subject group was higher than that of the control group because the incidence of adenoid hypertrophy in children generally increases with age.

They found that the kind of speech errors made by children with swollen adenoids were not the same as those present in children with speech disorders. Children with enlarged adenoids were more likely to substitute one sound for another and less likely to drop sounds, reflecting the fact that swollen adenoids, rather than the children's understanding of phonetics and language, were the cause of defects in speech. The sound "s" was particularly affected in these children. This sound requires a specific placement of the tongue, but children with swollen adenoids have reduced airway space and tend to drop their lower jaw and tongue to maximize their oral airway. As we've already seen, this affects the development of the face and leads to poorly aligned teeth and jaws.

It is also believed that enlarged adenoids can lead to changes in voice quality. The children in the study were found to have frequent nasalization. This is consistent with previous research that found adenoid hypertrophy could lead to hypernasal speech, alter the resonance characteristics of the airways, and cause changes in the dimensions of the vocal tract that can manifest as roughness in the voice.

Mouth breathing and SDB breathing in children has also been found to impact auditory processing—the ability to understand speech, distinguish sounds from one another, concentrate against background noise, and enjoy music.[57] Scientists in Brazil found that children with mouth breathing and OSA, as determined by polysomnography, displayed levels of auditory processing that were statistically significant when compared with children who had no airway problems.[58] The children with OSA performed less well in tests to determine auditory processing and nonverbal sequence memory.

We have already explored the impact of mouth breathing on the development of the face, jaws, and teeth. However, the problem extends further. Children with narrow or blocked airways tend to mouth breathe by default, and so they adjust the position of their head to get enough air in through their mouths. Information on the connection between mouth breathing and changes in posture in children is limited, but one 2018 study of children explains that problems in the positioning of the shoulders, including the shoulder blades and trapezius muscles, can occur in children who mouth breathe.[59]

While much research has focused on the position of the head, not looking any further down the spine, the fact is, the forward positioning of the head, which is necessary to draw air orally into the lower respiratory tract, will lead to further postural adaptations that can impact the whole body. Forward head posture requires the child to extend the upper cervical spine and flex the lower cervical and thoracic spine, leading to curvature in the lumbar spine. Over time, this causes muscle strain that pulls the lower jaw back, decreasing the airway even more.

The 2018 study recorded a significant reduction in forward head position and poor shoulder posture after adenotonsillectomy.[59] It would be interesting to see the results of a study that made the same comparison following upper airway development and nasal breathing training; it seems likely they would be similar and perhaps more sustainable.

## ADVICE TO PARENTS OF CHILDREN AND TEENAGERS

It is important to monitor your child for signs of mouth breathing. Take the opportunity to observe the breathing when your child is concentrating on homework, watching TV, or sleeping. It can be helpful to monitor the breathing of younger children after they have eaten, particularly if you suspect specific foods such as dairy or wheat may be triggering overbreathing.

Avoid overdressing your child, and keep your house cool and well ventilated. Encourage your child to play outside and to breathe through their nose as much as possible during physically active play. Notice if your child maintains an open mouth posture for significant periods. If the mouth is open for 40% of the time or more, you must act. If your child's nose is blocked, try using the exercise to decongest the nose. (You will find this exercise in Chapter Two.)

Look at the following list of questions. If your answer to any of these is "yes," your child might be displaying the harmful effects of SDB:

- Do you notice your child breathing through an open mouth?
- Does your child wake up with tangled sheets in the morning after a night of twisting and turning during sleep?
- Does your child hold his or her breath during sleep?
- Does your child have a stuffy nose on waking, or complain about his or her mouth being dry?
- Do you hear your child snoring?
- Does your child experience disrupted sleep?
- Does your child have nightmares, wet the bed during sleep, or wake up needing to use the bathroom?
- Is your child's breathing audible during sleep?
- Is your child tired on waking, or fatigued and struggling to concentrate during the day?

We have looked in detail at the many factors that lead to breathing pattern disorders. Nasal breathing not only prevents and relieves the many symptoms related to breathing pattern disorders and SDB but is also essential to the correct development of the jaws and face. The foundation of breathing reeducation for children and teenagers is restoring full-time nasal breathing with the lips closed, jaws relaxed, and tongue in the correct resting posture, both during wakefulness and sleep.

As the many studies have shown, the growth of the face and airways in childhood is often directly related to the way a child breathes. Enlarged adenoids or any other restriction of the airways causes the child to switch to mouth breathing because of the difficulty in getting enough air through the nose. While it may seem counterintuitive, this only exacerbates the nasal obstruction. Further, it causes poor development of the airways and can result in lifelong issues with breathing.

## MOTIVATING CHILDREN

In helping children and young people change their breathing habits, they need to understand the importance of breathing through the nose. When I work with young people, I ask them which reasons they consider to be the most important when it comes to breathing nasally. The most popular replies tend to focus around athletic performance and the development of a good-looking face. I find it best not to highlight the negative features of mouth breathing when talking to children. Instead, I find they respond well to hearing about the many benefits of nasal breathing. The following ideas may be helpful.

**Nasal breathing makes you more intelligent:** Explain to your child that intelligent people breathe in and out through their noses. Nasal breathing improves cognition, concentration, alertness, and energy levels because it promotes better sleep and delivers more oxygen to the brain. This helps your child focus better in class so learning will be easier and more enjoyable.

**Nasal breathing improves sports performance:** When children habitually mouth breathe, they tend to quickly become breathless during sports or physical exercise. This might make them reluctant to take part in healthy activities they would otherwise enjoy. Professional athletes, Olympians, Special Forces, and military personnel all use breathing techniques from the Oxygen Advantage to improve their performance during training.

**Mouth breathing causes crooked teeth and bad breath:** No teenager wants to have bad breath. Nasal breathing helps maintain a healthy mouth and prevents smelly breath.[3, 60] It can also avert problems in the development of the face, such as narrow jaws, crooked, overcrowded teeth, and small upper airways.

**Breathing through the nose helps you sleep better and gives you more energy:** Mouth breathing interferes with a good night's sleep, and you will have less energy to enjoy life. Also, children who sleep poorly are 10 times more likely to develop learning difficulties.[3]

**Mouth breathing is bad for posture:** Persistent mouth breathing during early childhood can lead to changes in posture as the head is thrust forward to optimize the oral airway. This, along with a tendency to breathe into the upper chest, will have a knock-on effect on the stability of the spine. These things may not be particularly motivating for children, but parents will understand their importance.

**Nasal breathing leads to good table manners:** If your child has a blocked nose, he or she may have difficulty eating. Nasal congestion makes it tricky to coordinate breathing and swallowing, so the child may need to stop chewing or chew faster to breathe through the mouth. This breathlessness may look like bad table manners as the child sniffs and gulps his way through each meal.[61]

In all cases, the best place to start is by encouraging nasal breathing both day and night. Children under five years of age may find it difficult to practice breathing exercises, so parents of young children must take preventive action to avoid the factors that contribute to overbreathing. Children tend to mirror their parents, even in their breathing habits. If you tend to walk around the house with your mouth open, puffing and panting, not paying attention to your breathing, your child will do the same. Equally, a child will struggle to learn if everybody else in the house continues with their own bad habits. I often see the behavior of parents interfering with the progress of their children in this way. You need to lead by example. Only then can you ensure success with breathing reeducation. Luckily, this is a win-win situation because everybody involved will enjoy the benefits.

Help your child understand what "breathing too much" means and that overbreathing is what causes tiredness, wheezing, coughing, and a stuffy nose. The best way to do this is by giving a physical demonstration. Ask the child to hold out a finger and blow a large puff of air onto their finger. Let them feel the strength and quantity of air on their finger. Explain that this is "big breathing." Then ask the child to blow a tiny amount of air onto their finger. This should be so light they can hardly feel it at all. Explain that this is correct breathing.

You can also ask your child to explain the ideas behind good breathing to other people in your household. This will allow your child time to reflect on his or her breathing. By listening to the storytelling and description your child gives, you will be able to tell how well the theory has been understood.

*If you are concerned about your child's breathing and want to explore maxillary expansion, there are healthcare professionals who can assist with gently widening the palate even in very young children. I would advise looking for a myofunctional therapist or specialist pediatric dentist. Contact AomtInfo.org to find a practitioner near you.*

## CHAPTER NINE
# THE BREATHING SECRET FOR HEALTHY BLOOD PRESSURE

---

Globally, 1.13 billion people are thought to suffer with hypertension, the majority living in low- and middle-income countries. In America in 2020, around 108 million people, or 45% of the adult population, have high blood pressure[1] and fewer than one in five sufferers have the problem under control.[2] The risk is higher for those who have reached retirement age. Under new guidelines published in 2017, nearly 80% of Americans aged 65 and older qualify as high risk for blood pressure.[3] In the United Kingdom, 2020 figures show that one in three adults have the condition, rising to one in two in people over 65—that's around 16 million people in total.[4]

High blood pressure is a problem that can affect anyone, regardless of income, race, gender, or age. The risk increases as you get older, with certain lifestyle choices, and if you have a genetic predisposition to hypertension. But whether or not you are likely to develop the condition often depends upon the health of your heart. The good news is that it is actually fairly straightforward to ensure that your heart stays healthy, simply by eating a sensible diet, maintaining a moderate exercise regime, and learning to breathe correctly.

## THE HEART AND HIGH BLOOD PRESSURE

The heart is the organ responsible for pumping blood around the body through the blood vessels. It operates all day, every day, beating approximately 109,000 times every 24 hours.[5] It pumps deoxygenated blood to the lungs where it can be replenished with oxygen, and it circulates oxygenated blood back around the body, supplying the brain, muscles, organs, and every cell with oxygen. In other words, the primary role of the heart is to distribute the oxygen brought into the lungs during inhalation, and to bring carbon dioxide back to the lungs where the excess can be breathed out.

As the heart pumps, blood pushes against the walls of the arteries, creating pressure. Like many of the body's homeostatic systems, this pressure is in constant flux. It is regulated by the movement-sensitive nerve endings called baroreceptors (which we read about in Chapter Four). Problems with blood pressure occur if the pressure rises and remains too high over a sustained period of time. This can damage the body in many ways, leading to heart failure, stroke, kidney disease, and a number of other health problems.[6]

High blood pressure is the buildup of pressure caused by a restriction to blood flow. Picture the scene: On a beautiful sunny day, you decide to water the flowers in the front garden. You attach the hose to the tap and turn it on halfway to provide enough water flow to spray the flowers with a fine mist. All is going well until your absent-minded neighbor unknowingly parks his car with a tire pressing firmly down on the hose. In an instant, the blockage reduces the flow to a trickle, while water pressure increases inside the hose.

The blood vessels work in a similar way. When arterial blood vessels are dilated, wide and relaxed, blood flows easily, circulation is good, and blood pressure is normal. However, when arteries are constricted due to age-related hardening or a buildup of fatty deposits along their inner walls, flow becomes restricted, and pressure begins to rise.

The main function of the heart is to pump blood back and forth from the lungs, around the body. When the blood vessels are restricted, the heart will increase the blood pressure to keep the blood moving, much as you might turn up the garden tap when the water coming out of the hose dries to a trickle. While this extra pressure may temporarily provide the body with an adequate blood flow, it puts extra strain on both heart and blood vessels, which over time is damaging. If the blood vessels remain constricted, circulation gradually gets worse, and blood pressure continues to rise.

Normal blood circulation is vital to health. The blood carries oxygen to everywhere it is needed, so if circulation is cut off to any part of the body, that area will become starved of oxygen. The sensation of pins and needles you might get if you sit with your legs crossed for too long is a mild example of what happens when blood flow becomes constricted. In the case of a "dead" leg, a few stretches and a short walk will quickly restore circulation, but when blood vessels are restricted on a long-term basis, the reduced blood flow will have a detrimental effect on the heart and brain. Ultimately, when circulation to any part of the heart is cut off, the lack of oxygen causes cells in the heart to die, and this can result in a heart attack. If there is insufficient blood flow to the brain so it gets too little oxygen, you may suffer a stroke.

Hypertension occurs when the heart is pushed to beat faster or more forcefully than it should. This can happen when the body contains a greater volume of blood than normal, when the arteries become too narrow, or when blood vessels harden and lose some of their elasticity. While genetic predisposition is a risk factor, a family history of high blood pressure is not definitive. In fact, understanding your inherited potential for hypertension can empower you to take the steps to avoid developing it.

Many lifestyle choices that promote healthy blood pressure are well within your control. These include:

- Eating a nutritious, healthy diet
- Avoiding foods known to increase blood pressure
- Taking adequate exercise
- Quitting smoking
- Addressing snoring and sleep apnea
- Managing stress
- Practicing slow breathing

Even with a family history of hypertension, the exercises in this book can help you avoid high blood pressure, often without the need for medication.

## MEASURING BLOOD PRESSURE

Blood pressure is typically recorded as two measurements: systolic and diastolic pressure. Systolic pressure, the higher of the two numbers, refers to the pressure of the blood when the heart is actively pumping blood. Diastolic, the lower figure, measures blood pressure between heartbeats when the heart is at rest. Blood pressure measurements are presented with the systolic number above or before the diastolic number, for example: 120/80 mmHg. The mmHg refers to millimeters of mercury, the units used to measure pressure.

When your blood pressure is taken, a healthcare professional places an inflatable cuff on your upper arm. Air is pumped into the cuff to increase the pressure around the arm. As the cuff becomes tighter, the pressure becomes sufficient to temporarily collapse the artery and restrict blood flow. The doctor or nurse then places a stethoscope on the artery and gently releases the pressure from the cuff, listening attentively for signs of blood flow while observing pressure levels. When the first pulse of blood flows back through the artery, the reading is noted. This is the systolic pressure.

The cuff is then gently released, and the sound and pressure of the blood flow is carefully monitored. At first, as blood begins to flow, it makes a turbulent noise, because the artery is still partially constricted. The diastolic reading is taken at the first moment the blood begins to flow effortlessly, without restriction.

One of the most confusing things about hypertension is that there may be no warning signs or symptoms until blood pressure reaches 180/110, yet once the condition has developed, it can last a lifetime. Unless your blood pressure is checked, you may not even know that it is high. When symptoms are present, they can include a persistent headache, blurred or double vision, memory loss, low libido, dizziness, nose bleeds, palpitations, nausea, vomiting, and shortness of breath.

The following table summarizes normal blood pressure levels for adults. It also shows which measurements put you at greater risk for health problems.

### Categories of blood pressure levels in adults, measured in mmHg

| Category | Systolic Pressure (First number) | And/ Or | Diastolic Pressure (Second number) |
|---|---|---|---|
| Normal | Less than 120 | And | Less than 80 |
| Prehypertension | 120–129 | And | Less than 80 |
| Stage 1 high blood pressure | 130–139 | And/ Or | 80–89 |
| Stage 2 high blood pressure | 140 or higher | And/ Or | 90 or higher |

*Blood pressure chart: what your reading means—MayoClinic.org*

If you are told that your blood pressure is 120 over 80 (120/80 mmHg), it means that you have a systolic pressure of 120 mmHg and a diastolic pressure of 80 mmHg. Hypertension is defined as blood pressure that is 140/90 or more for a sustained period.

## TAKING YOUR OWN BLOOD PRESSURE READINGS

Nowadays, anyone can measure their own blood pressure by purchasing a good quality blood pressure monitor or using a blood pressure cuff with a smartphone. Some people may find this provides more accurate measurements as they feel more relaxed at home than at the doctor's office. If you want to take your own blood pressure measurements, follow these simple steps:

- **Sit quietly** for a few minutes with your back supported and your feet resting on the floor. Roll up your sleeve and rest your arm on a table or armrest so that your elbow is at the same level as your heart.
- **Secure the blood pressure cuff over the bare skin of your upper arm and measure your blood pressure according to instructions.** After the first reading, leave the cuff in place. Take a break of one minute, then take a second reading. If the two readings are close, work out the average, and take that as your measurement. If not, take a third reading, and find the average of the three.
- **Repeat the procedure for the other arm.** It may sound odd, but it is useful to check the readings from both arms for consistency. Readings that differ by more than 10 points between the left and right arm may signify a buildup of fatty deposits in the arteries.[7]

To improve the accuracy of self-monitoring, it is important to bear in mind the following guidelines:

1. **Measure consistently:** Blood pressure fluctuates throughout the day, so try to measure around the same time each day. To assess accuracy, take two or three readings in a row and record the average. Do this at least once a month.
2. **Avoid coffee:** It's best not to drink coffee for at least two hours before measuring, as caffeine can cause a temporary but dramatic increase in blood pressure.
3. **Wait 30 minutes after exercise:** Vigorous exercise can temporarily increase blood pressure, so it's best not to take a measurement immediately after physical activity.

## BREATHING FOR LOWER BLOOD PRESSURE

The relationship between breathing and blood pressure was first documented in the 1930s in a handbook for physicians, *The Cure of High Blood Pressure by Respiratory Exercises*.[8] Since then, the fact that regular practice of slow breathing can help lower blood pressure has been widely acknowledged in medical literature.

Recent studies include a 2006 paper that compared the effects of mental relaxation and slow breathing on high blood pressure.[9] Researchers examined 100 participants during practice of 10 minutes mental relaxation and 10 minutes slow breathing. They concluded that slow breathing activated the parasympathetic response and resulted in a fall in systolic blood pressure, diastolic blood pressure, heart rate, and respiratory rate. In this study, slow breathing performed better than relaxation, causing a significantly greater reduction in heart rate and blood pressure.

Regular slow breathing practice also produces long-term benefits for blood pressure, as demonstrated in a 2009 study.[10] Sixty subjects aged between 20 and 60 years practiced slow breathing for three months. They showed improvements in both sympathetic and parasympathetic reactivity, which researchers deemed to be favorable for patients with high blood pressure.[10]

Research into the effects of mental relaxation and slow breathing exercises on patients with high blood pressure has repeatedly proven that these techniques successfully activate the parasympathetic response. The calming physical reaction reduces blood pressure, heart rate, and respiratory rate.

The value of practicing reduced breathing exercises and relaxation is reinforced by the fact that people with high blood pressure tend to have a stronger than normal response to stress. One study reported greater impacts from stress on people who already had high blood pressure. Scientists tested 115 people with a series of challenging activities such as mental arithmetic, thinking unpleasant thoughts, staring at a fixed point, and catching a dropped object. Participants who had high blood pressure at the start of the experiment experienced significantly higher respiratory rate, systolic blood pressure, and diastolic blood pressure in reaction to the exercises than those with normal blood pressure.[9]

There is no denying that stress is a significant trigger for increasing blood pressure or that people with high blood pressure are likely to have a stronger reaction to stressful events. However, what is less commonly understood is the potential value of light, slow, and deep breathing exercises for people with hypertension and how these exercises work to lower blood pressure, alleviate stress, and avert further health complications over both the short and long term.

Breathing reeducation is vital in the management of OSA, a condition closely linked with hypertension. Both OSA and hypertension are common and occur more frequently in older people. According to a 2020 paper, around 50% of OSA patients have high blood pressure, and between 30% and 40% of hypertensive patients have OSA, though their sleep disorder is often undiagnosed.[11] Nonobese OSA patients have a less responsive heart rate (low heart rate variability) and higher blood pressure, even in a resting state of wakefulness and in the absence of any heart problems. In terms of the impact of OSA on chronic stress, researchers cite a 2001 study, which demonstrates that hypoxia (where the body is starved of oxygen, as it is during apneas) induces prolonged activation of the nervous system's stress response.[12]

Interestingly, the activity of the sensors that regulate blood pressure changes with the different sleep-wake cycles.[13] The function of the baroreflex during sleep is state-dependent. The scientists suggest that baroreflex sensitivity increases slightly during light non-REM sleep, and there is a marked enhancement during deep non-REM sleep, the stage of dreamless, restorative sleep vital to well-being. A clear impairment of baroreflex control during non-REM sleep has been documented in patients with OSA and high blood pressure. It is thought that reduced baroreflex sensitivity along with a heightened sensitivity to blood $CO_2$ may amplify the sympathetic stress response to apneas, increase activation of the sympathetic nervous system during wakefulness, and create the conditions for daytime hypertension. Heightened sympathetic nerve activity is common in patients with OSA, and it also plays a major part in the development of treatment-resistant hypertension.

Since both OSA and hypertension are so common, they can often coexist independently of each other or, in medical terms, "comorbidly." Because high blood pressure is not always the result of OSA, traditional treatments for OSA may not alleviate hypertension. However, whether the two conditions exist side-by-side or one causes the other, both problems can be helped with the practice of light, slow, and deep breathing.

There has been research into blood pressure and using inspiratory muscle training devices and whether the benefits of slow breathing are enhanced by the adding an inspiratory load.[14] In a 2010 study, 30 patients with Stage I or II essential hypertension were divided into three groups. The first group practiced slow diaphragm breathing twice a day for eight weeks; the second practiced the same exercise using a loaded breathing device; the third group, a control, continued with normal activities. It is not recorded whether breathing in the second group was nasal or oral. The purpose of the breathing device, which in this experiment was loaded with 20 cm $H_2O$ (water), was to strengthen the breathing muscles in the same way that adding a load increases muscular strength in weight lifting. Because breathing muscles are largely passive on exhalation, this device works to strengthen the muscles used to inhale. (The SportsMask has the same purpose.) Resting heart rate and blood pressure were measured before and after the respiratory training period.

The results showed that both systolic and diastolic blood pressure decreased significantly with slow breathing exercises. Diastolic pressure decreased by 7 mmHg and systolic by 13.5 mmHg. With the inspiratory muscle loading devices, the reductions were even more marked. The improvement in systolic blood pressure was 5.3 mmHg more than it was with just slow breathing. Heart rate dropped by eight beats per minute with slow breathing and nine beats per minute with load-added breathing.

In a 2019 trial, 20 patients with isolated systolic hypertension (ISH)—a condition where the diastolic reading is normal, but the systolic reading is high—undertook a similar eight-week breath training program. In this new study, patients were asked to complete 60 breaths every day at a respiratory rate of 6 breaths per minute and at 25% of their maximal inspiratory pressure.[15] *Maximal inspiratory pressure* (MIP) is the most commonly used measure to evaluate inspiratory muscle strength.[16] Readings were taken of blood pressure and the response of patients' heart rates to static hand-grip and dynamic arm-cranking exercises.

At the end of the eight weeks, systolic blood pressure had dropped by 22 mmHg, diastolic blood pressure by 9 mmHg, and heart rate by 12 beats per minute. Sizable reductions in blood pressure and heart rate were also seen following the hand-grip and arm exercises. The loaded breathing exercises at six breaths per minute reduced blood pressure and improved the body's ability to manage both static and dynamic exercise in all participants.

Researchers concluded that this could reduce the negative impact of exercise for patients with high blood pressure, supporting the health of the heart.[15] In this experiment, the loaded breathing group was compared against a control group who practiced slow, deep breathing without the load. Blood pressure and heart rate were also lower in the control group after the trial, but as with the previous study, the differences were much less marked.

One noteworthy aspect of both of those studies is that the loaded breathing device required the patient to mouth breathe. A 2019 review published in *Frontiers in Physiology* studied the effect of adding inspiratory loads using both nasal and oral breathing.[17] Loaded breathing resulted in increased tidal volume. Nasal breathing promoted greater lung volume and inspiratory muscle activation compared with oral breathing. Resistance from nasal breathing is higher because the nostrils are so much smaller than the mouth, so much greater energy and muscle recruitment is necessary to generate the inhalation. The authors considered the effects of nasal breathing better for the respiratory system[17]. But what is really interesting is the suggestion that nasal breathing effectively adds a natural load to breathing. This means that slow breathing exercises carried out through the nose will have a positive impact on resting blood pressure without the need for special load-adding equipment.

In regard to the spikes in blood pressure experienced during intense exercise, the results of a 1990 study are relevant.[18] Scientists examined the effect of nasal breathing on systolic blood pressure in 10 healthy men during exercise. In this experiment, the participants wore nasal dilators, which increased nasal airflow by around 29%. With these dilators, all 10 men could cycle at maximum load without mouth breathing and with a much smaller increase in systolic blood pressure than normal. The reason for this moderation in blood pressure is not known, but researchers put forward the theory that facilitated nose breathing decreased respiratory work, relieving the load on the heart, which, in turn, lowered the systolic blood pressure during exercise.[18]

## DENISE'S STORY: A PROGRAM FOR CHANGE

Denise is in her fifties and lives in California. When I first met her, she had already spent 12 years suffering from constant fatigue, muscle pain, anxiety, brain fog, and high blood pressure. She experienced a range of symptoms including dizziness, constriction around the chest, and the feeling of never getting enough air.

Denise was worn down by her ill health and had little zest for life. In her search for help, she had spent thousands of dollars visiting many doctors, specialists, and other healthcare professionals. Recently, her chiropractor had suggested that she may have chronic hyperventilation. Shortly into my first Skype session with Denise, it was evident just how noticeable her breathing was. While sitting comfortably for 15 minutes, Denise displayed a fast breathing rate with each larger-than-normal breath. She was breathing from the upper chest, and I could hear each sharp intake of air as she spoke. Denise didn't suffer from asthma or any respiratory condition, yet her breathing during rest was as noticeable as that of any person with uncontrolled asthma I have seen. When she mentioned that this all started 12 years earlier, I suggested that she must have suffered from significant stress at that time. She replied, "Yes, I had a huge amount of stress."

Undoubtedly, the stress Denise experienced 12 years earlier had activated her sympathetic nervous system, resulting in a large increase in the volume of air she was taking into her body. Over weeks and months, her brain became accustomed to this larger volume of breathing and it became habitual. This contributed to the negative effects that were impacting Denise's quality of life, including chronic stress, high blood pressure, fatigue, and general ill health.

Denise's starting BOLT score was only 5 seconds. Given such a low measurement, I started her off with the *Breathing Recovery* while sitting exercise (see Chapter Two). This involved her holding her breath for up to 5 seconds after exhaling, breathing normally for 10 seconds, and then repeating. She was to continue this pattern for about 5 minutes before taking a rest.

The reason I asked Denise to practice this exercise first is that when the BOLT score is less than 10 seconds it can be challenging to maintain a tolerable air hunger during the reduced breathing exercise. This can add tension and stress to the experience, which is not necessary and can be avoided by beginning the practice very gently.

For the first week, Denise's program was as follows:

- Practice *Breathing Recovery* for 5 minutes every hour.
- Practice *Breathing Recovery* for 10 minutes before sleep.
- Breathe only through the nose at all times.

- If Denise sighed, she was to hold her breath for 5 to 10 seconds following the sigh.
- Tape her mouth at night using MyoTape or 3M Micropore tape.
- Avoid taking large breaths before speaking.

One week later, Denise's BOLT score had increased to 10 seconds, and she was already feeling much more in control of her breathing. She no longer felt that she was not getting enough air while at rest.

In weeks two and three, Denise began gentle, light, slow, deep breathing and relaxation. She downloaded some recorded relaxation exercises and played them twice daily, once before bed and again when she woke in the morning. By practicing relaxation to gently lower breathing volume toward normal, it is possible to begin the process of reversing years of stress. Denise also practiced gentle, light, slow, deep breathing for 10 minutes every hour to continue her progress throughout the day.

If you have high blood pressure, it's important to go slowly and gently when practicing reduced breathing exercises so as not to put added pressure on your body. Practicing light, slow, deep breathing stimulates the baroreceptors and activates the parasympathetic nervous system, bringing you into a relaxed state. Your BOLT score will increase each week as you continue to practice. This will help lower your blood pressure, making you less reliant on medication. If you are currently taking medication to control high blood pressure, it's important to consult a medical professional when your BOLT score reaches 20 seconds so that your medication can be adjusted to suit your current condition.

Over several months, Denise's high blood pressure and cholesterol both normalized, and she reported much higher energy levels. She also felt calmer than she had for many years. Her BOLT score increased to 28 seconds, which, considering it was only 5 seconds when she began, is remarkable. Denise's health improved, and her doctor altered her medication based on her progress.

Denise's ongoing routine is as follows:

- She practices 10 minutes of light, slow, and deep breathing exercises four times each day, with one session just before bed and one just after waking.
- She tapes her mouth closed during sleep to ensure nasal breathing at night.

- She practices *Breathing Recovery* whenever she feels anxious or stressed.
- She walks, with her mouth closed, for half an hour daily.
- She observes her breathing periodically throughout the day and avoids taking big breaths through her mouth.

The benefits of slow breathing and relaxation are twofold: the baroreceptors become more responsive to changes in blood pressure, and the BOLT score increases. The reason Denise's BOLT score improved so noticeably was that her sensitivity to blood $CO_2$ had decreased. There is an inverse relationship between sensitivity to $CO_2$ and the sensitivity of the baroreceptors[19]—those movement-sensitive nerve endings that work to regulate blood pressure. When the sensitivity to $CO_2$ is lower, which is the case in healthy breathing, the baroreceptors are stronger and more able to maintain blood pressure at healthy levels.

As we discussed in Chapter Four, there's a link between HRV and the baroreceptors. This means that better HRV leads to better-regulated blood pressure. Low HRV is a feature in adults[20] and children[21] with hypertension. Autonomic dysregulation is present in the early stages of hypertension[20]. Scientists suggest that because HRV provides an important window into the responses of the autonomic nervous system, HRV biofeedback may be valuable in treating hypertension.[22] A 2013 study into evidence-based applications for HRV biofeedback suggests that biofeedback could be helpful in strengthening the baroreflex.[23]

# CHAPTER TEN
# FREEDOM FROM RESPIRATORY DISCOMFORT

---

## WHAT IS ASTHMA?

No book on breathing would be complete without a discussion about asthma. But just what is asthma? The word *asthma* is borrowed from the ancient Greek ἄσθμα, âsthma, meaning "laborious breathing,"[1] shortness of breath,[2] or panting."[3] Reference to the condition can be found in ancient Hebrew, Egyptian, and Indian medical writings, and clear observations of patients experiencing asthma attacks exist as early as the second century CE.

The categorization of asthma was refined in the second half of the nineteenth century[2] when English physician Henry Hyde Salter published his book, *On Asthma and Its Treatment*, a volume that one 1985 article describes as "the best book on asthma to appear during the nineteenth century."[4] In this work, Salter, who was himself asthmatic, describes paroxysmal breathlessness of a "peculiar character" with periods of healthy breathing between attacks. This description perfectly captures a disorder in which the airways narrow due to inflammation and contraction of the smooth muscle. By the late nineteenth century, the medical community had accepted the view that asthma was a distinct condition with a clear set of causes and treatment requirements.

The Canadian physician, Sir William Osler, who is sometimes credited as the father of modern medicine, wrote about asthma in his 1892 textbook.[5] He described the symptoms of the disease as:

- Spasming of the bronchial muscles
- Swelling and inflammation in the airways
- Having distinctive, gelatinous mucus secretions
- Resembling hay fever, and being sensitive to atmosphere, climate, and allergens

- Running in families, often beginning in childhood and lasting a lifetime
- Sometimes triggered by fright, strong emotion, overeating, or particular foods

Asthma was treated predominantly by managing exacerbations with the use of bronchodilators taken in the form of oral inhalers. Over-reliance on this medication was believed to be a contributing factor in various epidemics of asthma death in the United States, United Kingdom, and Australia in the 1960s, and in New Zealand in the mid 1980s.[2] These deaths drew attention to shortfalls in asthma treatment and emphasized the extent to which asthma was still not clearly understood.

By the 1980s, doctors had more knowledge about the role of allergen exposure as an asthma trigger. However, although the primary characteristic of asthma—blocked or narrow airways—was well recognized and easy to diagnose, the causal mechanisms were still not fully understood.

While current thought questions whether inflammation is the root cause of asthma, it is certainly a factor in the disease. In *eosinophilic asthma*, inflammation occurs as part of an allergic or immune system reaction, which causes specific white blood cells called eosinophils to be released. An increase in white blood cells typically leads to an inflammatory response, causing the airways to thicken. The resulting fluid and mucus may result in bronchospasm and asthma symptoms.[6]

## THE CONGESTION CONNECTION

The nose and lungs form a single, unified airway. This means that where inflammation is present, it can travel from the nose to the lungs and from the lungs to the nose.[7] This is one reason people with asthma experience high levels of nasal congestion. The normal response to a stuffy nose is to begin breathing through the mouth. This, however, increases breathing volume, draws cold, unfiltered, dry air into the airways, and makes the symptoms of asthma worse. Habitual mouth breathing also affects sleep and causes or contributes to stress.

People with asthma often don't realize how much the condition can impact their overall health, but asthma can lead to fatigue, poor concentration, and anxiety. As you'll read in the next chapter, it can also have an enormous effect on things we would otherwise take for granted, such as the ability to enjoy a healthy sex life. As with other respiratory conditions and underlying breathing pattern disorders, when breathing is affected, so is the body and the mind.

For any child or adult with asthma, the switch to nose breathing and the practice of breathing exercises to normalize breathing volume can be life changing. When I work with a client, I expect their asthma symptoms to decrease by 50% in just two weeks. There will also be notable improvements in their sleep patterns, ability to focus, concentration, and levels of stress.

The airways of people with asthma are particularly prone to narrowing. This is due to a combination of factors including inflammation, increased mucus secretion, and constriction of the smooth muscle surrounding the airways. When the airways narrow, a feeling of breathlessness occurs. As the body tries to compensate for the lack of air, breathing becomes faster, and the volume of inhaled air increases. The sensation of air hunger may encourage the switch from nasal to oral breathing.

Normal breathing volume for a healthy adult is now between five and eight liters per minute.[8] This volume has actually increased. Twenty years ago, normal minute ventilation was between four and six liters, with six liters considered the upper limit. A minute volume of eight liters per minute implies a breathing rate of 16 breaths per minute, which is too fast. In my opinion, eight liters is an unhealthy minute volume, and it makes me wonder, has modern living changed our breathing patterns so much that it is now normal to overbreathe?

In contrast, in people with asthma, resting ventilation is typically between 10 and 15 liters per minute.[9-11] While it is common for the narrowing of the airways to cause breathing volume to rise, breathing too much air will itself cause the airways to narrow. Thus, overbreathing can easily become a vicious cycle.

The negative impact of overbreathing on compromised lungs is underlined in a paper published in the *Annals of the American Thoracic Society* in 2020. According to it, a body of research demonstrates the importance of low tidal volumes when ventilating patients whose lungs have been damaged by the COVID-19 virus. Scientist have found that, when lungs have been injured by infection and the patient has suffered acute respiratory distress syndrome

(ARDS) and respiratory failure, the injury can be compounded "if the size of the breath provided by the ventilator is too large or the pressure used to inflate the lung is too great."[12, 13] These patients must be treated with smaller breath sizes to prevent additional damage. However, this makes the sensation of air hunger much worse. Prolonged air hunger can cause feelings of anxiety and fear, and the paper points out that acute air hunger has been used as a very effective form of torture. In this extreme case, to avoid both damage to the lungs and psychological distress, researchers urge the use of opiates to treat the resulting breathlessness and sedatives to moderate feelings of anxiety.

More generally, a substantial 2016 study in *Allergy* demonstrated that mouth breathing was associated with the worsening of asthma. Even participants who did not have asthma experienced poorer lower lung function and more sensitivity to house dust mites when they mouth breathed. Researchers examined questionnaires completed by 9,804 people from Nagahama City in Japan and found that mouth breathing causes asthma to become more severe, possibly by increasing vulnerability to inhaled allergens. Scientists concluded, "The risk of mouth breathing should be well recognized in subjects with allergic rhinitis and in the general population."[14] A separate study found that habitual mouth breathing reduced lung function in people with mild asthma and exacerbated the symptoms of acute asthma.[15]

A diagnosis of poor lung function should be cause for concern, prompting better self-care, and positive action. In a trial lasting 30 years, scientists from the University at Buffalo found that men with the poorest lung function at the start of the study were over twice as likely to have died by the follow-up than men with good lung function. Women with the worst lung function were one-and-a-half times more likely to have died than their healthy counterparts.[16] In an interview for *Science News*, Holger Schünemann, lead author on the study said, "This observation suggests that those with lower lung function levels may need to pay particular attention to avoid negative effects, such as smoking, on their lungs."[17]

The term *dysfunctional breathing* describes abnormalities in breathing patterns that span a range of extremes from fast, superficial breathing to slow, overly deep breathing. A person with hyperventilation syndrome may breathe into the upper chest 18 to 40 times a minute. While the term *hyperventilation* is often used interchangeably with *dysfunctional breathing*, a slow breathing rate of 5 to 8 breaths with breathing that engages the diaphragm and the whole chest is also unhealthy. Both patterns result in an excessive volume of air entering the lungs each minute and may cause frequent sighing as the body tries to compensate for overinflated lungs and high tidal volume.

While disordered breathing is widely recognized, it is ill-defined and often coexists with asthma. One 2017 study, which used the *Nijmegen Questionnaire* (NQ), the preferred tool to screen for hyperventilation syndrome, estimated that 25% of studied patients with severe asthma also displayed dysfunctional breathing.[18] Given what we know about the accuracy of dysfunctional breathing screening, it is likely that the actual figure is higher.

Standard asthma drugs target bronchoconstriction, airway inflammation, and possible comorbidities (conditions that exist alongside asthma but are not necessarily the result of it). Nonpharmacological asthma treatments focus on diet, physical fitness, weight reduction in obese patients, and avoiding triggers. When asthmatics show overt signs of dysfunctional breathing, a program of breathing reeducation may be implemented with a trained physiotherapist.

Physiotherapists use methods including pursed lip, abdominal and cadence breathing. However, even more benefit can be gained when the breathing biochemistry is addressed with the practice of light, nasal breathing. One of the simplest ways to understand the BOLT score is in terms of breathlessness. A lower breath-hold time corresponds with more breathlessness during rest and more airway obstruction. Each five-second increase of the BOLT score reduces asthma symptoms such as exercise-induced asthma, coughing, wheezing, breathlessness, and chest tightness. The BOLT works the same way as a breath-hold measurement called the Control Pause, which is practiced in the Buteyko method—the breathing technique I learned from Dr. Konstantin Buteyko.

Scientists have studied the Buteyko method and its effect on asthma. The first trial of the Buteyko method for asthma in the western world was conducted at the Mater Hospital in Brisbane in 1994.[19] Nineteen people were assigned to learn the Buteyko method, while a 20-person control group followed the hospital's in-house program for asthma. After 12 weeks of practice in nasal and reduced volume breathing, the Buteyko group showed a 70% reduction in symptoms, a 90% drop in their need for rescue medication, and a 49% decrease in their need for inhaled steroid medication. The control group, who were taught physiotherapy exercises, experienced no improvement. The reason for this is likely to be that nasal breathing and reduced volume breathing are not taught during physiotherapy. At the start of the trial, all of the study particiopants breathed 14 liters of air per minute. At the end of the 12 weeks, the Buteyko group had reduced their minute ventilation to 9.6 liters, while the control group had minimal reduction.

Interestingly, end-tidal carbon dioxide ($CO_2$) remained low in both groups. At the beginning of the study, the Buteyko group showed an average of 33 mmHg and the control group 32 mmHg. After 12 weeks, the Buteyko group had slightly increased $CO_2$ to 35 mmHg and the control group to 33 mmHg. Although Dr. Buteyko's original theory regarding asthma revolved around $CO_2$, the science has moved on since his work in the 1950s. While the precise mechanism explaining the beneficial effects in the Buteyko group is not clear, the fact is that over the past 20 years, research into the impact of the Buteyko method on asthma has demonstrated positive results. Now, the *British Medical Journal* states in its physiotherapy guidelines for adults, "The Buteyko breathing technique may be considered to help patients to control the symptoms of asthma."[20]

## EXERCISING WITH ASTHMA

Many elite athletes who suffer from asthma favor swimming above other forms of exercise. This is no coincidence. During swimming, the face is immersed in water, and the weight of the body in the water exerts gentle pressure on the chest and abdomen. Both of these factors naturally restrict breathing volume. Even though the swimmer draws the breath in through the mouth, the amount of air that reaches the lungs per minute is still less than in other sports such as running or cycling. According to a 2018 paper, swimming causes much less post-exercise bronchospasm than running or cycling at the same intensity.[21] This is partly because the air is moist and warm. In an indoor swimming pool, the average air humidity is around 60% and the air temperature around 27° Celsius (80.6° Fahrenheit). Both factors can relieve asthma symptoms. The pressure of water on the chest wall helps with exhalation, and the accumulation of $CO_2$ caused by the controlled breathing necessary during swimming helps relax the airways.[21]

There is, however, a downside to swimming. Too much time spent in chlorinated pools can damage lung tissue,[22-25] a factor particularly problematic for people with asthma. This is important for very young children, especially if they are predisposed to asthma. One longitudinal study of 337 children with asthma and 633 controls (age-matched children without asthma) demonstrated that swimming pool exposure in early life is associated with a significantly higher risk of preschool asthma onset by the age of one year.[26] The 2018 paper found that 21.7% of the asthmatic children reported eye irritation in indoor swimming pools compared with only 9% of the control group, and that 5.5% of children, all of whom were sensitized to at least one inhalant allergen, experienced worse asthma symptoms in indoor pools.

A 2018 *Canadian Respiratory Journal* article found that asthma is highly prevalent among elite endurance athletes.[27] The study aimed to determine how common asthma and the use of asthma medication were in competitive recreational endurance athletes and the association of these factors with training. Researchers examined web survey responses from 38,603 adults who were participating in three Swedish endurance competitions that involved cross-country running, cross-country skiing, and swimming. They found that 12% reported asthma and 23% of those with asthma used inhaled corticosteroids and long-acting beta-agonists daily. Participants who were more likely to suffer from asthma were female, those with allergic rhinitis, a history of eczema, a family history of asthma, and those who cycled or trained for more than 5 hours 50 minutes per week.

The study found that the incidence of asthma among competitive recreational endurance athletes was higher than in the general population. A significant number of the athletes used asthma medications. The study describes a distinct phenotype of asthma specific to elite athletes. "Sports asthma" is defined by "exercise-induced respiratory symptoms and airway hyper-responsiveness without allergic features." This kind of asthma is more common in athletes taking part in water and winter sports.[27] Researchers also found that around 70% of swimmers and skiers suffered with allergic rhinitis.

The athletes in the Swedish study included those at international and high national competitive levels as well as professional and semiprofessional sportspeople who trained for a significant number of hours per week. A high training volume was found to impact asthma more than the age of the athlete, suggesting that training may prevent remission of asthma in adults. Cycling was found to be the sport most closely associated with asthma, regardless of fitness. In fact, a high prevalence of asthma has previously been reported among Olympic cyclists.[28] This may be because cycling requires long training sessions with high-volume breathing. Also, training often takes place outdoors, frequently on roads where the cyclist is exposed to vehicle exhaust fumes, tire particles, and pollen, all of which may contribute to asthma symptoms.

Fortunately, by practicing the breathing exercises described in this book, it becomes possible to continue nasal breathing at a higher intensity of exercise. This reduces mouth breathing, which is one of the primary triggers for exercise-induced asthma.

## SLEEPING WITH ASTHMA

Sleep is often very difficult for asthma sufferers. Asthma symptoms commonly worsen overnight,[29] particularly in the early hours of the morning, and nighttime exacerbations are extremely common. The detrimental effect of poorly controlled asthma on sleep has long been recognized,[30] but in recent years there has been a growing interest in the way asthma interacts with sleep and sleep disorders. People with asthma frequently suffer with sleep disturbance and poor-quality sleep, particularly when asthma is severe. Lack of sleep or impaired sleep quality is linked with worse asthma control. Poor sleep impacts quality of life and can affect physical and mental resilience.

As someone who suffered noticeable asthma symptoms and poor sleep for over 20 years, I am intrigued why such a strong connection exists between asthma severity and sleep-disordered breathing. I believe that if researchers were to investigate uncontrolled asthma during sleep, they might uncover clues for the treatment of sleep apnea.

It is my experience from working with thousands of children and adults with asthma, that people with asthma have a low breath-hold time. In adults, the typical BOLT score is between 10 and 15 seconds, and children with asthma can normally hold their breath for around 20 to 40 paces. This low breath-hold time, which is indicative of high chemosensitivity to $CO_2$, corresponds to a phenotype of sleep apnea called high loop gain. High loop gain results in unstable breathing during sleep, from total stopping of the breath to an exaggerated gasping for air when breathing resumes. The exercises in this book are ideally suited to people with high loop gain and can be used to develop stable breathing patterns.

When asthma is uncontrolled, breathing generally becomes faster and harder. When we breathe faster, we are more likely to wake during the night, resulting in poor sleep quality. This ties in with the arousal threshold phenotype in sleep apnea. In addition, inflammation of the lungs during uncontrolled asthma can migrate to the nose, resulting in nasal stuffiness. The feeling of air hunger when breathing through the nose inevitably results in mouth breathing. This, in turn, narrows and increases turbulence in the airways, causing sleep disruption.

Finally, faster and harder breathing through an open mouth is generally from the upper chest. Breathing fast from the upper chest is inefficient, uneconomical, and the worst way to breathe as it inhibits oxygen transfer from the lungs to the blood, reduces lung volume, and results in easier collapse of the upper airway, causing the breath to stop during sleep.

Scientists believe that sleep disturbances in asthmatic patients may relate to sleep disorders including obstructive sleep apnea[30]. A substantial body of research also indicates that nocturnal symptoms, including coughing and breathlessness are accompanied by variations in airway inflammation and anatomical changes that may be impacted by circadian rhythms.[29]

Persistent coughing is another factor likely to disrupt sleep. Coughing wakes the sleeper out of deep sleep, causing poor quality of sleep and fatigue the following day. Symptoms of asthma frequently worsen at around four o'clock in the morning, when the incidence of asthma-related sudden death is also most common.[29] In one survey of 7,729 asthma patients, 74% awoke at least once per week with asthma symptoms, 64% suffered nocturnal asthma exacerbations at least three times a week, and around 40% experienced symptoms every night.[31]

Circadian rhythms are the autonomous, self-sustained natural processes that regulate the sleep-wake cycle.[29] They make it possible for the body to anticipate environmental changes and optimize survival. For example, the sleep-wake cycle enables us to rest at night and be active during the day. Lung function fluctuates in any 24-hour period in healthy people, but in people with nighttime asthma symptoms, these changes are much more profound, with the difference in breathing volumes between wakefulness and sleep exceeding 15%.[29]

One reason asthma symptoms are worse at night and in the early morning is that mouth breathing during sleep can add to breathing volume. If breathing during the day is poor, breathing during sleep will also be uncontrolled. Even without the circadian fluctuations in lung function and inflammation, poor breathing patterns and sleep-disordered breathing can lead to nighttime breathing difficulties. For this reason, it is not advisable to sleep for more than eight hours. While nocturnal asthma symptoms frequently cause sleeplessness and daytime fatigue,[32] correct practice of breathing exercises during the day will help reduce overbreathing at night.

Uncontrolled asthma results in hard, fast, upper chest breathing. The solution to improve asthma control and quality of sleep lies in light, slow and deep breathing. There are several techniques you can try that can greatly improve asthma control and sleep quality:

1. Pay attention to your asthma symptoms before you go to bed. If you are wheezy or have noticeable symptoms as you head off to the land of nod, it's likely you will wake up during the night with an attack. If you are experiencing symptoms before sleep, it's best to remain awake until they are under control or sleep sitting upright. If you have been prescribed a steroid medication, make sure to take it before you go to sleep, and **always practice your breathing exercises to reduce symptoms before going to bed**.
2. Practice light, slow, and deep breathing to achieve a tolerable air hunger for 15 minutes before sleep.
3. Avoid sleeping on your back. This is the worst position for over-breathing. As there is very little restriction to breathing, you are likely to breathe more deeply during the night. The lower jaw is also more prone to drop down, causing mouth breathing. Sleep on your side or abdomen instead.
4. Wear the Buteyko belt over your nightshirt during sleep. The Buteyko belt is a specially designed tool that imposes a resistance to the breathing muscles, lowering the risk of hyperventilation during sleep. I often wear the belt during sleep and find that it improves my quality of rest. Tighten or loosen the belt to create a tolerable air hunger. You can purchase a Buteyko belt online.
5. Make sure your bedroom has a good circulation of fresh air.
6. Only breathe through the nose while asleep. Wearing MyoTape will help bring the lips together to ensure nasal breathing. If the

nose is very stuffy, wear a nasal dilator such as Mute Snoring. MyoTape can be ordered from MyoTape.com.

7. Work to improve your everyday breathing patterns by addressing breathing from all three dimensions—light, slow, and deep.

8. Achieve a higher BOLT score. Every 5-second improvement to your BOLT score will result in more light, slow, and deep breathing. Ideally, to improve asthma control and sleep quality, the BOLT score needs to stay above 25 seconds.

Once you have begun to normalize your breathing volume, addressed underlying breathing pattern disorders, and increased your BOLT score, you will find you enjoy better sleep, and this will have a positive impact on your energy levels and quality of life.

## PREVENTING AN ASTHMA ATTACK

Generally, an asthma attack does not come out of the blue. You will usually experience warning signs such as increased tightness of the airways, a blocked nose, and wheezing or coughing. When you feel the first symptoms of an attack, it can be very helpful to perform the following exercises to help control your breathing. Use these exercises to prevent or lessen symptoms at the onset of the attack. Once an asthma attack is underway, it is very difficult to maintain control of breathing using exercises. Medication or medical attention may be necessary.

## EXERCISES

Performing *Breathing Recovery (sitting or walking)* when you first observe the onset of asthma symptoms can help reduce the severity of an attack or even head it off completely. However, it is important not to create too strong an air hunger during this exercise as it will cause a pronounced increase in your breathing after the exercise.

### Breathing Recovery, Sitting

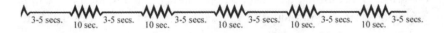

3-5 secs.   10 sec.   3-5 secs.   10 sec.   3-5 secs.   10 sec.   3-5 secs.   10 sec.   3-5 secs.   10 sec.   3-5 secs.

- Take a normal quiet breath in and let it out.
- Following an exhalation, hold the breath for between 3 and 5 seconds.
- Do not try to hold your breath for longer than this. It will only increase your breathing and exacerbate the asthma attack.
- Maximum breath-hold time should be no greater than **half your BOLT score at the time of practicing.**
- Leave 10 seconds between each breath hold, and don't try to interfere with your breathing during this time.
- Repeat the small breath hold, followed by a rest of 10 seconds, during which you should breathe normally through your nose.
- Continue until the attack has passed.

### *Breathing Recovery, Walking*

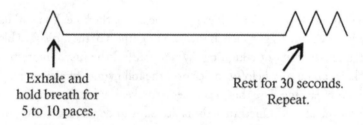

Exhale and
hold breath for
5 to 10 paces.

Rest for 30 seconds.
Repeat.

Instruction:

- Exhale through your nose.
- Pinch your nose with your fingers to hold your breath, and walk for 5 to 10 paces, holding your breath.
- Stop walking.
- Breathe in through your nose, and rest for about 30 seconds while standing still.
- Repeat up to 10 times.

If you are practicing at home, you can repeat this exercise 6 times, five times per day. Holding the breath for up to 10 paces is very suitable for anyone with severe asthma, COPD or panic disorder. It is also ideal if you have disproportionate breathlessness, anxiety, a racing mind, or a low BOLT score.

During an asthma attack, incomplete exhalations can cause air trapping or breath stacking. It is often harder to breathe out than to breathe in. If you experience this feeling of overinflated lungs, it is helpful to practice breathing out slowly and completely. This is not easy to do when your breathing is fast and labored, but it can be practiced between the exercises to help stop your symptoms. Follow these steps to ease the feeling of overinflated lungs:

## EXHALATION BY RELAXATION

- Breathe in gently and hold your breath for half a second.
- Concentrate on relaxing the chest, shoulders, and abdomen.
- Slowly exhale through your nose. Do not force your breath out in any way. Gently breathe out, slowly and completely. The natural elasticity of your diaphragm, lungs, and ribs will return the breathing muscles to their resting positions, resulting in a full, passive exhalation.
- Breathe in as normal.
- Repeat the exercise several times over the course of 10 minutes or until the attack has passed.

This exercise can be used at any time, whether you are suffering from breathing difficulties or not. It will help to normalize breathing through relaxation. Many people with asthma find that they truly begin to understand the benefits of reduced volume breathing the first time they successfully use the exercises to overcome an asthma attack.

## EXERCISE TO STOP A COUGHING ATTACK

Coughing is one of the most common symptoms of asthma. Although some people are more prone to bouts of coughing than others, a 2018 study states, "Cough alone may sometimes be the sole presenting symptom of asthma." Some asthmatics have normal lung function[33] and experience coughing and bronchial hyperreactivity (sensitivity to airway-narrowing stimuli) without any shortness of breath or wheezing.[34] Scientists have found that, on average, 25% of patients with chronic cough have a type of asthma called cough variant asthma. These people tend to respond to traditional asthma therapy.

A prolonged episode of coughing can be particularly difficult to stop. Much like other asthma symptoms, coughing attacks tend to be more frequent at night or in the early morning. Persistent coughing is very disruptive to breathing, so it is important to reduce its effects and prevent an attack taking hold.

Coughing is a reflex action caused by irritated airways. It's the body's way of clearing the airways of mucus and other irritants. Overbreathing can make the airways dry and inflamed, triggering a cough, and this, in turn, can lead to further overbreathing. When you cough, you take in a deep breath followed by a forced expiration of air. This action causes cooling and drying of the airways and a loss of $CO_2$, which inevitably leads to another cough and another forced expiration. If you don't stop the cycle, you will soon find yourself having a coughing fit.

The following approach can help you stop an attack of coughing:

- Try to suppress the cough if possible. You will experience a ticklish feeling in your throat, but after a while, the urge to cough should decline. Swallowing will help curb the need to cough.
- Don't try to force out mucus. Instead, reduce your breathing, and allow the mucus to come up naturally. It can then be swallowed to dissolve harmlessly in the acid of the stomach or be spat out if the circumstances are appropriate.
- Try to cough only through your nose.
- Perform *Breathing Recovery, Sitting* of between 3 and 5 seconds until your cough has passed.

The main point to remember is that the deep breathing and forced exhalations that occur during coughing will only perpetuate the cycle. Being conscious of this will help reduce the attack.

It is important to note that breathing exercises will only help alleviate a coughing fit when applied during the early stages of an attack. If symptoms have been occurring for more than five minutes, they will be a lot more difficult to control using breathing exercises, especially if your BOLT score is less than 20 seconds. If breathing difficulties continue for as long as five minutes, take your medication. If you are having a severe attack, take your medication immediately. If your symptoms do not respond to your medication within a few minutes, seek medical attention.

## BLOWING YOUR NOSE

Another common symptom of asthma is a blocked nose. If you are prone to nasal stuffiness, you will continue to experience symptoms until your BOLT score is at least 25 seconds. The normal reaction to nasal congestion is to repeatedly blow your nose, in an effort to get rid of mucus and clear your sinuses. But blowing your nose too much can actually aggravate the problem, inflaming the airways and increasing production of mucus. This makes feelings of congestion worse, and so you find yourself caught in a self-perpetuating and distressing cycle of excess mucus and nose blowing.

To help decongest your nose without increasing your breathing volume, follow these guidelines:

- Only blow your nose when it feels absolutely necessary.
- If you must blow your nose, do so gently.
- Spend five minutes reducing your breathing or practicing the nose unblocking exercise (see Chapters Two and Three).

## OVERCOMING RHINITIS AND HAY FEVER

Severe asthma is associated with a number of conditions that can make disease management more difficult and affect treatment outcomes[35]. These "comorbidities"—illnesses that exist independently of but alongside asthma—often mimic asthma symptoms and contribute to poor disease control.

Asthma and rhinitis are closely connected, and the risk of allergic rhinitis (AR) is higher in those who have had allergic asthma in childhood.[36] The global prevalence of allergic disease has increased considerably in recent decades,[36] with a significant cost both economically and in terms of well-being. One 2020 paper reported that 17.8% of 8,000 participants, aged between 20 and 69 years, had allergic rhinitis,[37] otherwise known as hay fever. The same article states that incidence of AR is highest during childhood and steadily decreases with age. A 2018 review of adults in Tehran found that 28.3% of those studied had AR.[38] And a 2013 paper from the World Allergy Organization reported that allergic rhinitis is the most common form of noninfectious rhinitis, affecting between 10% and 30% of adults and up to 40% of children.[39]

Allergic rhinitis is defined as an inflammatory and antibody-mediated disease.[40] Symptoms occur when airborne allergens are inhaled, but diagnosis depends on how often symptoms are triggered. If rhinitis occurs due to pollens, it will be classified as seasonal; if dust mites are the cause, it is perennial, and, if it is brought on by a specific allergic environment, it is intermittent.[40] This differentiation helps doctors to find the most appropriate treatment strategies. AR is also considered to be intermittent or persistent, according to the duration of symptoms. People with persistent rhinitis may suffer significantly impaired quality of life, loss of productivity and workdays, missed school time, and reduced ability to learn.

One of the most obvious and problematic symptoms of rhinitis and allergic rhinitis is nasal congestion.[41] It can be triggered by allergens such as dust mites, pollen, and spores, by an oversensitive immune reaction, or by nonallergic reactions such as the common cold, and it can interfere badly with sleep. People who have difficulty breathing through the nose are almost twice as likely to suffer sleep problems,[42] meaning that persistent nasal congestion can leave them feeling tired much of the time.

A 2020 study summarizes the main underlying mechanisms that link allergic rhinitis and altered sleep patterns as follows:

- Inflammatory cytokines related to allergic rhinitis cause feelings of fatigue.
- The symptoms and underlying physiological changes that occur in AR indirectly affect sleep.
- Sleep can be negatively impacted by dysfunction of the autonomic nervous system.[43]

Nasal congestion is known to affect sleep and contribute to sleep disorders, including snoring and OSA. By decongesting the nose using the exercise from Chapter Two and normalizing breathing patterns, you are likely to experience better sleep, less daytime tiredness and improved quality of life.

## RHINITIS AND THE AUTONOMIC NERVOUS SYSTEM

Scientists believe that an imbalance of the autonomic nervous system (ANS) plays a role in the poor quality of sleep experienced by people with allergic rhinitis. One pathway by which the ANS impacts rhinitis is a powerful autonomic reflex called the *trigemino-cardiac reflex* (TCR). The trigeminal nerve is the fifth and most complex of the cranial nerves. It innervates the face and takes care of actions including chewing and biting.[44]

TCR helps reduce the heart rate in challenging situations. It is known to cause apneas. An exaggerated form of the reflex may contribute to sudden death and sudden infant death syndrome.[46] One 2017 review explains:

> The amount of influence that the autonomic system exerts on the heart, manifesting either as arrhythmias or as OSA-induced brady-cardia and hypertension, does suggest the possibility of the TCR playing a role in sudden death.[45]

Another paper, also from 2017, concludes that TCR could link rhinitis and sleep disorders.[46] TCR triggers parasympathetic overactivity and sympathetic inhibition, leading to the sudden onset of bradycardia (slow heart rate) hypotension (low blood pressure), apnea, and gastric motility (contractions of the smooth muscle of the stomach). Autonomic imbalance also contributes to the onset and development of rhinitis.

While the extent of autonomic dysfunction in allergic rhinitis and sleep still needs further research, it is certain that constant nasal congestion, uncomfortable breathing, and poor quality of life can influence autonomic imbalance in the form of chronic stress. This has a direct effect on sleep. AR is associated with symptoms, including congestion, nasal discharge, sneezing, palatal itching, fatigue, and mood changes. Its most common behavioral complications are tiredness and sleep disturbance caused by an inability to breathe properly. Studies have also acknowledged compromised mental health, including anxiety and changes in emotional reactivity.

A higher incidence of anxiety, and, in some cases, depression, has been observed in people suffering from respiratory allergies. Anxiety itself can produce an exaggerated inflammatory response due to an overactive fight-or-flight mechanism. It has been suggested that high levels of anxiety can develop as a direct result of chronic illness, creating a self-perpetuating negative feedback loop. In a 2009 study, scientists demonstrated anxiety and reduced social interaction in rodents with experimentally induced rhinitis. They concluded that allergic rhinitis could influence behavioral responses.[47]

During allergic rhinitis, inflammatory mediators, including histamine, are released. These have a direct influence on the central nervous system and contribute to disturbed sleep and daytime tiredness. Histamine can affect the regulation of the sleep-wake cycle, and this may lead to a sleep condition called arousal disorder. Allergic rhinitis also causes reduced levels of certain cytokines called interleukins that are vital in activating immune responses, such as inflammation, and may be important in stimulating restorative sleep and improving circadian rhythms.[43]

While it may not be news to anyone who suffers with the condition, scientists have proven that rhinitis can have a negative impact on feelings of well-being. One 2020 study reported that the quality of life in children with allergic rhinitis was directly related to the severity of their symptoms.[48] Researchers noted that parents often overestimated the quality of life experienced by their children in this situation, and therefore, that it is of great importance to ask children how they feel rather than rely on parental perception.

## CAN NASAL BREATHING RELIEVE RHINITIS?

Healthy nasal breathing can minimize symptoms of rhinitis and moderate a range of conditions that lead to nasal congestion. The high concentration of nitric oxide in the sinuses is instrumental in keeping the nose and lungs free of disease and inflammation. It is likely that the reduction in inhaled NO caused by mouth breathing during sleep contributes to the negative effects of nocturnal mouth breathing[49]. When we breathe nasally, NO is released into the nasal cavity[50] and carried down to the lungs in concentrations that are between 5 and 20 times higher than during mouth breathing.[51] When nasal breathing is combined with slow breathing, this allows an even greater concentration of NO to be carried into the lungs. As the BOLT score increases, breathing becomes slower, and so it is likely that a higher BOLT score leads to improved uptake and use of NO.

Numerous studies demonstrate that nasal nitric oxide is found in much greater amounts in people with untreated symptomatic seasonal rhinitis, and that when AR is treated with nasal steroids, NO levels return to normal.[52] This strongly suggests that quantities of NO are released as part of the body's immune response, which fits with what we know about the role of NO as a first line of defense against infection. The increased level of NO in rhinitis patients is so marked that nasal NO measurement has become a more-or-less standard way to assess nasal inflammation and the response to anti-inflammatory medications.

This function of nasal NO is noted in various studies, including a 2019 paper that examines the clinical uses of exhaled NO measurement in the management of asthma and allergic airway inflammation. Researchers in that trial concluded that when stimulated as part of the inflammatory response,[53] special enzymes called nitric oxide synthase produce NO at a slow rate but in large quantities. This causes the concentration of NO to increase many times, and it is why NO is viewed as an important inflammation biomarker in the respiratory tract.

What's interesting in terms of breathing exercises is that nasal NO has been found to increase sharply during 30 seconds of breath holding.[54] This may be one mechanism by which techniques including the BOLT, yogic breathing, and the exercises in this book significantly relieve the symptoms of various respiratory complaints.

## THE ROLE OF $CO_2$

Another reason breath-holding and reduced breathing may be helpful in rhinitis is the role of $CO_2$. One 2008 study, which examined the application of intranasal $CO_2$ ($CO_2$ administered directly into the nose) in seasonal allergic rhinitis, found that the gas produced a statistically significant improvement in nasal symptoms. The trial involved 89 participants, 60 of whom received treatment with $CO_2$. The other 29 were given a placebo. Two 60-second intranasal $CO_2$ treatments resulted in relief of allergic rhinitis symptoms within 10 minutes and which lasted for 24 hours.[55]

Intranasal $CO_2$ was also shown to reduce symptoms of seasonal allergic rhinitis in a 2011 trial designed to evaluate the effect of $CO_2$ on symptoms caused by nasal allergens.[56] In a small study with only 12 participants, subjects were exposed to 20 seconds of $CO_2$ before breathing a filter paper "sham" allergen followed by two increasing doses of either grass or ragweed allergens. Researchers collected secretions from both nostrils and tested for histamine and eosinophils to evaluate the nasal reflex. In this study, both nose and eye symptoms were recorded. After the $CO_2$ treatment, participants experienced a significant reduction in symptoms including sneezing and runny nose. When the subjects received a placebo treatment, their histamine levels increased significantly on exposure to the allergens, but in those participants who had been treated with $CO_2$, no increase in histamine was found.[56]

Researchers concluded that $CO_2$ not only resulted in a reduced reaction to allergens, it suppressed reflex responses, indicating that it had some positive effect on the way the brain processed its reaction to allergens. These findings have been reiterated more recently in a 2018 review, published in *The Journal of Allergy and Clinical Immunology*, which described the efficacy of $CO_2$ in treating allergic rhinitis.[55]

The most common treatments for rhinitis and hay fever include trigger avoidance, decongestants, corticosteroids, allergy shots, and surgery. While these may offer therapeutic benefits, they are often effective only for as long as treatment continues. Breathing reeducation, however, harnesses the power of gases intrinsic to respiration in a natural, noninvasive way that has been proven to reduce symptoms.

It's important to understand the extent to which mouth breathing contributes to nasal congestion, and the prevalence of habitual mouth breathing. This can be illustrated by the fact that patients who undergo nasal surgery to correct mouth breathing often retain unhealthy breathing habits and therefore continue to experience symptoms. This point is easily illustrated by "empty nose syndrome" (described in Chapter Three). It was also my own experience before I learned about the therapeutic benefits of functional breathing training.

## NASAL BREATHING AND RESPIRATORY INFECTION

We already looked at the connection between nitric oxide and respiratory illness in Chapter Three. However, I'd like to add that over the years, I have observed many students experience a significant reduction in head colds and chest infections after they changed to light nasal breathing. Unfortunately, it is often those people who are most vulnerable to chest infections, those with asthma, bronchiectasis, bronchitis, and cystic fibrosis, who mouth breathe because they feel that they cannot get enough air through their nose.

Nasal breathing serves to filter the air before it enters the body, but as we discussed, nasal NO also has intrinsic qualities that form a first line of defense for the immune system. Optimal protection of the lungs takes the coordinated action of multiple cell types, and the tissue cells of the airway secrete a variety of antimicrobial substances as well as NO.[57]

Respiratory infections, such as cold, flu, and more recently SARS and COVID-19, commonly travel from person to person in droplets of mucus or saliva. The virus disperses when an infected person sneezes or coughs and droplets are expelled into the air and onto surfaces. Droplets from these airborne illnesses can travel several feet in a cough or sneeze and stay suspended in the air for up to 10 minutes making it easy for infection to spread.[58] Health guidelines for preventing the transmission of these infectious illnesses center on hand washing, catching sneezes in a tissue or elbow, and staying home from work if you are unwell. Pandemic responses have also seen people using protective facemasks to shield them from viruses or to protect those around them if they have symptoms.

Concerns about the impact of influenza-type viruses on the elderly and those with compromised respiratory systems have been particularly pressing during the COVID-19 outbreak. Ageing often involves a progressive decline in immune responses, rendering vaccines less effective and increasing susceptibility to infection.[59] Lower respiratory tract infections are thought to contribute to the development of asthma and are known to exacerbate asthma symptoms. One 2019 study suggests that asthma in the elderly is a distinct, more severe variant that may be linked with the deterioration of immune function in the airways.[59]

The respiratory tract can be colonized with bacterial, fungal, and viral microorganisms. These are collectively known as the airway "microbiome"[60] and may play a significant role in the development, persistence, and outcome of chronic inflammatory diseases, including asthma and COPD.[59] The presence of respiratory viruses during childhood has been recognized as a major risk factor for asthma in adolescents and adults. Viruses like rhinovirus, parainfluenza viruses, and respiratory syncytial virus represent the most common causes of asthma exacerbation.

While the spread of any infection is alarming, it has been consistently demonstrated that nasal breathing leads to better overall health. It also makes logical sense, given that nasal NO offers an initial defense to airborne viruses, that breathing through the nose can support the body's natural resistance to infection, pathogens, and allergens. While nasal breathing does not guarantee

that you will never experience another cold, bout of flu, or asthma exacerbation, it becomes ever clearer that this small change in daily habits can make
a genuine difference to quality of life and health.

# CHAPTER ELEVEN
# SEX AND BREATH, AN INTIMATE CONNECTION

---

The term *peak performance* used in the context of breathing techniques doesn't generally refer to your prowess between the sheets. Yet sex is one of our most fundamental physical activities. It may not use as many muscles as a gym workout, but it still requires exertion. Sexual function relies on a healthy body. It can be dramatically affected by poor breathing patterns, like every other area of health, with sometimes devastating impacts on quality of life, self-esteem, and relationships.

You may be slightly taken aback to find this boldly titled chapter in the middle of a book about breathing and health. Until relatively recently, sex was taboo. Just like money, it's something we all have in varying amounts, but nobody talks about it. It may, in all honesty, never be a topic you casually bring up over dinner. Even if it isn't still viewed as "dirty," our perceptions of other people's sex lives can certainly cause us to wonder if we've been getting it wrong for years. Fortunately, I see from my coaching that attitudes to sex are changing, and people are more open than ever to educating themselves about the body in a holistic way.

In writing this chapter, I am approaching the subject of sex in response to many questions from readers and clients over the years. The information is not based on my personal experience but is included to show the wide application of functional breathing and other breathing techniques for healthy sex. If you want to read more detailed personal accounts, there are several books mentioned that are perfect for further exploration.

For sure, I am no expert on sex or the topic of breathing during sex. My wife will be the first to tell you that! But on a more serious note, the science shows that sexual function can be an important indicator of heart health and that respiratory illness, which I work with a lot, can create a distressing impediment to a healthy sex life. You may still feel uncomfortable broaching this subject with your healthcare professionals, but I hope this chapter can help you open up that often-difficult conversation around sex and chronic conditions and perhaps give you some useful insights and vocabulary to ask the right questions for your own health.

Ancient practices, such as Taoism and Tantra, actively use the breath to harness what they consider to be the spiritual power of sex. In these traditions, the breath is seen as a connecting life force. As Jolan Chang points out in *The Tao of Love and Sex*, diaphragm breathing is basic to almost all forms of meditation.[1] Kundalini Tantra yoga focuses on raising the sexual power to nourish the vital centers known as the chakras, and its breathing exercises are designed to heighten and channel sexual energy.[2] In Tantra and Taoism, sex is perceived as something more than a stimulating erotic act. It is used to achieve and experience different states of consciousness and to promote a healthy body and a long life. In contrast, restricted breathing is seen as creating a sort of internal "contraction" that blocks feelings and emotions and makes it difficult to control the mind.

Healthy breathing helps provide the energy for sex. In the same way that it supports overall health, improves sleep, and reduces stress and anxiety, the breath can directly and indirectly affect sexual function and sexual pleasure. When breathing patterns are unhealthy or respiratory illness is present, it is common to experience breathlessness, fear of breathlessness, or worsening respiratory symptoms during sex. This can cause particular problems for people with chronic conditions like asthma and COPD. Sex is active. It uses the heart, lungs, and muscles, and causes the heart rate and blood pressure to rise.

If you have struggled with sex, you are not alone. The inability to enjoy a "normal" sex life is a feature of many common health conditions. If you suffer with ongoing respiratory symptoms, chronic stress, a bad back, or sleep-disordered breathing, chances are that your sex life is below par. Snoring is not sexy, and stress can switch off your libido. However, don't despair. Not only can these issues be managed and improved by practicing the exercises in this book, some schools of thought claim that the breath can provide the gateway to the best sex you've ever had.

## (DON'T) TAKE MY BREATH AWAY

We've talked a lot about the importance of nasal breathing and the problems that mouth breathing can cause, so it shouldn't be too much of a surprise to find that nasal breathing during waking and sleeping is important for sexual function too. The first reason for this relates to carbon dioxide ($CO_2$). When we breathe through the mouth, we overbreathe, causing blood $CO_2$ levels to drop below normal. $CO_2$ has vasodilatory properties, meaning it helps the blood vessels dilate. This contributes to the relaxing of the muscles around the penis and erectile tissues. When the concentration of blood $CO_2$ is low, the smooth muscles responsible for blood flow to the penis, clitoris, and vagina contract. Blood can't flow as easily, and it becomes more difficult for the erectile tissues to become, well . . . erect. This can mean, for example, a dip in sex drive for women during the second part of the menstrual cycle, when increased progesterone creates a drop in blood $CO_2$.

Nitric oxide also plays an important role in sexual health. NO has vasodilatory properties and enables the dilation of blood vessels that lead to the sexual organs, without which erection is impossible. It also plays a role in delaying ejaculation.[3] In 1998, the Nobel Prize in Physiology or Medicine was jointly awarded to three US researchers who demonstrated the role of NO as a "signaling molecule" in the cardiovascular system—the gas is produced by one cell but can pass through cell membranes to regulate the function of other cells. The researchers pinpointed the widening effect of NO on blood vessels, an insight applied in the treatment of male impotence. This research led to the development of drugs, including Viagra.

Viagra (Pfizer's brand name for the drug sildenafil, a PDE5 inhibitor) was first developed in 1989. It had been designed to compete with nitroglycerin as a treatment for heart-related chest pain. However, Viagra caused men to have erections, so it became marketed as a solution for erectile problems, slated to enhance sexual prowess in men. This product seemed to solve a real problem for the 30 million men in the United States with erectile dysfunction.[4]

Although the NO responsible for blood flow to the sexual organs is produced in the cells rather than traveling down the airways, research has, nevertheless, identified nasal breathing as directly important for sexual wellbeing. A 2011 paper published in the *American Journal of Rhinology and Allergy* found that men who mouth-breathed as a result of nasal polyps were more likely to experience erectile problems than men who breathed through the nose.[5] Before their mouth breathing was treated by surgically removing the polyps, 34% of the men had reduced sexual function compared to only 3% in the control group. After the polyps were removed and nasal breathing was restored, only 10% of the men continued to have problems. An earlier study reported that

67.5% of men who mouth-breathed experienced sexual difficulties, including erectile dysfunction, premature ejaculation, and lower sex drive.

Nasal breathing also helps engage the diaphragm, encouraging deep belly breathing. This is important because of the role of the pelvic floor muscles in sex. For men, the muscles of the pelvic floor, which are connected to the diaphragm, help maintain an erection by exerting internal pressure on the veins of the penis so that enough blood remains in the penis to make it fully rigid.[6] Pelvic floor muscles, including the pubococcygeus muscle, also play a role in orgasm.[7]

Over the last 20 years, researchers have explored the relationship between the pelvic floor muscles and the diaphragm.[8] They found that the muscles of the pelvic floor contract and relax during inhaling and exhaling at the same pace as the diaphragm. The pelvic floor becomes more active during the sudden increase of intra-abdominal pressure (IAP) that happens when we cough or sneeze. In fact, these muscles have been found to be essential to the interaction of the diaphragm and abdominal muscles for maintaining IAP. A recent study found that men who practiced breathing exercises to improve diaphragm function after prostate surgery experienced greater improvement to pelvic floor muscle endurance than men who practiced only pelvic floor strengthening exercises or abdominal muscle exercises. The men who practiced diaphragm exercises also had greater improvement in urinary continence after six months.[8]

Studies have demonstrated the effectiveness of pelvic floor muscle exercises in treating men with erectile dysfunction, [9] even suggesting that the exercises produce benefits comparable to PDE5 inhibitor drugs like Viagra.[6] Regarding women, Arnold Kegel made the connection between pelvic floor muscle tone and "sexual feeling" in the vagina way back in 1952.[10] Scientists have likewise found direct links between overactive bladder and poor sexual arousal in women[11]. However, no trial has yet explored whether diaphragm breathing exercises might be beneficial when it comes to sexual arousal. Nevertheless, a new approach to the treatment of premature ejaculation was devised in 2006.[12] Functional sex therapy, which incorporates aspects of functional movement and breathing, was shown to be more effective than traditional masturbation-based techniques.

While Viagra or equivalent drugs may seem like the perfect solution for men with erectile dysfunction, there are strong arguments for exploring more natural alternatives. A 2003 study that importantly but rather unusually examined the impact of Viagra on men's sexual partners found many problems. Not only were women experiencing physical symptoms such as cystitis from prolonged penile-vaginal sex, often in the absence of other sexual stimulation and foreplay, the "blue pill" put a heavy weight of expectation on the partner, sometimes leaving little room for the respectful, engaging interaction essential to healthy sex.[13] Rather as an afterthought, researchers asked the question:

> Will the sexual script of Viagra lovemaking actually be flexible and
> worry-free, or will Viagra-sex be all about worshipping the penis, since
> no one spending upwards of $10 to have an erection will ignore it?[14]

The implications behind this question are not insignificant. Popping a blue pill is quick and easy, but with the focus purely on a rather penis-centric idea of performance, it cannot be without problems and may actually prove damaging to vulnerable partners.[13] In fact, in homosexual men, the drug has been linked with increased sexual risk-taking.[15]

Fortunately, a growing weight of scientific evidence indicates that functional breathing practice can provide long-term benefits for sexual function through better oxygenation and improved diaphragm function. Unlike quick-fix pharmacological solutions, this has the bonus of overall improved health, physically, mentally, and relationshipwise.

Nasal breathing is also important in our sexuality through its connection to our sense of smell. Research has confirmed that the olfactory system plays a significant role in choosing a partner and in empathic functioning. Scientists examining people with impaired olfactory function found that the sense of smell influences various aspects of our sexuality.[16] A 2018 study explored the link between odor sensitivity and sexual desire, experience, and performance in 28 men and 42 women. Researchers found that the enjoyment of sex was enriched by olfactory input, and women who were more sensitive to smell reported a higher number of orgasms during sex. Odor sensitivity correlated with pleasure experienced during sex, perhaps because the perception of certain body odors enhances the recruitment of reward areas in the brain.[16]

This connection between our sense of smell and the way we interact with others, including our sexual partners, was also examined in a study from

2017. Scientists assessed the reliability of social judgments made via olfactory cues to discover the difference between responses to natural body odor and perfumes/deodorants, and between whole-body olfactory impressions and armpit odor presented on a t-shirt. Participants wore ear plugs and an eye mask to ensure that their impression of the person they were "meeting" was confined to their sense of smell. The results showed that people make consistent social judgments about others based on body-odor alone."[17]

We don't yet know the full function of human body odor or the role it plays in sex, but it is known that nasal breathing activates the olfactory nerve.[18] According to another 2017 paper, "airflow rhythm in the olfactory system can regulate the physiological and brain states, providing an explanation for the effects of breath control in meditation, yoga, and Taoism practices."

On the other hand, smell can also be a big turn-off. Kissing, which should be a delightfully pleasurable experience, can be rendered unbearable by bad mouth odor. However, bad breath is not always the result of poor oral hygiene. It is also a symptom of mouth breathing. Bad breath in the morning can be the result of mouth breathing during sleep. When we sleep with the mouth open, saliva dries up and bacteria proliferates, producing the dreaded "morning breath," even in people with otherwise meticulous oral hygiene. If you have a dry mouth when you wake, it is likely that you mouth breathe during your sleep. It is also likely that you have a buildup of plaque on your teeth and tongue.[19] Fortunately, it is easy to restore nasal breathing during sleep simply by taping your mouth with MyoTape—though you may want to wait until after you've had a cuddle to apply the tape.

## WHY STRESS IS A BIG TURN "OFF"

While nasal breathing directly enhances sex drive and performance due to increased blood flow to the penis and clitoris, functional breathing also helps reduce stress and promote better sleep, which, of course, impacts sexual function. Despite the once widely held belief that most sexual dysfunction has its roots in mental health, it's now known that sexual problems such as erectile dysfunction are caused by physiological factors in more than 80% of cases.[20] Nevertheless, chronic stress can and does create emotional and cognitive changes that prevent us from responding to sexual cues.[21] Stress has a powerful negative impact on all of the body's systems and can cause many problems that show up as physical or biochemical imbalances. If you are exhausted, stressed out, depressed, or have a poor body image, you will find yourself in the mood for sex much less often, and this can impact your relationships and further undermine self-esteem.[22]

To understand the impact that stress can have on sex, we need to look back to the autonomic nervous system (ANS). Remember that breathing, stress, and the ANS are interconnected, as we have already discussed (Chapter Four). The ANS controls functions that include heart rate, respiratory rate, and sexual arousal. It consists of the two main branches, the sympathetic and parasympathetic nervous systems, commonly known as fight, flight or freeze, and rest and digest (or "feed and breed"). Ideally, those two branches function in balance. However, when sympathetic activation is too high or too constant, we experience chronic stress. In that state, the body's evolutionary mechanisms prioritize survival over sex and sexual desire.

Under normal circumstances, sex can be a great way to relieve stress. It causes the release of mood-enhancing hormones, including endorphins. It can be great exercise, which is uplifting, in itself. However, stress can create a vicious cycle. Imagine this scenario. You've been working hard all week and want to enjoy some quality intimate time with your partner. Your mind is elsewhere, still going over a problem you didn't manage to fix. You're too stressed and can't get aroused or can't get an erection. Your partner asks what's wrong, but because you haven't realized how stressed you are, you brush the question aside and push yourself to perform. You can't or it's unsatisfying. The next time you want to be intimate, the episode replays in the back of your mind. Anxious not to repeat the embarrassment and discomfort, the inevitable happens. The more you try, the worse things get. Anxiety about your ability to perform in bed quickly becomes habitual, causing erectile dysfunction, lack of arousal, or even aversion when you think about having sex. This is one of the main reasons some men and women begin to avoid intimacy altogether.

While many of the situations we discuss in this book are primarily health-related, sex is more than just a physical experience. Any health concern can impact quality of life, but sex has a unique place in our closest relationships, as an emotional outlet and as a marker of personal identity. It is hardly surprising that we can form negative feelings around sex that trigger automatic physical responses that prevent sexual function.

For many men, erectile dysfunction begins as a stress response. Stress on top of stress triggers a vicious cycle of events. Unfortunately, because sexual arousal is controlled by the ANS, it doesn't respond to attempts at conscious control. However, there are ways to mediate the ANS to address the issue from a body-to-brain perspective. These include slow diaphragm breathing exercises at six breaths a minute and mindful breathing—the simple practice of paying attention to the breath.

It may be helpful to understand what the ANS does when it comes to sex and why it's such a problem when things are out of whack or when the ANS is affected by stress. First, the ANS is responsible for the dilation of the blood vessels that cause erection of the penis or clitoris. In men, this dilation is largely facilitated by nitric oxide.[23] Erection depends on nerve impulses from the ANS directing blood flow to the penis. It also requires the autonomic constriction of a circular muscle called a sphincter, which ensures that blood doesn't flow back out of the penis. The ANS also controls stimulation of secretions from the vagina or prostate. It mediates smooth muscle contractions of the vas deferens during ejaculation, or rhythmic contractions of the vagina during orgasm, and contractions of other pelvic muscles that accompany orgasm in both sexes.[23]

The processes differ between men and women. The female sex hormone *estrogen* is associated with increased synthesis and release of acetylcholine,[24] the neurotransmitter produced by the vagus nerve. In women, acetylcholine floods into the pudendal artery during vasodilation. Relaxing this artery, which supplies blood to the genitals, is essential to engorge the clitoris and vagina during sexual stimulation. Researchers believe that when relaxation of this artery is compromised, it can contribute to female sexual dysfunction.[25] Women who are stressed experience lower levels of genital arousal, even when psychological arousal is high. Women are reputed to be gifted with the ability to multitask, but research has found that arousal decreases in women who are distracted due to stress.[21] The practice of mindful breathing can help with the ability to stay present during sex and attend to physical and emotional sensations. Research has shown that mindfulness enhances sexual arousal.[26]

When the ANS is out of balance and sympathetic activation is high, the body is not able to function normally. Stress floods the body with cortisol and disrupts other hormones. Cortisol is needed for the regulation of blood pressure and the normal functioning of the body's systems, but too much of it can affect the normal biochemical functioning of the male sex organs.[27] Stress can affect testosterone production,[28] resulting in lower sex drive, erectile dysfunction, and impotence. It can also negatively affect sperm production, maturation, and make the body more vulnerable to infection. Infection in the prostate, urethra, and testes can all prevent normal sexual function in men.[27]

In women, stress can affect menstruation, increase symptoms of PMS, reduce sexual desire, negatively impact pregnancy health and postpartum adjustment, and worsen symptoms of menopause. It contributes to the exacerbation of diseases such as polycystic ovarian syndrome and can disrupt estrogen and progesterone levels, along with other hormones that support fertility. Sexual arousal relies on a variety of functions, including vaginal blood flow and engorgement of the labia, clitoris, and vestibular bulbs. These physiological responses are triggered by neurons that are controlled by the parasympathetic nervous system,[29] which can be suppressed by stress.

Research, paradoxically, shows that moderate sympathetic activation may boost sexual arousal in women.[30] The genitals are largely innervated by a nerve that, rather unusually, contains both sympathetic and parasympathetic neurons[31] (if you're dying to know, it's called the *major pelvic ganglion*). Scientists believe that this sympathetic activity may increase arousal by enhancing focus and attention on erotic cues, increasing blood flow, decreasing digestion, and directing more blood to flow to the genitals.

Alessandro Romagnoli is an Oxygen Advantage Master Instructor in Italy and France. He works as a psychologist, specializing in cognitive neuroscience. He has a wealth of clinical and scientific experience that allows him to help a broad range of clients, from people with severe psychiatric conditions to high-level professional athletes. I asked him to bring some insight to the topic of breathing and sex. He explained:

> Breathing techniques can be helpful in the treatment of sexual dysfunction because the breath can influence not only the physiological aspect but also the state of mind, and even the quality of the relationship. For example, slowing down the respiratory rate before intercourse would be tremendously beneficial, reducing any feelings of inadequacy and stress.

Ultimately, the ANS must be in balance to function optimally. Despite the relationship between sympathetic activation and stress, both the parasympathetic and sympathetic branches of the ANS contribute to sexual arousal. The male sexual response, in particular, reflects a dynamic balance between exciting and inhibiting influences of the ANS.[32] Interestingly, a 2002 study in *Cardiovascular Research* found that the human heart is more geared toward sympathetic mediated responses in men and parasympathetic responses in women.[24]

## VAGUS NERVE—SECRET TO DEEPER ORGASMS?

The parasympathetic nervous system (PNS) plays a significant role in in sexual function, as it does in general health. Elevated heart rate variability (HRV) has been linked to better erectile function in men.[33] HRV, which is used as a measure of parasympathetic or vagal tone, can also be used to predict female sexual dysfunction. In a study of 84 women aged between 18 and 47 years, low HRV was identified as a risk factor for sexual dysfunction. The study recorded measurements of respiratory sinus arrhythmia (RSA) before, during, and after sexual arousal. Researchers found significant differences in vagal activity between women who were sexually functional and women who experienced dysfunction, suggesting that vagal tone could provide a potential mechanism through which to treat sexual dysfunction.[34] This implies that sexual dysfunction could be alleviated by stimulating the vagus nerve— which can be done by practicing slow breathing at six breaths per minute.

Research from 2015 reached a similar conclusion from a different starting point. In a study of women who had survived childhood sexual abuse, their HRV was compared against women who had no history of trauma. It was found that when women were treated to reduce autonomic imbalance, their sexual well-being improved. Over time, as HRV became better regulated, the women showed increasing improvements in sexual arousal and orgasmic function.[35]

The vagus nerve is implicated in female orgasm and in ejaculation for both men and women. In women, vaginal orgasm is physiologically different from clitoral orgasm.[36] While sensory input from the clitoris travels to the brain via the pudendal nerve, information from the vagina and cervix travels via the pudendal, pelvic, hypogastric, and vagus nerves. The vagus nerve is stimulated during heterosexual sex as the penis connects with the cervix. This stimulation appears to be linked to better cardiovascular and psychological function and increased vagal tone.[36] Research by Beverly Whipple and Barry Komisaruk, authors of *The Science of Orgasm*, demonstrates that the vagus nerve plays a role in deep orgasms in women.[37] So much so that it is possible for a woman who has a completely severed spinal cord and no feeling in her lower extremities to experience orgasms, even in the absence of any connection between the external clitoris and the brain.[36]

More recent research has shown that much of the clitoris is internal, with four-inch roots reaching into the vagina.[38] This would indicate that vaginal and G-spot orgasms are, in fact, also clitoral and come from stimulating the internal parts of the clitoris. It is certainly the case that if the vaginal walls had as much sensation as the clitoris, childbirth would be impossibly painful. Just the tip of the clitoris has over 8,000 nerve endings, double the number found in the penis.[39] However, it is hardly surprising that understanding of female orgasm is limited and conflicting, because it wasn't until 2009 that the first sonographic mapping of an erect clitoris was carried out. Without this knowledge, much study of the female anatomy and female sexual satisfaction has assumed that penile stimulation is necessary to orgasm—only adding to an unhealthy culture around female sexuality that may help explain why 1 in 10 women has never had an orgasm.

Looking at it from a different direction, the ancient Tantric idea that restricted breathing creates a type of internal contraction, blocking feeling and emotions, was confirmed in 2008 by scientists who made a link between the way a woman walks and her experience of, or potential for, vaginal orgasm. The researchers speculated that chronic muscle tension impacts sexual function by impairing feeling and functional movement, possibly representing mental or emotional blocks. The paper cites a study of men in which it was found that a method of therapeutic manual tissue manipulation known as Rolfing decreased postural problems in the pelvis and increased cardiac vagal tone, which indicated better parasympathetic function. Research from 2004 similarly linked physical therapy with better orgasmic function in women,[40] and another review from 2007 indicated that problems in the muscles of the pelvic floor are closely related to sexual dysfunction.[41] The 2008 paper concludes,

> The discerning observer may infer women's experience of vaginal orgasm from a gait that comprises fluidity, energy, sensuality, freedom, and absence of both flaccid and locked muscles.[36]

This raises the question, could the diaphragm—which is central to breathing, integral to the core, vital for stability of the spine and pelvis, and connected to the vagus nerve—also play an important role in the ability to achieve satisfying orgasms?

Significantly, that all-important vagus nerve also innervates the voice box and throat, and it is directly connected to the cervix and uterus.[42] Research into this area is incredibly sparse, but one paper explores the involuntary vocal noises we typically make during sex, linking the more powerful sounds with hyperventilation. It is the first study to examine blood sensitivity to $CO_2$ during intense sex. It suggests that the metabolic changes occuring in the brain during hyperventilation may deepen states of sexual trance.[43] The researchers observe that changes in breathing patterns during sex are similar in both men and women. However, accelerated breathing is more accentuated in women. Anecdotal evidence also suggests that women are more vocal during sexual intercourse.[43]

*The Multi-Orgasmic Woman* describes the use of the breath to extend female orgasm by contracting the pubococcygeus muscle and expressing pleasure with the voice, explaining that, according to Taoist wisdom, the throat and vagina are connected.[44] As you gain better control of your sexual energy, "you will be able to extend your orgasm through one long out-breath, a quick intake of breath, and then another one or two breaths." The book states that if the throat is open, the genitals will be "open to pleasure."[44] In the book *The Multi-Orgasmic Man* by Mantak Chia and Douglas Abrams, we learn that the ability for men to control ejaculation and have more than one orgasm also begins with strengthening and deepening the breath[45]. If you are interested in exploring the Taoist techniques for sexual pleasure more deeply, those books, along with *The Multi-Orgasmic Couple*, provide an approachable and informative resource.

As we know, hyperventilation alters levels of blood $CO_2$, and $CO_2$ moderates the rate of blood flow in tissues, especially the brain. Hyperventilation also induces changes to the blood's acid-base balance, which increases the affinity of blood hemoglobin for oxygen. This further decreases the amount of oxygen available for the cells and tissues. Blood flow to the brain can decrease by as much as 50% during hyperventilation.[43] At the same time, metabolic activity in the brain changes. Functional magnetic resonance imaging (fMRI) studies show that oxygen consumption is predominantly reduced in the neocortex gray matter and much less in the limbic structures. The limbic systems in the brain are responsible for our emotional responses, while the gray matter influences attention, memory, thought, and motor control. The study suggests that this may explain the role of hyperventilation in intensifying emotional states and changing behavioral control during sex.

The study also suggests that changes within the nervous system induced by hyperventilation could lead to altered states of consciousness. This involves a shift in the pattern of activity between different structures within the brain. The result is something that scientists describe as an "arousal dissociation," which may result in a more primitive form of brain function. This brain "state," which involves activation of pleasure responses, less self-control, a decrease in abstract thinking, and an increase in emotionally guided thinking is known to occur during dreams, hypnagogia (the state of consciousness just before we fall asleep), and in states induced by hallucinogenic drugs.[43] Hyperventilation may be used instinctively in this context to intensify experiences of sexual excitation, sexual trance, and orgasm.[43]

Tantra.com founder, Suzie Heumann, speculates that for women, opening the mouth and chest cavity with slow, deep breathing may connect with the vagus nerve to greatly enhance orgasmic capacity.[46] Heumann writes,

> When women emit deep, low sounds from their abdomens and with their mouths wide open this can sometimes lead to longer lasting, powerful orgasms and even female ejaculation.[46]

Since it has been found that people who are more susceptible to hypnotic trance have a higher autonomic responsiveness and higher levels of brain to body vagal activity,[47] Heumann's suggestion that a highly activated vagus nerve can produce "out of body pleasure" may not be far from the truth.

## WHEN SEX IS DYSFUNCTIONAL

Sexual function is defined in Western medicine as a state of physical, mental, and social well-being as it pertains to sexuality. It requires a positive and respectful approach to sexuality and sexual relationships, and it involves the possibility of pleasurable, safe sexual experiences. Sexual function is about more than just frequency or duration of sex. It includes sexual desire, arousal,

satisfaction, orgasm, lubrication, and the workings of the sex hormones[22]—all
of which can ultimately be affected by breathing.

While sexual problems can include lack of desire, pain, inability to
orgasm, erectile dysfunction, aversion, difficulty with vaginal penetration,
premature or delayed ejaculation, lack of arousal, or inappropriate, unwanted
arousal, there is no universally accepted definition of sexual dysfunction.
For women, it encompasses ongoing or recurring decrease in sexual desire
or arousal, the feeling of pain during sex, and an inability to reach orgasm.
For men, it's generally the inability to "get it up" or early ejaculation. Few
men know (or take advantage of the fact) that orgasm and ejaculation are
two quite distinct functions.[3]

Hormonally speaking, there is plenty of evidence to indicate a relationship
between sexual function and testosterone production in men. On the other
hand, the relationship with estrogen in women is less clear. What most of
us know about female hormones and sex is limited to how it relates to pregnancy (or trying not to get pregnant) and worries about vaginal dryness, pain
during sex, and changes after menopause. Lack of knowledge and a paucity
of research into female sexual function adds to the pressure on women to
stay "youthful" and the unhealthy prejudice that postmenopausal women
are sexually redundant. On the other side, lack of understanding about the
physiological aspects of sexual function leaves men feeling emasculated.
Neither of these common reactions reflect the truth.

Sexual dysfunction is a problem that can affect anyone, particularly as
we get older and when other health conditions are present. Global prevalence
of sexual dysfunction is high. Studies have identified that as many of 57.8%
of men and 41% of women suffer from lack of desire, anxiety about sexual
performance, and orgasmic dysfunction. A 2003 study of 1,793 Australians
reported sexual dysfunction in 55% of men and 60% of women. However,
while prevalence is high in both sexes, there has been no breakthrough in
the treatment of women equivalent to the PDE5 inhibitor (Viagra) for men.
Although PDE5 inhibitors can increase clitoral blood flow in postmenopausal
women, and some women report heightened arousal, these drugs have not
been found to be consistently effective.[25]

Overall, male sexual function has been extensively documented and is
well understood. In contrast, in women, the problem has been much understudied.[25] Ironically, sexual dysfunction is also considered more complicated

in women due to the combination of anatomical, psychological, physiological, and social-interpersonal factors that contribute.[25] However, it seems likely that this perception is colored by the lack of research.

In middle-aged and older men, factors such as high blood pressure, diabetes, cardiovascular disease, and obesity (all affected by breathing issues) clearly contribute to poor sexual performance. Substance use (including smoking), thyroid conditions, anxiety, and depression can also play a part. Erectile dysfunction is normally caused by problems with blood flow to the penis, hormones, or nerve supply. When the arteries harden due to cardiovascular disease or hypertension, blood is less able to flow to the penis, and it becomes difficult to achieve or maintain an erection.[48]

As with men, female sexual disorders are affected by health and by psychosocial factors. Several studies have made the connection with cardiovascular disease in women, indicating that treatment of sexual dysfunction purely as a matter of lifestyle may underestimate its importance as an indicator of health. A 2008 study claimed that 87% of middle-aged women with heart failure reported some level of sexual dysfunction,[49] 76% had problems with dryness, and 63% struggled to orgasm.

Cardiovascular and respiratory health are important from a purely physiological perspective too. One early study, published in 1966, recorded a peak coital heart rate of between 140 and 180 beats per minute and a mean increase in blood pressure during sex.[50] Even earlier research, from 1956, found a similar outcome.[51] Peak coital heart rates at orgasm approached 170 beats per minute in both men and women.

Respiratory rates and tidal volumes were also recorded in this early trial. Both measurements increased significantly in all subjects, with some participants demonstrating a breathing rate of more than 60 breaths per minute and a peak minute volume comparable with that during moderately intense physical exercise.

A study of middle-aged men from 1970 compared the increase in heart rate during sex with that seen after climbing two flights of stairs.[52] Body oxygen consumption was equivalent to 60% of the subject's $VO_2$ max.

While the clinical implication is that sex imposes a modest physiological cost, with maximal heart rates lasting around 15 seconds, this cost is significant for anyone with heart or lung conditions.

Diabetes (see Chapter Fourteen) can affect the blood vessels and the nerves that supply the penis. On average, men with diabetes experience erectile dysfunction 15 years earlier and are four times more likely to suffer from it than men without diabetes. Sexual dysfunction in diabetic women has been less well studied,[25] but recent research shows they are more prone to sexual dysfunction than healthy women,[25, 53] suffering with lower sex drive, vaginal dryness, little or no arousal, difficulty achieving orgasm, and reduced sexual satisfaction.

Obesity is linked to several types of sexual dysfunction in men and women, both due to health reasons and to the poor body image that often accompanies excess weight.[23] For people with epilepsy (see Chapter Fifteen), hyperventilating during sex can directly cause seizures.

The study of female sexual dysfunction is challenging, due to its multifaceted nature and to preconceptions that labeled women as "frigid" or "neurotic" until alarmingly recently. It is also more difficult to overtly define arousal in women, and the understanding of the female orgasm is limited. Even today, the problem has largely been investigated in terms of comorbid conditions such as diabetes and high blood pressure, making it necessary to interpret results in terms of those disorders. Traditionally, women with sexual problems were treated with psychological therapy, whether the underlying cause was mental or physical, and there have been few medications available. Since female sexual function was first addressed in research only 50 or 60 years ago, it's hardly surprising that treatment options can, at best, be described as inadequate,[25] which makes the benefits possible through effective breathing all the more important.

For both men and women, sex changes as we age. Scientists directly compared the effects of aging on erectile dysfunction with the impact of various comorbidities typically associated with aging and found that age alone increased the risk of sexual dysfunction. Researchers reported that poor health, diabetes, and urinary incontinence increased the risk of sexual problems in all age groups.[54] In women, too, aging can, of itself, cause problems. As we get older, the likelihood of developing decreased energy and strength, cardiovascular disease, diabetes, arthritis, cancer, and other health concerns is greater. Relationships can change if one or both partners develop chronic medical problems, and the inevitable physical decline of the aging body must be accepted and accommodated if we are to maintain a satisfying sex life.[55]

Aside from the direct impact of poor physical and mental health, hundreds of common medications also cause sexual dysfunction. These include depression medications, particularly SSRIs (serotonin reuptake inhibitors) such as citalopram, fluoxetine, and sertraline, and blood pressure drugs including beta-blockers.[48] One study found that while SSRIs caused more incidence of sexual dysfunction in men, the dysfunction experienced by women using the drugs was more intense.[56]

Many hormonal birth control methods can cause side effects, including decreased sex drive and vaginal dryness. *The Multi-Orgasmic Woman* offers a detailed overview of contraceptive methods and intimate problems such as urinary tract and yeast infections that may impede sexual function in women.[44] The book is a valuable resource for any woman wanting to gain better understanding and control of her sexual health.

Sexual function can be a useful measure of how well other systems are working. Throughout this book, we examine how dysfunctional breathing impacts general physical and mental health and longevity, as well as specific conditions. By making positive changes to health through better breathing, your sex life can be improved.

## BREATHLESS: SEX AND RESPIRATORY DISEASE

If you have a respiratory disease, the connection between it and sex is much more obvious. If you suffer from asthma or another chronic respiratory condition, sex can quite literally leave you breathless. A 2019 study explored problems of sex and intimacy in patients with severe asthma, revealing a huge number of constraints facing people with respiratory symptoms.[57] Some of these had to do with expectations, fear, and embarrassment, while others directly related to physical exacerbations. This study, which describes the experiences of nine patients in detail, is the first to really address a problem that affects millions of people worldwide.

An earlier study had raised the issue of postcoital asthma and rhinitis.[58] The paper describes the case of one male patient whose acute severe asthma after sex resulted in several emergency department visits and hospitalization. Patients with COPD also struggle with breathlessness during sex, a feeling that may be worsened by hyperventilation.[59] Erectile dysfunction and low testosterone levels have been reported in men with respiratory diseases such as COPD,[60] asthma and obstructive sleep apnea syndrome (OSA). In patients with COPD, breathlessness, coughing, muscle weakness, and diminished physical activity all contribute to decreased sexual activity.[61] In these situations, anxiety around respiratory symptoms adds another burden on both the sufferer and the spouse or lover.

A study of patients with *rhinoconjunctivitis*—an allergic condition characterized by nasal congestion, runny nose, sneezing, postnasal drip, red eyes (conjunctivitis), and itching of the nose or eyes—found a significant relationship with sexual dysfunction in women and erectile problems in men. In both genders, sexual function was much better in patients who had received treatment for nasal and conjunctival symptoms than in those patients who were untreated.[62]

The 2019 asthma study gives the most detailed account of the problems facing asthmatics. Each of the nine people interviewed felt that a good sexual experience required some physical effort,[57] yet even moderate exertion limited their performance due to worsening symptoms. Intimacy was made difficult by asthma, even to the extent that kissing caused a flare-up of breathlessness. One participant described having to stop in "full flow" because of feeling unable to breathe. They described feelings of exhaustion that came from living with asthma and taking high-dose corticosteroids. Sleep deprivation caused marital strain in one case, as the participant's partner interpreted attempts to get enough sleep as an evasion of intimacy. Patients felt they had to organize equipment or remember to use inhalers or nebulizers, detracting from any spontaneity. While some could accept this as being part of their condition, others found it distressing and a barrier to intimacy. One commented that her inhaler pump was almost like a third person in the relationship because it was necessary to maneuver around it during sex.

There was also a genuine fear that sexual climax might induce severe bronchospasm requiring emergency medical intervention. This added level of anxiety reduced sexual satisfaction. The embarrassment caused by having to explain the reason for the exacerbation to paramedics and healthcare professionals was a major consideration. Some devised positive coping mechanisms, including using pillows as props and finding positions that didn't lead to exacerbations—the "Asthma Sutra." Emotional intimacy has more elements than the purely physical expression of sex, but all of the participants found that the physical act of sex was restricted by their asthma. Certain positions caused feelings of suffocation, especially for women, and men perceived their sexual performance to be dampened by the need for physical exertion.

Emotionally, the patients experienced frustration and guilt, and felt pressure to perform. Often part of the problem was feeling they couldn't broach the subject with their partner. Five of the female participants (83%) described giving their partners permission to sleep with other women because they felt so guilty over being unable to offer sexual satisfaction in the relationship and feared losing their partner altogether. Many felt that they should not impose their asthma-related concerns on their partners. Others reported an emotional weight being lifted when they did manage to explain the situation and receive support. Insights into self-image uncovered feelings of self-loathing in all participants and problems balancing the dual role of the partner as a carer and a lover: "One minute they're wiping your bum and then the next minute you're ripping each other's clothes off. It does vary." Two of the participants described how this conflict in roles had caused the breakdown of previous marriages.

Weight gain due to long-term corticosteroid use and difficulty exercising because of symptoms also had a negative impact on body image and feelings of sexuality. Even things most people take for granted, such as wearing sensual underwear, were problematic due to feelings of restriction on the chest wall. All participants voiced some element of struggle on a daily basis.

Despite the significance of these issues in the day-to-day lives of people with severe asthma, no healthcare provider had ever initiated discussion of sexual intimacy during medical appointments with any of the participants. Two even described negative reactions when they tried to raise their concerns. One commented, "I actually brought it up, and I thought the counsellor was going to run out of the room screaming!" Seven of the participants felt that the topic was too intimate to raise but would welcome the chance to talk about it with a specialist nurse if the opportunity were offered.[57]

The study confirms that fatigue has a significant impact on sexual quality of life for people with severe asthma. The finding that the fear of exacerbation was so present during sex is new, as is the discovery that embarrassment about having to call an ambulance was generally worse than anxiety about the asthma exacerbation itself. Intimacy, from kissing to full sex, produced breathlessness and feelings of suffocation, and spontaneity was difficult. All these factors added pressure to the sufferer's relationship, presenting a huge emotional burden on top of the physical limitations. The study concluded that it is essential for their quality of life that healthcare professionals openly address sex and intimacy with asthma patients.

The breathing exercises in this book have been shown, time and time again, to reduce asthma symptoms and prevent asthma exacerbations. If asthma is affecting your quality of life, relationships, and sexual pleasure, it's time to take back control. You can read much more about using breathing exercises to control your asthma in Chapter Ten.

## SLEEPING TOGETHER

Sex and sleep are interesting bedfellows—quite literally both are typically done in bed—but the connection goes far deeper than this. We've already discovered that sexual function is indicative of health, and we also know that sleep is fundamental to physical and mental well-being. A healthy sex life will help decrease stress and improve sleep; conversely, quality sleep is essential for sexual health.

We've explored how stress can affect sex drive and sexual function for physical and psychological reasons. Fatigue, sleep disturbance, and sleep deprivation, by themselves, can simply make us too tired for sex. The impact this can have on self-esteem, intimacy, and relationships is all too apparent in the study of patients with severe asthma. According to a 2002 paper, being "too tired" is the primary reason people lose interest in sex.[63] Conversely, 2015 research from scientists at the University of Michigan Medical School reported that the more sleep people had, the more likely they were to feel like sex the following day.[64] If all that you and your partner are doing is actually sleeping together, it's time to look at the quality of your sleep.

Whenever you can improve the quality and quantity of your sleep, you are likely to improve the quality and quantity of your sex life. We have already looked in detail (in Chapter Seven) at sleep-disordered breathing and ways we can ensure better sleep and better health through improved breathing. However, it is worth examining the statistics here. One research paper found that about 50% of men aged between 18 and 70 years who have moderate to severe sleep apnea also suffer from erectile dysfunction.[65] Another study found that 69% of participants with sleep apnea also had erectile problems.[66] The link may be partly hormonal. Men with sleep apnea have lower levels of testosterone.[65] Since we already know an overactive fight-or-flight response inhibits testosterone production, this makes a lot of sense.

For men, it is absolutely normal for erections to occur during sleep. Night-time erections often go unnoticed, perhaps only becoming obvious first thing in the morning as "morning wood," but to use its medical name, nocturnal penile tumescence (NPT) is actually an important marker of heart health,[67] vascular tone,[68] and parasympathetic function.[69] Medical science frequently uses NPT as an indicator of sexual or hormonal well-being,[70] especially when diagnosing the causes of erectile dysfunction. If a man has frequent nightly erections but is unable to achieve or maintain an erection during sex, it is likely that blood flow and nerve responses in the penis are healthy. In this instance, erectile dysfunction may have a psychological basis. If, however, he has no NPT and is unable to function sexually, it is more likely that the root cause is physical. This differentiation allows doctors to treat the problem effectively.

Nocturnal erections usually occur during rapid eye movement (REM) sleep.[71] The reason that they are most apparent in the morning is that we tend to wake up at the end of a REM sleep cycle. Equally, testosterone levels tend to be higher in the morning. It is thought that erections of this type may differ in some way physically from those caused by arousal. Research has reported cases of men who experience pain with NPT but never with erections related to sexual arousal.[72]

It is common for a man to have three to five of these nocturnal erections, each lasting 30 minutes or longer, during eight hours of sleep.[73] Contrary to what many people believe, these are not the result of sexual stimulation, thoughts, or dreams. Young men, who have higher testosterone levels, tend to experience more NPT, and incidence declines in men during their forties and fifties. This gradual decrease is normal too, but if these erections stop altogether, this can be a sign of a hormonal imbalance, high blood pressure, or other potentially serious health problem. We know, for example, that the production and stability of sex hormones can be strongly affected by dysfunction in the autonomic nervous system caused by stress. Research found that men with a condition called hypogonadism,[74] which causes diminished function of the gonads and testes (or the ovaries in women), experienced more NPT after they were given testosterone therapy.

Scientists have demonstrated that NPT can be affected by quality of sleep.[75] Poor or disturbed sleep prevents us from entering the REM sleep cycle when nocturnal erections usually occur. We know that sleep-disordered breathing results in less restful sleep. Men with sleep apnea and erectile dysfunction experience more nocturnal erections when they use a CPAP machine to improve their sleep than those whose OSA is untreated.[76] Mouth breathing at night is a significant anatomical risk factor for OSA, increasing the incidence and severity of upper airway collapse[77] and therefore contributing to erectile dysfunction. This underlines how important it is to ensure nasal breathing during sleep—something that can be easily achieved by using MyoTape. (You can read more about CPAP compliance in the chapter on sleep.)

One of the hallmarks of sleep apnea is recurrent hypoxia throughout the night. In hypoxia, not enough oxygen makes it to the cells and tissues in the body. This can happen even when blood flow is normal. It is related to many factors, including heart and respiratory failure, sleep apnea, smoking, COPD, diabetes, high blood pressure, and clogged arteries.[78] Significantly, all of these disorders are characterized by erectile dysfunction and by a reduction in sleep-related erections.

In one study, scientists used high altitude to reproduce symptoms of hypoxia in healthy men and assessed the results in terms of penile rigidity.[78] The level of inspired oxygen decreases incrementally as altitude increases. Researchers followed three mountain climbers in their early thirties over a 26-day stay at altitudes ranging from 2,000 to 5,600 meters above sea level. At altitudes over 4,450 meters, the rigidity of erections decreased almost completely, confirming that hypoxia negatively impacts erectile function. We already know that slow, nasal breathing significantly improves oxygenation due to the fact that more air reaches the small air sacs of the lungs. This is yet another reason why nasal breathing during sleep is so important.

Nitric oxide, which we harness by breathing through the nose, is also essential both for vascular health and erectile function. In one study, scientists state that "maximal attention should be placed on measures known to improve vascular NO production."[6] This includes the use of PDE5 inhibitors and exercises to ensure normal functioning of the pelvic floor muscles. These two approaches are complementary rather than competing as they work on entirely different aspects of erectile function.[6] As we've discussed, normal functioning of the pelvic floor relies on a fully operational diaphragm, and it is nasal breathing during wakefulness and sleep that promotes deep breathing from the diaphragm rather than fast, upper chest breathing.

For women, sleep apnea and insomnia have been linked to sexual dysfunction and decreased sexual satisfaction. This is certainly the case after menopause, but there are also a few studies of younger women that examine this connection. A 2017 study of postmenopausal women found that those with higher insomnia scores were less satisfied sexually. Also, women who slept less than seven or eight hours a night were less likely to have sex with their partners at all.[79] Researchers concluded that shorter sleep and worse insomnia was associated with decreased sexual function in these women.

Despite the many decades of sexual revolution, studies of younger women still often focus on fertility[80] (or infertility) rather than on sexual satisfaction in relation to common disorders such as poor sleep. One study examined female sexual function in terms of sexual desire, sexual arousal, lubrication, orgasm, sexual satisfaction, and intercourse pain in women aged between 18 and 45 and found significant links with sleep quality.[81] There was a marked inverse relationship between daytime sleepiness, insomnia, poor sleep quality, and sexual function. Sexual desire was highly dependent on good sleep, while poor lubrication, orgasm, and satisfaction were all associated with sleep disorders. Pain during intercourse also increased when sleep was inadequate. Sexual function decreased incrementally with each reduction in sleep quality and with each increase in the time it took to fall asleep.

Another study explored factors in sexual function and infertility in women with endometriosis[82]—a common condition where tissue similar to the lining of the womb starts to grow outside the womb. The authors found that sleep quality was a primary contributing factor in sexual dysfunction for these women. As sleep quality, anxiety, depression, and pelvic pain worsened, sexual function decreased.

Again, as we have found in various chronic conditions, quality of sleep can make a huge difference to how "in control" we feel. When sleep is restorative, everything is a little bit easier. We feel mentally stronger, more resilient, and less sensitive to pain. By making the switch to functional breathing day and night, it is possible to experience significant improvements in sleep, in quality of life, and in sexual function.

## LEARNING FROM ANCIENT WISDOM

It may sometimes seem like there is a constant focus on sex. As the old marketing adage says, "Sex sells." Adverts on the station platform, magazine articles, self-help books, films, talk shows, and gossip columns are all obsessed with sex and sexuality. Even in a culture where attitudes to sex and gender are changing, the sexual narrative, an almost competitive, heteronormative view of sex is ever-present. Ironically, our fast-paced, thrill-seeking, consumerist world paradoxically creates an environment where it is difficult to fully enjoy a healthy, truly pleasurable sex life. As with breathing and sleep, the real power of sex is in the quality, not the quantity.

Phallocentric attitudes have narrowed our view of sex to center on the release of seminal fluid, an end goal which is largely irrelevant and leaves men and women unsatisfied and disconnected. Sex has become functional. Despite all our advancements as a species, our relationship with sex is far less healthy than it was thousands of years ago, and our understanding of it is less assured.

For instance, ancient Taoism teaches that men can control ejaculation by using the breath. This makes no sense if you equate "coming" with orgasm. However, Taoism also tells us that ejaculation and orgasm are two different things. If this sounds far-fetched, research from 2015 confirms it to be true. Male orgasm and ejaculation are, in fact, two distinct physiological processes.[3] Orgasm is "an intense transient peak sensation of intense pleasure creating an altered state of consciousness associated with reported physical changes." Ejaculation is "a complex physiological process that is composed of two phases (emission and expulsion)" and influenced by complex hormonal and neurological pathways. Although male sexuality is very well studied, much about this topic is still unknown. However, even less is known about the "mythical" female orgasm.

Taoism and yogic cultures embrace sexual function and orgasm in a way that many people never experience. They view sex as wholesome and life-preserving, not a taboo laden with concepts of guilt, sin, voyeurism, and exploitation. By using the breath to guide and build sexual energy, they access a health-giving resource. In this mindset, where sex is part of the human experience and not separate from it, erotic ecstasy is a tool for spiritual development and physical and mental well-being. Although research is limited, these concepts are to some extent being examined and contextualized in scientific literature. Increasing credence is being given to the idea that the ancient sages may have been onto something.

For example, a 2019 paper in *The World Journal of Men's Health* looks at yoga for managing premature ejaculation.[83] The study describes the connection between health and sexual function, including the links with diabetes, heart disease, and chronic illness. It mentions that while psychological disorders such as anxiety, depression, and stress are often associated with premature ejaculation, medications used to treat these conditions can come at a significant cost to sexual function.[83] The integrated approach of yoga therapy has been found to be effective in the management of many of these diseases. At its core, yoga involves a deep integration of mind and body, without which it is difficult to enjoy a fulfilling sex life. This study examines yoga in relation to breath control and pelvic floor muscle strength, which we know are vital to mental and physical health and to functional movement, something many other papers have touched on concerning sexual dysfunction.

There are many forms of yoga. Of the better-known types, Tantra yoga is generally perceived to focus on sex, although, in fact, Tantra is more accurately about connection, either with the self, a partner, or the divine. Scientists have supported the potential applications of Tantric practices as a holistic, accessible way to treat aspects of sexual dysfunction, such as mental blocks, premature ejaculation, erectile dysfunction, and intimacy issues.[84] Another branch of yoga called Kundalini can be used to intensify sexual pleasure[85] and to produce orgasms without ejaculation in men, resulting in sex that can last longer and involve multiple orgasms. A specific concept for conservation of semen, known as *Bindu Samrakshana*, was described in a fifteenth-century yogic treatise, *Hatha Yoga Pradeepika*.[86]

Unfortunately, modern perceptions concerning these practices have limited their therapeutic use. For instance, you may have heard of Tantric sex in association with the musician Sting. If you mention his name, the question of marathon sex is likely to come up. It turns out that claims he enjoyed seven-hour lovemaking sessions with his wife Trudie Styler were originally a joke. However, in an interview for *Inside the Actor's Studio*, he told host James Lipton that the concept of Tantric sex has its roots in a very serious belief system:

The idea of tantric sex is a spiritual act. I don't know any purer and better way of expressing a love for another individual than sharing that wonderful, I call it, "sacrament." I would stand by it. Not seven hours, but the idea.[87]

A 2011 article in the South African information website, *Independent Online* described the prevailing male attitude to yoga as akin to "declaring yourself a New Age hippy and wearing crystals."[88] Nevertheless, between 2012 and 2016, the number of men practicing yoga in the United States rose from 4 million to 10 million.[89] Yoga was long believed to be a traditionally male-only practice, although historians now argue that women played a central role in its development.[90] Now, in Western society, yoga for men is a rapidly growing trend with some classes being marketed as "Broga."[91]

Yoga has many benefits for everyone. Most yoga practices focus on the breath and have some element of pelvic floor muscle activation. Yoga improves nervous system function and hormonal balance and reduces age-related decreases in testosterone. It eases stress, suppresses the sympathetic nervous system, and promotes parasympathetic activation. Stimulation of the parasympathetic nervous system through yoga practice is believed to improve ejaculatory control, providing a nonpharmacological alternative to treatments such as fluoxetine for premature ejaculation.[92]

Yoga builds strength, stamina, flexibility, and muscle tone. It increases stability in the core muscles, improves control of pelvic and perineal muscles, and requires a focused interaction of breathing and movement. It is thought that the deep breathing, better cardiopulmonary efficiency, and mindfulness that develop through regular yoga practice may also improve ejaculation control due to better awareness that ejaculation is about to occur.

The 2019 study from *The World Journal of Men's Health* also reports that focused attention on abdominal breathing is associated with a marked increase in whole blood serotonin. A heightened level of serotonin is believed to improve ejaculatory control—SSRI antidepressants can cause delayed ejaculation in some men.[93]

The researchers suggest that yoga can provide the following benefits for men who experience premature ejaculation:

- Seated postures, in particular, relax the muscles of the pelvic region. Poor control of the pelvic floor muscles is implicated in premature ejaculation, urinary incontinence, and erectile dysfunction.

- Inverted postures improve the circulation to veins in the pelvis and perineum, enhancing the flow of blood to the sexual organs. (Recall that one value of nitric oxide is in increasing blood flow to the erectile tissues. This is the function that is enhanced by sexual performance drugs like Viagra.)

- Controlled breathing practice (*Pranayama*) is very effective in reducing heart rate and improving cardiovascular health. Specifically, diaphragmatic breathing reduces sympathetic activation and stimulates the vagus nerve, reducing anxiety. The study observed that after a five-minute practice of a *Pranayama* breathing technique, involving a respiratory rate of six breaths per minute, systolic and diastolic blood pressure markedly decreased.

- A yogic cleansing practice called a *Kriya*, which is done by exhaling forcefully and inhaling passively, both through the nose, may help delay ejaculation. A similar Tantric breathing technique, involving rapid exhalations through the mouth, can be practiced as orgasm approaches to trigger changes in blood chemistry that are believed to delay ejaculation.

- Meditation and mindfulness improve sexual well-being by increasing relaxation, body awareness, and autonomic nervous system balance.

Many treatment options are available for men who are confident enough to approach their doctor about premature ejaculation. Unfortunately, those treatments can cause side effects and affect sexual satisfaction. However, a lot of men never seek help at all due to the perceived stigmas around sexual dysfunction.[83] Yoga, as a nonpharmacological intervention or as a compliment to standard medical treatments, has been established in empirical studies as effective, although there is scant research into which techniques or postures may be most helpful. Even so, it is widely recognized that alternative methods, such as functional breath training and yoga, provide low cost, accessible alternatives that may benefit men who are uncomfortable discussing sexual problems with a healthcare professional. Breathing techniques also help bring focus onto the mind-body connection—an aspect missing in standard sex therapy—enriching the sex life. The 2019 study concludes that integration of these techniques into contemporary sex therapy could have a positive influence on different facets of human sexuality.[83]

## REACHING YOUR PEAK

Orgasm is characterized by certain physiological features including hyperventilation up to 40 breaths a minute, tachycardia (a very fast heart rate), and high blood pressure. A faster heart rate was found to be indicative of "real" (as opposed to fake) orgasm in men during heterosexual intercourse.[3] Orgasm also produces powerful, highly pleasurable contractions of the pelvic muscles. Intense sexual pleasure has been equated with trance states[94] and can even result in synesthesia—a light show akin to your very own fireworks.[95]

It is possible to train the breath to experience powerful orgasms. While orgasm is often associated with losing control, ancient practices like Tantra emphasize that control is of the utmost importance. If your goal is sexual ecstasy, you must first learn to master your sexual desire. For men, this involves a practice of forceful exhalation called *Kapalbhati* as orgasm approaches,[96] changing the blood biochemistry, and delaying ejaculation by reducing blood flow to the genitals. But there's more to it than prolonging sex. These techniques are part of a spiritual practice that may seem at odds with the Western idea of sex. In discussions of spirituality, some writers avoid the topic of sex altogether, but across a number of spiritual traditions, the concept of sexual energy is considered fundamental to spiritual growth.

In Tantra and Taoism, sexual energy is no less than the manifestation of our vital life force. The erotic sculptures in ancient Hindu temples display rapture rather than lust in the upturned faces of the lovers.[97] Descriptions of spiritualized sex involve extended intercourse and a sense of timelessness that makes them very different from everyday sex. Normally, we follow an automatic series of behaviors, movements, and fast breath patterns in which the desire to express love becomes sidelined in the search for physical pleasure.[97] These ancient practices teach us to take time and to reach new peaks.

In his book *Nature, Man and Woman*, Alan Watts describes how sex can give rise to extraordinary spiritual experiences.[98] He explains that, at its height, sexual love is one of the most complete experiences of which humans are capable, but that "prejudice and insensitivity have prevented us from seeing that in any other circumstances such delight would be called mystical ecstasy." The whole purpose of Tantra is to generate a transcendental state. In a 1981 edition of *Yoga Journal*, Dio Urmila Neff concludes that "Generating spiritual ecstasy may have been . . . [along with procreation] . . . the original purpose for sexual delight. It may indeed be our most precious grace."[97]

Whether you are interested in exploring the more esoteric concepts at play here or just want to enjoy a better, healthier sex life, for yourself or as a couple, these techniques all begin with the breath. *Prana* is the ancient word for breath—or life force. As the ancient yogic text *Shiva Samhita*, says,

> The wise man does not talk about the capacity of uttering words, about sight, hearing, or meditation; he speaks only of the different types of prana that makes all these things possible. Because everything else is nothing but manifestations of prana.[99, 100]

## WORTH WAITING FOR

Consciously controlled breathing has considerable benefits. Better oxygenation gives you more energy, so tiredness doesn't curtail your enjoyment or arousal. Sex that lasts longer before orgasm generally results in a more intense orgasm and greater satisfaction. Awareness of the breath can help you to overcome resistance, relax the muscles, and ease difficulty, for example during anal sex.[101]

According to Urmila Neff, the way you breathe during sex has "everything to do with its duration." Both Tantra and Taoism recommend deep nasal breathing from the diaphragm rather than fast, upper-chest mouth breathing. In discovering the functions of the vagus nerve and the diaphragm, we have learned that there is a direct relationship between the emotions and the breath, and this is thought to extend to sexual arousal too. While the breath is constant and normally unconscious, we can choose to change its depth and rhythm. By deliberately directing the breath, it is possible to modulate the emotions and temper sexual excitement.

Another connection lies in the idea that the breath is a rhythmic extension of the nervous and glandular systems. This idea of rhythm throughout the systems and its place in the sexual experience has recently been studied in the context of sexual trance.[94]

There are various methods that can be used to stop ejaculation, but the consensus is that fast breathing contributes to orgasm while slow breathing helps delay (and intensify) it. The first and most basic way in which breathwork can contribute is that it makes us more aware of the breath and more attuned to the body. This is significant because unless you have a certain awareness of your body, you are likely to employ any method of delaying orgasm too late. Also, until you become accustomed to working with the breath during rest, you will find it very difficult to adjust your breathing during sex.

For men, tantric breathing for "sexual continence" has two basic principles: first, rhythmic breathing through the nose to slow the metabolism and activate the parasympathetic nervous system, and second, breathing explosively through the mouth, which is important for the expression of feelings.[102] In yoga and Tantra, slow nasal breathing is used to control sexual energy. The fast breathing generates an explosive external orgasm—the faster the breath, the more effectively it works. When breathing is slower, we receive more vital energy. When it speeds up, we emit more energy. A daily practice of diaphragm breathing is essential to controlling ejaculation and increasing erotic sensation in the body.

In the book *The Multi-Orgasmic Man*, authors Mantak Chia and Douglas Abrams explain that because quick, shallow breathing increases the heart rate, and a fast heart rate is synonymous with orgasm, deep, slow breathing to slow the heart will control arousal and delay ejaculation.[45] The book describes how some men breathe quick, shallow breaths (the yogic *breath of fire*) while others find that holding the breath for a few moments on a deep inhalation lessens the urge to ejaculate.

In Tantra, once you have reached the goal to no longer ejaculate, you need to continue with the breathing exercises to learn how to channel your sexual energy into conscious mental energy. Diaphragm breathing massages the prostate and other internal organs, and it relieves the sense of pressure many men experience when they don't ejaculate. This tension in the genital area is common for men who are new to sexual continence practice. It is caused by a buildup of sexual energy in the pelvis. If this energy is not diverted, it causes irritability, anxiety, and confusion. At this stage, diaphragm breathing is used to guide the sexual energy up through the spine. Retaining sperm is not the only aspect to developing the ability to experience multiple whole-body orgasms: sexual energy must be transformed, and that is done with the breath.

## BACK TO BASICS AND THE THREE DIMENSIONS OF BREATHING

Learning any of these techniques begins with integrating light, slow, deep nasal breathing. It forms the basis for healthy breathing and is developed in the exercises in this book. Once you are familiar with how a healthy breathing pattern feels, you will be much freer to enjoy more specific breathing techniques. Becoming aware of your own breathing and that of your partner opens the way to many avenues of exploration. For instance, deep, mindful breathing can provide a way to relax and get in the mood before foreplay. By becoming conscious of the breath as you bring air into your belly, you can bring your awareness to the breath as it travels right down into the genitals. This awakens the area, infuses it with energy, and stimulates vasodilation, increasing blood flow to your sexual organs. While there are plenty of advanced methods out there, which are best approached with a qualified teacher, there are also simple things you can do for better sex.

When you breathe through your nose, you enjoy greater oxygen uptake, harness nitric oxide, and engage your core for better movement. Diaphragm breathing activates muscles that stretch between the coccyx and pubic bone. These are the muscles that contract during orgasm. By improving your BOLT score, you are less likely to get out of breath. Just as increasing the BOLT score can help alleviate breathlessness during exercise, reducing your sensitivity to blood $CO_2$ will help improve your stamina during sex. This can be especially valuable in the control of asthma symptoms and in alleviating the fear of exacerbations. It may also provide relief for people with epilepsy, because hyperventilation during sex is known to trigger seizures for some.[103] In this context, *Breathe Light* exercises and breath holding following an exhalation to improve the blood biochemistry should first be practiced outside of the bedroom.

It's common to tense up and hold the breath as orgasm approaches, but scientists have proven that hypoxia reduces sexual arousal.[104] This tendency to hold the breath can often be caused by self-consciousness. Opening the mouth in the lead up to orgasm means you're going to make more noise.

Many of us are conditioned by perceptions of how sex should sound. We alter our sexual groans and grunts into moans and sighs, perhaps to reflect what we've heard in erotic films. But it's important not to imitate the sounds you think are expected. This can repress orgasm and create tension in the breath. Instead, if you continue breathing deeply when the orgasm begins, you will enjoy a full-body sensation.

The idea of breath holding during sex may become a little confused with the idea that some people use behaviors such as asphyxiation or hanging to induce arousal. Unfortunately, the severity of these "games" to become aroused may gradually increase as tolerance to hypoxia develops, so these practices sometimes result in accidental death. A 2016 study reports that the mechanisms by which these methods create heightened pleasure for some people are complex and unclear,[104] and, although this relates to breathing practices and sex, there is not enough evidence to explore them here.

## PRACTICING ORGASMIC BREATH

Breath retention is a feature of the Tantric practice of *healing breath*.[105] This exercise has a ratio of 1:4:2 for inhalation, breath hold, and exhalation. The retention is four times longer than the inhalation, and the exhalation is twice as long. Breathe in for one second or heartbeat, hold for four seconds or four beats of the heart, and exhale for two seconds or two heartbeats. To practice this, you can gradually increase the length of the inhalation, maintaining the ratios between in-breath, retention, and out-breath. It is important not to practice too intensely to begin with. If you get dizzy or feel your heart beating too fast, stop the practice and breathe normally.

The exercise asks that you don't count mentally, because this takes the focus away from the breath. Instead, count using the heartbeat, or practice while walking, using the paces to keep track. In other words, practice the breathing during everyday life so that you feel the benefits during sex. The objective is to slow the breathing and to instill a profound level of calmness in the mind. This exercise is for men to practice in the lead up to orgasm to delay ejaculation and for women to deepen their orgasm. The best way to ensure you are able to bring your attention to the breath during sex, when you are bound to have your mind elsewhere, is to practice the breathing exercises for developing control of your breathing during day-to-day life.

Breath retention is also used in the yogic practice of orgasmic breath, *sushumna nadi Pranayama.*[106] This exercise is designed to pull energy from the base of the pelvis up through the chakras, filling the body with life force. It involves working the muscles of the pelvic floor and focusing on the breath and the physical body to reach a meditative or orgasmic state. It uses a technique of reduced mouth breathing similar to sipping through a straw. According to Courtney Avery, creator of the San Diego sexual-health-based yoga business Intimate Health, LLC, "the more you practice meditation, the more you train your brain to come into an orgasmic state." When you add breathwork and activation of the muscles, "magic happens."

With practice, it becomes possible to bring yourself to full-body orgasm using only the breath and muscle engagement. You should avoid practicing this technique during menstruation or if you are experiencing pelvic pain.

- Sit comfortably in an upright posture and breathe normally.
- On your next inhalation, purse your lips as if you were sipping through a straw.
- Breathe in through your pursed lips and engage your pelvic floor muscles. Keep your buttocks relaxed and your muscles engaged.
- Continue to breathe in as if you are sipping, while being aware of the muscles and the energy that is lifting through the spine.
- Pull in your lower abdominal muscles and tuck in your belly button.
- Relax and widen your chest and shoulders.
- Lengthen your neck and tuck in your chin.
- When you feel "full up" with air, seal your lips and hold your breath, engaging all the muscles along the length of your spine.
- When you are ready to release, slightly open your mouth. Visualize the energy pouring from the top of your head down the front of your body, gently softening your muscles as it flows down.
- Relax your neck, shoulders, belly, and abdominal muscles.
- Finally, release the pelvic floor muscles and surrender.
- When you have finished, relax, and breathe normally for a few breaths, remaining in a state of calm relaxation.
- Repeat the exercise up to 13 times.

The key lies in practice. By beginning to explore the breath by yourself, you can prepare to share new experiences with your partner. Try practicing nasal breathing before jumping into bed. Pay attention to your pelvic floor muscles. It allows you to engage those muscles and heightens sensation in your genitals, increasing pleasure.

You can also experiment with exercises that synchronize your breath with your partner's. You can do this sitting face to face, holding hands, hugging, touching foreheads—anything, as long as you are physically connected. You can try lying down and embracing. Again, the practice uses gentle breath retention:

- Exhale all the way out.
- Slowly inhale together, breathing from the diaphragm.
- Pause together at the top of the breath, feeling full of life-giving energy.
- Gently exhale together, all the way out.
- Pause again at the bottom of the exhalation, feeling safe and empty.
- Slowly inhale.
- As you breathe, imagine the breath carrying energy throughout your body.
- Repeat the exercise as many times as you like.

This exercise simply involves mindful breathing, exhaling and inhaling through the nose, breathing from the diaphragm, and gently bringing your breath into sync with your partner. If you want, you can continue this as you make love, exploring how the calm feeling of breathing together enhances intimacy.

# CHAPTER TWELVE
# YES, BREATHING IS DIFFERENT FOR WOMEN

---

## AN UNHELPFUL BIAS

Historically, in most physiology literature and, indeed, across every field of science, research has predominantly focused on male subjects. This gender bias can be seen in many areas of study and in trials using both humans and animals.[1-5]

However, it is now known that gender differences do affect breathing control and vulnerability to some respiratory diseases. For example, women recover better after a severe episode of hypoxia. There are also differences in sleep apnea[1] and heart rate variability.[6] The reasons are not properly understood, but the disparity between sexes might explain many otherwise contradictory findings. It has been said that where the influence of gender is disregarded, the progress of scientific knowledge can only be held back.[7]

Another anomaly is that, when women take part in studies, researchers often fail to account for the fluctuations in hormone levels that occur during the menstrual cycle.[1, 8] This is despite the fact that the menstrual cycle is one of the most important biological rhythms that modulate the physiological processes of a living being. Airflow and gas exchange are known to be among the many vital functions that change during the menstrual cycle[9]. Studies have demonstrated, for example, that women's ventilatory responses to hypoxia and hypercapnia vary throughout the 28-day cycle directly parallel with hormonal fluctuations.

In all honesty, I avoided this topic in my own work for many years, largely because as a man I didn't feel qualified to discuss it. However, I am aware of the growing frustration that women's health, particularly in regard to menopause, has been brushed under the carpet for too long. I wanted to address this by sharing research and connections to the three dimensions of breathing that might be helpful. In my coaching, I work with as many women as men, and their experience with breathwork is incredibly informative. Also,

I always aim to be guided by the questions people ask me and to find ways to answer them. In putting this and the next chapter together, I am grateful for the guidance, assistance, and experience of two female medical doctors, along with help from several other brilliant women.

## THE MENSTRUAL CYCLE

There are several "phases" to the menstrual cycle, which are important to recognize in understanding the issues surrounding breathing in women. Some are familiar, but the changes through the month are mainly invisible. Unless you are trying to conceive (or trying not to), you may not have given much thought to how the cycle works. The different stages and events in the cycle are:

- **Menstruation:** This is your "period." The lining of the uterus sheds and you bleed. During this time, levels of estrogen and progesterone are low[10].
- **The follicular phase:** This is the time between the first day of your period and ovulation. Estrogen rises as your body prepares to release an egg.
- **The proliferative phase:** The lining of your uterus builds up again after your period.
- **Ovulation:** The egg is released from your ovary midcycle. Estrogen levels peak just before this happens and drop shortly after.
- **The luteal phase:** This is the time between ovulation and the start of menstruation. Because this is the stage when the body prepares for a potential pregnancy, progesterone is produced, peaks, and then drops. This is the phase most associated with hyperventilation as progesterone levels fluctuate.
- **The secretory phase:** The lining of the uterus produces chemicals that will either support an early pregnancy or prepare the lining to break down and shed during your next period.

## WAYS BREATHING IS DIFFERENT FOR WOMEN

The regulation of breathing is complex and affected by many factors, including gender. In 1905, it was first found that the resting pressure of blood $CO_2$

was around 8% lower in women than in men,[1] and this finding has since been confirmed. On average, women have lower ventilation than men, in part due to smaller airways, rib cages, and lung volumes, as well as diaphragms that are around 9% shorter.[11] Ventilation was first linked to levels of sex hormones in 1904 when Adolf Magnus-Levy, a pioneer in the study of human metabolism, observed that women hyperventilate during pregnancy[1]. Later, it was found that women also hyperventilate during the luteal phase of their menstrual cycle, and research confirmed that the cyclical variations in ventilation are no longer present in postmenopausal women.[1] This last fact clearly links changes in breathing to fluctuations in sex hormones.

A 2006 study reported that the female hormone progesterone, which is known to stimulate breathing, might contribute to respiratory changes seen at different times of the menstrual cycle.[12] General respiratory function is known to be influenced both by the different phases of the menstrual cycle and by common hormonal and metabolic states.[11] This can have an impact on health.

When the first occurrence of menstruation is early (early menarche), the likelihood of poor health in later life increases, with a higher risk of illnesses, including asthma, cardiovascular disease, and compromised lower lung function.[11] The instances of poor respiratory health in girls who reach puberty early may be due to factors such as higher body mass index, which can cause early menarche. However, research suggests that early onset of puberty may affect airway and lung development, because to some extent, puberty signals a termination of growth.[13]

The menstrual cycle influences disorders as varied as epilepsy, bipolar disorder, migraine, and rheumatoid arthritis.[13] Respiratory symptoms such as breathlessness, coughing, and wheezing vary considerably over the 28 days. These become worse between days 10 and 22 (the midluteal to midfollicular phases),[13] possibly due to the influence of hormonal changes on the airways.[13] This explains why asthma severity fluctuates during the menstrual cycle, and why irregular menstruation is associated with a higher risk of asthma.[13]

Increasingly, evidence indicates that sex hormones can either contribute to disease pathology or serve as protective factors against lung disease. They regulate the development of the lung and airways in unborn babies, and it is thought that they play a part in the varying adverse effects of antenatal smoking on lung function. The lung function of adult men is more severely affected by exposure to smoking in the womb than that of women. Scientists also believe that sex hormones may cause changes in the growth pathway of the lungs in response to in utero exposure to smoking.[14] This would suggest that males and females have a different susceptibility to inflammation from an early stage of development.

Breathing pattern disorders are also almost twice as common in women, possibly due to the hormonal influences we've already touched on. Progesterone stimulates the respiratory rate, meaning that in the luteal phase of the menstrual cycle $CO_2$ levels drop by around 25%.[15] When $CO_2$ levels are already low, any extra stress can cause breathing to speed up even more, and this creates a range of symptoms that are commonly interpreted as premenstrual syndrome.[16]

In 2000, a study in the *Journal of Orofacial Pain* reported increased respiratory rates during the luteal phase of the menstrual cycle, when progesterone levels increase.[17] At the same time as breathing increased, pain thresholds lowered. This indicates that cyclical respiratory changes may also influence pain perception.

## PAIN CONDITIONS AND BREATHING IN WOMEN

### FIBROMYALGIA

Fibromyalgia predominantly affects women,[18] and it changes during the menstrual cycle. In 2007, researchers found that several participants fulfilled the diagnostic criteria for fibromyalgia during the luteal phase of their cycle, but not during the follicular phase. As pain is the most common diagnostic measure of fibromyalgia, this is another indicator that pain perception differs depending on the concentration of sex hormones in the body.

Dysfunctional breathing can aggravate pain associated with fibromyalgia, especially in tender areas of the upper body.[19] This can lead to fatigue and difficulty carrying out normal daily activities. A 2017 paper assessed the impact of an eight-week functional breathing program on 18 patients with fibromyalgia.[20] Thresholds for pain tolerance increased in all the participants after one month, which means that pain was reduced. Sleep quality, duration, and efficiency also improved as a result of the breathing practice.[20]

A 2018 study examined the effects of breathing exercises on pain tolerance in tender points and on the quality of life for fibromyalgia patients.[19] The trial involved 35 women aged between 34 and 67 years, all with fibromyalgia. The women were randomly assigned to a breathing exercise group or to a control group. The breathing exercise participants practiced for 30 minutes every day for 12 weeks. At the end of the 12 weeks, the women who had practiced breathing exercises showed significant improvements, experiencing much lower levels of pain and fatigue and becoming more able to engage with daily life. The researchers concluded that breathing exercises provide a "real and effective intervention" for women with fibromyalgia.

A 2019 trial, also examining fibromyalgia, looked at the effectiveness and safety of patient self-management in the form of unsupervised breathing exercises.[19] After 12 weeks, during which 51 women practiced the exercises, no statistical differences were found between supervised and unsupervised participants. There were, however, added improvements in pain in those women who had practiced the exercises under supervision, suggesting that proper guidance in performing breathing exercises is beneficial.

Faulty breathing does not cause fibromyalgia. However, it does play a significant role in the development and persistence of chronic pain conditions.[15] For instance, biomechanical overuse combined with the biochemical changes typical of breathing pattern disorders can have a significant impact on pain and fatigue.[21] In fact, most people with fibromyalgia show signs of severe dysfunctional breathing. Because breathing is already dysfunctional, these women are constantly teetering on the brink of symptoms. Any further cyclical drop in $CO_2$ is likely to push the body over the edge. That is why pain often becomes much worse during the luteal phase of the menstrual cycle. It is also why the worst symptoms could be alleviated or even eliminated with correct breathing habits.[22]

Research shows that 27% of people with fibromyalgia hyperventilate, and 60% of fibromyalgia patients suffer with *dyspnea* (breathlessness).[23] Also, breathlessness is far more prevalent in the patients with the highest levels of pain.[24]

Naturally, fibromyalgia can trigger anxiety. This is not to imply that symptoms are "all in the mind," but anxiety about the condition and anxiety triggered by dysfunctional breathing itself can certainly aggravate pain and fatigue. Because pain causes anxiety and increases the breathing rate, it is likely that by normalizing the breathing pattern, pain symptoms would reduce.

Once a pattern of dysfunctional breathing exists, a variety of triggers can create a vicious cycle, causing pain, fatigue, and other symptoms, including anxiety and panic attacks. These, in turn, contribute to poor breathing patterns. Poor oxygenation of the tissues during hyperventilation contributes to the development of myofascial trigger points.[21] And because the working of the diaphragm is linked to the functioning of the pelvic floor, dysfunctional breathing exacerbates stress incontinence, other genitourinary symptoms, and pain in the pelvic region—all common in fibromyalgia. The fascia around the psoas muscle—a hip-joint flexor that runs from the lumbar spine through the pelvis—connects directly to the diaphragm.[25] Women who suffer with chronic pelvic pain often have poor functional movement and tend to breathe predominantly into the upper chest.[26]

Many people with chronic pain suffer with medically unexplained symptoms. They may be diagnosed with fibromyalgia, chronic fatigue, or "bodily distress syndrome."[27] Low blood $CO_2$ and feelings of air hunger are typical of all these patients.[28] As a result, scientists believe that levels of $CO_2$ should be assessed as part of the patient evaluation.[24] At the very least, it needs to be recognized that a significant number of fibromyalgia patients hyperventilate. Given that hyperventilation is considered at the severe end of breathing pattern disorders, it is logical to assume that a much higher number have poor breathing patterns.

Leon Chaitow, after 50 years clinical experience working with fibromyalgia patients, estimated that more than 90% breathe dysfunctionally.[15] Functional breathing training is an efficient and cost-effective treatment to achieve reduced levels of pain and fatigue. The ability to fully exhale is at the root of functional breathing. Without this understanding, it is not possible to inhale correctly. Chaitow cautions that this is not a quick fix. Between 12 and 26 weeks of work may be needed, and it takes patience to achieve behavioral change.[15]

In chronic pain conditions, it is particularly important to take things slowly in the beginning. Approaching breathing exercises too intensively can actually set you back. Begin the practice gently. If you suffer with fibromyalgia, your sensitivity to $CO_2$ may be very high. This can trigger too much air hunger, muscular tension, and feelings of panic. As your tolerance to $CO_2$ increases and your BOLT score improves, these feelings will ease.

## TEMPOROMANDIBULAR JOINT DISORDER

In Chapter Six, on pain, we looked at temporomandibular joint disorder (TMD) and its relationship to dysfunctional breathing. However, there is evidence that a link also exists between the condition and female sex hormones.

Gender differences in pain sensitivity are sometimes dismissed as matters of psychosocial and social conditioning[29]. Increasingly, however, it is believed that hormonal and other biological factors contribute[30,31]. Temporomandibular joint disorder is around 1.5 to 2 times more prevalent in women[32] and can be much worse than in men. Anatomically, women produce much higher levels of pressure in the temporomandibular joint when clenching than men[33]. It was traditionally thought that abnormalities in the alignment of the jaws and teeth are the primary cause of TMD, but if this were the case, the condition should be just as common in men as women. The estrogen hormone, estradiol (E2), which is the primary female sex hormone,[34] has been found to be a risk factor for temporomandibular pain in rats.[35] Incidence of TMD in women is thought to peak between 20 and 40 years, coinciding with reproductive function and decreasing in menopause when estrogen production declines.[36]

Hyperventilation during the second part of the menstrual cycle can contribute to temporomandibular pain. This is partly due to hyperventilation-induced adaptations in posture and to changes in the blood acid-base balance. For instance, the respiratory alkalosis that occurs when blood $CO_2$ drops is known to trigger muscle pain, while overbreathing can cause a forward head posture.

Postural adaptations including a forward-thrust of the head and rounded shoulders are common among people with dysfunctional breathing patterns. This often begins in childhood due to open mouth breathing caused by swollen adenoids. Equally, there is a chicken-and-egg scenario where poor posture from sedentary desk work can adversely impact breathing.[37] According to a 2019 article on the website *Spine Universe*, which describes sitting as "worse than smoking" in terms of health, 70% of people spend six or more hours a day sitting down.[37]

A forward head posture contributes to TMD because it reduces "freeway space." Freeway space is the distance between the upper and lower teeth when the jaw is in its rest position. When the head is pushed forward, the back teeth connect and pressure on the temporomandibular joint increases. Restoring freeway space is considered important in treating TMD.[29]

As with other pain conditions, symptoms of TMD fluctuate cyclically in line with the menstrual cycle. In the luteal phase of the cycle, estradiol and progesterone are released. Both hormones cause blood $CO_2$ levels to fall,[38] affecting the amount of air breathed per minute.[12] The pain associated with temporomandibular disorder increases toward the latter part of the menstrual cycle, peaking in the first three days of menstruation when progesterone levels increase and then decline. A second spike in pain coincides with ovulation,[36] when estrogen levels fluctuate. The worst pain corresponds with low or changing estrogen levels.[36] While the influence of sex hormones on pain is still relatively unstudied, the general consensus is that changes in breathing patterns across the menstrual cycle likely contribute to temporomandibular joint pain.

## MIGRAINE

Temporomandibular joint disorder is a risk factor for migraine[39] and tension headache.[40] At the same time, psychological conditions such as depression and anxiety are common to people with temporomandibular pain, migraines, and tension headaches.[41] It has been suggested that rather than the problem in the jaw causing the headache or migraine, these disorders develop and progress via the same underlying imbalances in the central nervous system.[39] This may be why relaxation techniques that influence the nervous system are effective for the relief of both migraine[42] and tension headaches.[43]

A case described in the *Journal of Neurology, Neurosurgery & Psychiatry* in 2004 demonstrated that hyperventilation,[44] both during rest and following physical exertion, "may cause severe, acute, 'explosive' headaches" and that these could be prevented with relaxation exercises and physical therapy. The precise cause of the headache in this case study was not identified, but researchers suggested that breathing exercises may prevent excessive hyperventilation after exercise, although they "would not prevent physiological exercise induced hyperventilation." They suggest that hyperventilation should be considered in all patients whose headaches are triggered by exertion.

It is important to remember that you can prevent exercise-induced hyperventilation by practicing nasal breathing while exercising and by improving your BOLT score. You can also make a conscious effort to bring your breathing and heart rate under control after exercising with a slow breathing practice.

Hypercapnia (high blood $CO_2$) has been found to stop the onset of migraines by increasing cerebral oxygenation—by dilating the blood vessels in the brain. Researchers in a 2018 pilot study tested to find out whether a self-administered partial rebreathing device would be effective for migraine patients.[45] A partial rebreathing device is exactly what it sounds like—a machine through which the patient "rebreathes" exhaled air, which has higher levels of $CO_2$ than room air. To some extent, the same effect can be achieved by wearing a face mask or covering.

Eight women and three men with an average age of around 35 took part in the trial. They each self-administered either the rebreathing device or a placebo in response to migraine attacks. The results showed that the partial rebreathing device increased end-tidal $CO_2$ by 24% and maintained oxygen saturation at over 97%. The intensity of headache symptoms after two hours was significantly less with the rebreathing device. What's more, the device became more effective the more it was used, with even better results with consecutive treatments. There were no adverse reactions, and side effects were nonexistent or mild. The researchers concluded that induced hypercapnia presents a promising alternative or add-on treatment for migraine patients and further work should be done to investigate the benefits in a larger population.

The fact that the efficiency of the rebreathing device increased from one treatment to the next corresponds with what we know about reduced-volume breathing. Regular practice of breathing exercises to increase levels of $CO_2$ results in reduced sensitivity to $CO_2$, and lighter, slower breathing, as evidenced by a higher BOLT score.

The 2018 hypercapnia study was preceded nearly 40 years earlier by an investigation into the relationship between migraines and blood $CO_2$.[46] A 1980 paper described the effects of $CO_2$ on blood vessels and circulation in the brain, noting that anesthetists "regularly hyperventilate patients to reduce brain volume during neurosurgery." The researchers hypothesized that, if migraine falls into two categories, dilatory and constriction-based, retaining $CO_2$ during sleep could trigger migraines by dilating the blood vessels, or hyperventilation provoked by "excitement, anxiety, or expectation of physical or sexual activity" could trigger migraines by constricting the blood vessels.

The results showed that hyperventilation occurred at the peak of the migraine, making the attack seem worse than it was. The researchers suggested that not only was the perception of the migraine heightened but symptoms were increased by the constriction of the blood vessels caused by the hyperventilation. This suggests that $CO_2$ may play a part in the onset and persistence of migraines.

In 2015, another paper in *Medicine* found a correlation between sleep-disordered breathing and migraine in adults but not in elderly people.[47] While more research is needed, it is thought that poor breathing patterns during sleep could be either a trigger or a predisposing factor for the development of migraines.

None of these papers mention the connection between the incidence of migraine and the menstrual cycle.[48] Various other studies have identified an increase in the risk of migraine without aura on the first two days of menstrual flow, a reduced risk coinciding with the time of ovulation, and much more prolonged headaches three to seven days before menstruation.[48] (Aura is a common neurological symptom of migraine usually involving visual disturbances such as flashing lights before the eyes, tunnel vision, and temporary blind spots.)

In one 2004 study, researchers observed that women were 25% more likely to suffer from a migraine in the five days before their period, with the risk increasing to 71% in the two days before, peaking on the first day of menstruation and on the next two days. This was confirmed in 2007 when scientists found that the highest occurrence of migraine coincided with the first three days of a woman's period.[49] Menstrual migraine is linked to increased menstrual disability and distress—a fact that recently led to the development of specific diagnostic criteria for menstrual migraine.[48]

Pure menstrual migraine and menstrually related migraine are slightly different. To characterize the migraine type, menstruation is defined either as bleeding as part of the normal menstrual cycle or as the withdrawal of progesterone in women who take combined oral contraceptives or cyclical hormone replacement therapy. Pure menstrual migraine is a migraine without aura that occurs on the first day of menstruation or the two days either side of it, in two out of three cycles, with no incidence at other times in the cycle. Most women will suffer from menstrually related migraines—a migraine without aura that occurs at other times of the month.[48]

Interestingly, the estrogen steroid hormone estradiol, which is implicated in temporomandibular joint pain, is also a factor in the onset and progression of menstrual migraines. Scientists claim that by maintaining levels of estrogen during the luteal phase of the cycle, it is possible to prevent menstrual attacks.[50] This is particularly relevant for women who take hormonal contraceptives or those with irregular periods. It has been suggested that continuous hormones in place of the usual "three weeks on, one week off" (known as a 21/7 regimen) may prevent the estrogen withdrawal that triggers the headache. This idea is based more on clinical practice than on research trial data,[50, 51] but this does not detract from the validity of the evidence.

In one study, a 168-day placebo-free regime of hormonal contraceptives, where hormones were taken at regular levels every day, helped relieve headache severity and improve work productivity and day-to-day function, compared to the normal 21/7 pattern. In a placebo-free contraceptive regime, the same levels of hormones are taken every day without a "break." In another trial, a transdermal contraceptive (a patch worn on the skin to prevent ovulation), when used for 84 days consecutively, resulted in fewer headaches compared with the standard 21/7 contraceptive regimen.[53]

Research into menstrual migraine is limited. It should be noted, however, that women who suffer from migraine with aura should not take combined hormonal contraceptives due to an increased risk of ischemic stroke.[54] More study of the link between sex hormones and migraines, and of the possible genetic predisposition in some women is needed to develop more targeted diagnosis and treatment. Nonetheless, it is important to understand that the functions of the sex hormones are not confined to the reproductive system—they are active in the nervous systems too.

## PELVIC FLOOR DYSFUNCTIONS

Another aspect of pain and function specific to women is the connection between the breath, pelvic floor function, and sacroiliac joint stability.[55] The sacroiliac joint connects the pelvis to the spine, essentially supporting the weight of the upper body. The pelvic floor and the diaphragm are structurally and functionally connected by fascia and muscles,[56] especially the pubococcygeus—the muscle that controls urine flow[57] and contracts during orgasm.[58]

The skeletal and muscular systems of the pelvis have been described as a unit forming the base of a lumbopelvic "cylinder" with the diaphragm at the top and the transversus abdominis at the sides.[59] The spinal column runs through the center of this cylinder, supported by elements of the lower back, psoas, and abdominal muscles. Because the psoas fibers merge with the diaphragm and the pelvic floor, stiffness or dysfunction in any of these muscles is likely to affect the ability of the diaphragm to function normally, impacting the stability of the spine.

Analysis of over 38,000 telephone interviews showed that middle-aged and older women were more likely to experience back pain alongside breathing difficulties. It also showed that problems with both incontinence and back pain might be due to physical limitations of functional movement, posture, and respiration in the trunk.[60] The fact is, if the muscles of the pelvic floor are dysfunctional, compensatory muscle activity may interfere with the activity of the pelvic floor, compromising spinal stability and possibly resulting in urinary incontinence. The results of a 2007 study into pelvic floor and abdominal muscle function in women indicated that women with incontinence actually have *increased* activity in these muscles.[60] Researchers concluded that their finding "challenges the clinical assumption that incontinence is associated with reduced pelvic floor muscle activity."

Women with chronic pelvic pain frequently breathe into the upper chest. They have poor coordination in basic functions such as sitting, standing, and walking, and very stiff muscles in the lower back and hips. In a 2007 interview, Dr. Leon Chaitow explained that, when normal diaphragm breathing is restored and the pelvic floor muscles are relaxed, it is relatively easy to reestablish function in the pelvic floor.[61] Dysfunction in pelvic muscles affects the stability of the spine and pelvis, while hyperventilation contributes to problems with motor control.

Normalizing imbalances in the joints and soft tissues, along with postural and functional breathing training, has the potential to modify, relieve, or eliminate symptoms, including chronic pelvic pain. Chaitow explains that manual deactivation of trigger points and physical relaxation exercises, combined with breathing rehabilitation, "offer a practical way forward."

Conversely, because the pelvic floor mechanism can affect diaphragm movement and the function of the lungs, the authors of a 2015 study also suggest including pelvic-floor-strengthening exercises in breathing rehabilitation programs.[62]

Many chronic symptoms relating to the urethra, bladder, lower bowel, and prostate can be caused, maintained, or aggravated by active myofascial trigger points in the muscles of the pelvic area.[61] When these trigger points are helping stabilize hypermobile joints or enhance the stability of the pelvic floor, their deactivation may ease pain at the cost of stability. It is therefore necessary to first address the underlying causes of the instability. As we discovered in the chapters on functional movement and pain, trigger points can be the result of psychological stress. They are a sign of autonomic imbalance, and the autonomic nervous system can be regulated through the practice of slow, light diaphragm breathing. It is also important to remember that the respiratory alkalosis intrinsic to hyperventilation encourages the development of myofascial trigger points.

Trigger points, clenched pelvic floor muscles, and hyperactivity of the muscles can sometimes be caused by psychological issues, including a history of abuse or assault, or by excessive tone created by a background of athletics, dance, or badly taught Pilates. When a psychosexual or psychosocial element is present, appropriate therapeutic support is necessary alongside breath and bodywork.[61]

## FEMALE HORMONES, LUNG HEALTH, SLEEP, AND ANXIETY

There is evidence that some respiratory illnesses behave differently in women than in men. Asthma, for instance, is more common in women. However, its prevalence changes with age.[11] In childhood, more boys have asthma than girls, but once puberty hits, women are more susceptible, and their symptoms fluctuate through the menstrual cycle.

Up to 40% of women report premenstrual asthma symptoms that can lead to severe attacks.[11] One study of girls aged between 8 and 17 years found that girls who begin menstruating earlier tend to develop more severe asthma after puberty.[63] The fact that respiratory symptoms change as hormone levels fluctuate indicates that sex hormones contribute to the onset and persistence of asthma.[1, 64] This theory is further confirmed by the fact that 20% of asthmatic women suffer from worse symptoms during pregnancy[11] and that female sex hormones can make the severe form of asthma even worse.[65]

A 2009 study compared respiratory function in women with and without asthma over the course of the menstrual cycle. In all women, forced expiratory volume and blood gas transfer varied through the menstrual cycle, peaking during menstruation and declining to the lowest point in the early luteal phase when progesterone was at its highest. Forced expiratory volume is an important measure of lung function, measuring the volume of air that can be forced out in one second after taking a deep breath. The cyclical respiratory changes occurred by way of very different physiological mechanisms in women with asthma compared to healthy women. In asthmatic women, cyclical variations in gas exchange were due to differences in the functioning of the alveoli[66]. These changes were consistent, regardless of inhaled corticosteroid or hormonal contraceptive use.

As hormone levels fluctuate over the 28-day cycle, blood vessels in the lungs are constantly forming and disappearing. This impacts the way the lungs take in oxygen because it affects ventilation perfusion. These findings begin to provide insight into the way asthma presents in women, why difficult-to-control, severe asthma is more common among women, and why exacerbations occur in the luteal phase. Female sex hormones also contribute to asthma exacerbations in women who are overweight because obesity causes imbalances in the levels of estrogen and progesterone.[67]

Another factor in the way asthma presents is the size and collapsibility of the airway[11]. Men tend to experience much more airway collapsibility, while women are more prone to inflammation in the airways.[68]

In one 2010 study, hormone replacement therapy (HRT) was linked with a high number of cases of newly diagnosed asthma in menopausal women.[69, 70] Some research also shows that menopausal women who are given hormone replacement medications experience worse asthma. One trial assessed 184 women aged between 34 and 68 over the course of 10 years and found that E2 (estradiol/estrogen) replacement therapy increased the incidence of asthma.[71] However, more recent papers contradict this finding, specifying that women are more likely to experience airway obstruction if they do not take HRT.[72] While the literature is limited and sometimes confusing, these findings begin to paint the picture that certain features of asthma are unique to women, including the much greater prevalence of symptoms that are severe or difficult to control and the phenomenon of premenstrual asthma exacerbations.[66]

COPD (chronic obstructive pulmonary disorder) is a condition in which patients have ongoing hypercapnia and hypoxia due to impaired lung gas exchange. It causes dysfunctional muscles that are easily fatigued, have reduced strength and endurance, and a tendency to atrophy.[73] COPD has traditionally been thought of primarily as a disorder affecting older men, but recent years have seen an increase of incidence and a significant rise in mortality in women.[74] This is thought to be, at least in part, due to smoking.

While the number of smokers is decreasing across North America and Europe, more women than ever are smoking in developing countries where the health risks are less known. For instance, a 2009 study found that only 38% of smokers in China knew that smoking could cause heart disease,[75] and even in developed countries, there is a degree of ignorance. Women are also more likely to be exposed to passive smoking than men, they develop COPD with less smoking history than men, and their decline in lung function is faster.[11] It is interesting that the resilience shown by females against maternal smoking compared to males reverses in adulthood.

COPD is an umbrella term rather than a specific disease. There are differences in the way it manifests in women. Emphysema, a debilitating "end state" of COPD, in which the alveoli become damaged and the patient requires constant oxygen, is more common in men. Women tend to display more reactive airways—irritation, inflammation, and infection—and more pronounced narrowing of the airways[11]. Long-term oxygen therapy is more effective in women, and women have a much greater improvement in lung function once they stop smoking. Estrogen is involved in maintaining cell structures and in the elasticity of the lungs that keeps the airways open.[76] Cigarette smoke has an antiestrogen effect,[77] and this may contribute to impaired lung function in women who smoke or inhale secondhand smoke.[76, 78]

In 2019, a study investigated whether female sex hormones contribute to COPD.[79] Researchers found that women who had used oral contraceptives were less likely to be hospitalized or to die with COPD. However, women who had started their periods later than 15 years old and those who experienced early menopause were more at risk. Early onset of puberty, which is a risk factor for asthma,[63] had an impact on lung function (how well the lungs work) but not on COPD. Women with a history of polycystic ovary syndrome (PCOS), ovarian cysts, HRT use, and surgery to remove the ovaries and/or fallopian tubes were all at higher risk of COPD, although their lung function was likely to be better. This corresponds with the finding that women were less susceptible to emphysema than men. Remember, COPD is an umbrella term, and symptoms can affect breathing to a greater or lesser extent. Scientists concluded that a variety of aspects of reproductive health throughout a woman's life can contribute to COPD-related hospitalization and death or to lung health. More work is needed to understand the complex links between COPD and sex hormones in terms of HRT,[11, 79] ovarian cysts, PCOS, and hysterectomy.

According to a 2018 clinical review, lung cancer mortality is increasing in women but not men. The number of women who die each year from lung cancer is greater than the combined female mortality rate for breast, uterine, and ovarian cancer.[11] A woman who doesn't smoke is three times more likely to be diagnosed with lung cancer than a nonsmoking man, indicating a possible hormonal influence. However, women have a better prognosis, in terms of chemotherapy and surgical response, and a higher five-year survival rate.

Pulmonary hypertension—high blood pressure in the blood vessels that supply the lungs—is more common in women and occurs around 10 years earlier in women than in men. Again, more research is needed to understand the role of the sex hormones, and to discover if and how estrogen increases female susceptibility to lung disorders.[11]

While there are differences between women and men across many respiratory conditions, it is still largely unknown whether these disparities are behavioral, social, environmental, or biological. To date, most research has simply concluded that more work is needed to ascertain the role of hormones in lung health.[11, 80]

## SLEEP-DISORDERED BREATHING

We have already discussed snoring, insomnia, and sleep apnea in detail (Chapter Seven), but here again, there are differences between men and women in sleep-disordered breathing, and these are worth mentioning. There is a higher prevalence of sleep apnea in men, perhaps due to a greater collapsibility of the airways.[11] But once women reach menopause, there is about a

200% increase in the incidence of sleep apnea.[I] This occurs independently of other risk factors, indicating that female sex hormones, thought to have a protective effect on the airways and ventilatory drive, could guard against sleep apnea in premenopausal women.[II]

Young and middle-aged women are far less prone to apneas than men, but older women experience much more sleep disturbance. Reduced levels of progesterone and estradiol (estrogen) contribute to the incidence of sleep-disordered breathing.[81] Replacement of these hormones decreases apnea frequency compared with untreated postmenopausal women.[82] Premenopausal women with severe obstructive sleep apnea have much lower progesterone than healthy women and women with mild OSA.[83] The gender differences in the prevalence of sleep apnea decreases after menopause, indicating that the menopausal status itself plays a part in OSA. Progesterone is known to improve the tone of the upper airway muscles.[II] Levels of the hormone decrease after menopause, which is one reason why postmenopausal women become more susceptible to sleep-disordered breathing. A 2015 study found that progesterone reduces sleep apnea in menopausal women.[84]

Another contributing factor is a change in the way body fat is distributed. After menopause, women are likely to have more body fat, and this tends to be concentrated in the upper body, where fat on the tongue, neck, and abdomen is a common anatomical factor in sleep apnea. Fat on the throat narrows the airway, causing increased resistance to breathing and greater airway collapsibility. Fat on the tongue takes up space in the mouth and may encroach on the airway. Extra weight on the belly reduces the amplitude of diaphragm movements, causing a decrease in lung volume and more frequent collapse of the upper airways during sleep.

The results of a 1988 study comparing incidence of sleep-disordered breathing in obese men and women found that obese women have an increased chemosensitivity to hypoxia and hypercapnia when compared to women of a healthy weight. Breathing is often noticeable in overweight women, even at rest. Fast, upper chest breathing with no pause after the exhalation and feelings of breathlessness are typical. While it would make sense that the increased sensitivity to blood $CO_2$ could be caused by oxygen desaturation and poor breathing during sleep, the same change in chemosensitivity in relation to body fat load is not present in obese men.[85]

Similarly, pregnancy increases the incidence of OSA by around 8% due to increased neck circumference, greater nasal congestion, and pharyngeal edema, a swelling in the tissues of the throat. In the later stages of pregnancy, there is also less room for the diaphragm to function, reducing lung volume and triggering upper airway collapse. As a result of these considerations, snoring is considered a primary risk factor in pregnancy-induced hypertension.[86] (We will look in more detail at OSA during pregnancy in the next chapter.)

## ANXIETY DISORDERS

Women are between two and three times more likely to develop panic disorder than men.[1] This susceptibility may be linked to sex hormones. Women with panic disorder experience a worsening of their panic symptoms and anxiety during the premenstrual phase of their cycle.[87, 88] Studies in rats have shown that withdrawal of progesterone increased susceptibility to panic-related anxiety, indicating that the lower levels of progesterone in the days before the period may be a trigger.[89] Numerous studies link low progesterone to feelings of anxiety.[87] Progesterone is a respiratory stimulant. High levels of the hormone can cause hyperventilation, but when levels drop very low, it is thought this can increase the perception of breathlessness.[90] While the weight of evidence points to a higher prevalence of anxiety disorders in women, the research is incomplete. This comes back to the male/female research bias and the fact that the bulk of the literature has focused on male rodents.[91]

Scientist have demonstrated an increase in panic symptoms, often interpreted as hot flashes, and anxiety in women experiencing the menopausal transition. This suggests that panic disorder may be linked to fluctuations in sex hormones.[92] Since studies have linked the onset of panic symptoms with heightened sensitivity to blood $CO_2$, it makes sense that the hyperventilation, which occurs at certain points in the menstrual cycle, may produce cyclic exacerbations of anxiety. When all the connections between hyperventilation, hormones, and panic disorder are taken together, it makes sense that sex hormones could contribute to anxiety in women. One recent paper concluded that it is important for future research to study anxiety in females so that results can be more accurate and applicable to women.[91]

## WOMEN'S HORMONES AND SPORTING PERFORMANCE

Another consideration when exploring the topic of breathing in terms of gender is the impact of sex hormones and anatomical factors on physical exercise. It is known that while women are capable of outstanding athletic achievement, they generally have to work harder to breathe during intensive exercise than men.[93, 94]

A 2020 study demonstrated that gender affects the respiratory aspects of physical exercise. The research team hypothesized that the smaller airways in females, when compared with the airways of height-matched males, produced more turbulent airflow during exercise. Turbulent airflow causes the air molecules to move in different directions, much like water bubbling round pebbles in a running stream. This creates more resistance, making breathing more difficult.[94]

Five women and six men took part in the trial, during which they each performed two exercise tests, gradually intensifying their workout on a stationary cycle until they reached maximum intensity. During the tests, participants breathed through a mouthpiece, inhaling either normal room air or a mixture of oxygen and helium. Respiratory effort was monitored via a small tube inserted into the nose and throat. In this experiment, the helium mix was designed to mimic the lower levels of resistance in the larger male airways. The helium mixture was less dense than the room air and moved in a more direct manner, with all the molecules flowing in the same direction.[94] This is called laminar airflow.

The results showed that women breathed much more air when they inhaled the helium and oxygen mix, but this change in breathing volume was not accompanied by an increase in the work of breathing. When breathing room air, the female participants had to breathe much harder than the men to overcome the turbulent resistance. When they breathed the helium and oxygen mix, the airflow was more laminar, and there was no difference between the males and females in ventilatory exertion. The study concluded that smaller airways increase turbulent flow and that is why women have to breathe harder during exercise.[94]

In an article in *Neuroscience News*, Paolo Dominelli, who was on the research team for the study, explained,

At rest, the rate of air flow is very low, so even though women have smaller airways than men, air flow is still laminar. As exercise intensity increases, you breathe faster, and at some point the airflow goes from laminar to turbulent. Air flow in men's airways will also eventually turn from laminar to turbulent, but this requires a higher rate of air flow than is required in women.[93]

It is important to understand that while the differences shown in this study relate to size and gender, with men typically having larger airways, airway size varies significantly between individuals.[93] For instance, people of both sexes who have set-back jaws or other craniofacial abnormalities caused by childhood mouth breathing, pacifier use, tongue-tie, and other factors will have smaller airways in adulthood, leading to a lifetime of sleep problems and reduced athletic ability.

Other differences may also have an impact on sporting performance in women. In 1993, a review published in *Sports Medicine* examined the impact of sex hormone fluctuations, due to the natural menstrual cycle and use of oral contraceptives, on the performance of female athletes.[95] Previous research had reported that the best days for athletic performance were generally those immediately after menstruation and the worst were in the premenstrual stage and the first few days of menstrual flow. However, those studies were limited by lack of accuracy as to where in the cycle the women were.

There was also an inherent bias, because many of the women already associated premenstrual symptoms such as weight gain, mood swings, and fluid retention with poor performance. Their perception of performance was therefore already less positive at that point in the cycle. Those premenstrual symptoms have also been linked with an increase in musculoskeletal injuries during the premenstrual and menstrual phases. In the days before menstruation, women were shown to experience compromised reaction time, neuromuscular coordination, dexterity, and judgment, but other potential confounding factors such as nutrition, blood sugar levels, and hyperventilation may cloud these findings.

Swimmers demonstrated worse performance times during the premenstrual phase and better times during menstruation and on the eighth day of the cycle. The women's perception of exertion during very intense exercises increased premenstrually and during the first few days of menstruation.[95] In cross-country skiers, the best performance times were recorded in the days just after ovulation and immediately following menstruation. To get the most out of training, loads should be adjusted for female athletes to account for changes during the menstrual cycle.

Studies using estradiol and progesterone levels to determine where a woman was in her cycle did not find any marked differences across the 28 days in response to either maximal or less intensive exercise, though a small decrease in aerobic capacity was observed during the luteal phase. However, in 2003, it was confirmed that breathing capacity was much higher in men than women[1]. During the follicular phase of the cycle, ventilation, tidal volume, and peak inspiratory flow were 21% lower in women during wakefulness and 22% lower during sleep. At the same time, no difference was found between men and women in blood flow to the respiratory muscles during exercise or rest, or during different phases of the menstrual cycle.[95]

A 2019 study investigated the effects of the menstrual cycle on running economy.[96] Eleven female athletes were assessed for oxygen consumption and blood gas exchange at rest and while running. Scientists concluded that gas exchange during exercise is better in the luteal phase than the follicular phase but that this is independent of running speed. It was also demonstrated that the menstrual cycle has no effect on body composition or physiological variables at rest.[96]

Again, research into this area is sparse. Perhaps most relevant to female athletes is knowing that hyperventilation is likely during the luteal phase, between ovulation and menstruation. By paying attention to the breath, working to normalize breathing volume, and reducing sensitivity to $CO_2$, it should be possible to moderate these naturally occurring phasic differences in breathing.

Another point worth mentioning is that, in extreme circumstances, women's sporting ambitions can impact their health and hormones in an unhealthy way. Excessive running or training places considerable stress on the body. This can cause an imbalance in the autonomic nervous system, affect the immune response, and put strain on the heart. When bodyweight and body mass index fall too low, estrogen will drop, and this can result in a lack of bone mineral density. Just as menopause is a risk factor for osteoporosis (something we explore in the next chapter), so is any condition that causes estrogen production to decline, because estrogen inhibits bone resorption.[97] Estrogen is a primary hormonal regulator of bone metabolism in women and men.[98]

When estrogen drops too low, fertility is impacted and menstruation ceases. This is the same for women with eating disorders. In fact, eating disorders and obsessive exercise combine to form the basis of a specific condition called relative energy deficiency in sport, or REDS. This can be an easy trap to fall into, especially for women with perfectionist, high-achieving personalities. If you feel your running is becoming obsessive and weight loss is tipping over into an eating disorder, it is important to speak with a specialist as soon as you can.

In an article for the UK website *Momentum Sports*, endurance runner Katherine Wood writes openly about her 10-year battle with anorexia nervosa and REDS.[99] Wood was a competitive runner and swimmer as a child and teenager, but as she went through puberty, she struggled to balance her nutritional input with the energy output required in her training. She rapidly transitioned from unintentional weight loss to full-blown anorexia that left her in hospital. Her periods stopped.

As her running career progressed, Wood pushed herself harder and further. She achieved success after success. But she was training compulsively, ignoring injuries and signs that her health was failing, and losing weight fast. She began to have repeated bacterial infections on the skin of her legs. Blood tests returned signs that her muscles were starting to break down, but she experienced a sense of failure if she didn't keep up her intensive training.

Eventually, she turned to Renee McGregor for help. McGregor is a sports and eating disorder therapist and cofounder of #TRAINBRAVE, an initiative aimed at raising awareness of eating disorders in athletes. In the first consultation, Wood was devastated to be told that she had to stop exercising immediately and that her heart could give way at any moment if she didn't. In the following months, she found it incredibly difficult to increase her food intake while not exercising at all. Scans revealed that her bone density was so low she was classed as osteopenic. She struggled to get a prescription for HRT; a lack of understanding of sports-related eating disorders among general medical providers meant she had to seek private healthcare.

In her article, she issues this caution against underfueling and overtraining, "Periods stopping is NOT a sign that you are training hard enough, it is a sign you are training TOO hard and your body is not coping. Please do not ignore these signs."[99]

# CHAPTER THIRTEEN
# FEMALE SEX HORMONES AND THE BREATH

---

## PMS AND CYCLIC HYPERVENTILATION

Premenstrual syndrome (PMS) manifests with similar or identical symptoms to chronic hyperventilation syndrome.[1] A 2006 study found that women with PMS experience a much greater decline in blood carbon dioxide ($CO_2$) in the premenstrual phase than women who do not experience symptoms. The symptoms appear as progesterone increases and blood $CO_2$ decreases. When the luteal phase ends, progesterone decreases, $CO_2$ levels normalize, and the symptoms disappear. The study concluded that women with PMS have a higher-than-normal sensitivity to $CO_2$, perhaps caused by progesterone, resulting in "pronounced hyperventilation"—and that the hyperventilation is responsible for the symptoms.[2]

Breathing plays a role even from the perspective of physical pain experienced. Not only is pain perception heightened by low $CO_2$ levels, the drop in $CO_2$ also causes constriction of smooth muscles. Since the uterus is comprised of smooth muscle, this can directly contribute to pain experienced as menstrual cramps.[3]

The authors of the 2006 study suggest that since the breath can be easily manipulated using a variety of techniques, including respiratory and biofeedback training, it would be promising to explore this phenomenon in more detail to understand the mechanisms underlying PMS and find more effective ways to treat it, at least for some women.[2] Their conclusion points to the relevance of the techniques in this book. Science has yet to adequately catch up, but existing research does point to the fact that women can control symptoms of PMS by changing their breathing patterns to restore slow, light, nasal breathing.

In the same study, researchers noted that selective serotonin-reuptake inhibitors (SSRIs), commonly used as antidepressants and for alleviating the symptoms of PMS, cause an increase in blood $CO_2$ levels. Serotonin is a chemical messenger that has many complex functions. It is known as the "happy chemical" because it contributes to feelings of well-being. During the luteal phase of the menstrual cycle, fluctuations in estrogen and progesterone increase serotonin neurotransmission.[4] But according to 2015 research, women who suffer with PMS or premenstrual dysphoric disorder (PMDD—a more severe form of premenstrual syndrome) appear to have an abnormal serotonin reaction to luteal hormonal changes[5]. Also, it has been shown that changes in the serotonin system may be indirectly related to breathing abnormalities[6] and treatment with SSRIs may improve respiratory responses to $CO_2$.[7]

The connection between PMDD and panic disorder has been receiving growing attention. Patients with both conditions experience high rates of panic attacks, and PMDD and panic disorder may share the same underlying pathology.[8] The link between menstruation, depression, and mood swings is commonly acknowledged and frequently stereotyped, but the symptoms of PMS and PMDD are no joke. At clinically significant levels, they are severe enough to interfere with daily life.

We have explored the connection between headaches, menstrual migraines, and hyperventilation, but there seems to be yet no scientific literature examining the cyclical occurrence of depression, panic symptoms, irritability, and mood swings in terms of hormone-induced respiratory changes. This is despite the clear relationship between mood disorders, dysfunctional breathing, and autonomic imbalance, and the fact that it is not always possible to distinguish between depression and PMDD.[9]

According to a 2017 advisory document from a New Zealand pharmacovigilance team, symptoms including depressed mood, feelings of hopelessness, difficulty concentrating, lack of energy, decreased interest in usual activities, hypersomnia, and insomnia are included in the diagnostic criteria for both disorders. However, differences in the regulation of the stress response between women with depressive disorders and those with PMDD may suggest two distinct conditions. It is believed, for instance, that premenstrual symptoms are not particularly influenced by familial or environmental factors while a history of anxiety disorder, traumatic events, and smoking can all contribute.[9]

## EMMA'S STORY

Emma is in her early thirties. She is highly active, enjoys eating a healthy diet, doesn't smoke, and rarely drinks alcohol. She has a sedentary job with an 8- to 10-hour day, but she walks between four and five kilometers, works out every day, and sleeps well for seven or eight hours every night. Despite the care she gives to her health, Emma found herself struggling with PMS symptoms that gradually became more and more difficult to cope with.

Emma had been taking an oral contraceptive since her late teens. In her late twenties, she took a break from her pill. After three years with no hormonal contraceptives, she began to take a combined contraceptive pill. This was when her "hormonal rollercoaster" began. At first, Emma chalked her PMS symptoms of mood swings, fatigue, bloating, and brain fog down to the particular pill she was prescribed. Her doctor switched her to a different combined pill. For the next three months, Emma's symptoms were constant. She was bloated all the time, her mood was low, she had problems with her digestion, and her energy levels were "on the floor." Despite her regular exercise regime and healthy diet, she gained two kilos in body weight. She was in a constant state of stress.

After much research, Emma switched to a more localized contraceptive, opting to have an IUD inserted. The IUD is different from an oral contraceptive in that the release of hormones is much more direct so that the hormones are not constantly circulating in the bloodstream. Next, she prioritized her well-being to combat the debilitating PMS symptoms she had been experiencing. Synthetic hormones were still being released into her body, even with the IUD, so she wanted to do everything she could to support her health while her system adapted to the new contraceptive.

In the following months, she did several things that significantly improved her condition:

- She began taking daily supplements of diindolylmethane (DIM), magnesium, and a vitamin B complex. DIM is a natural supplement found in vegetables including kale, broccoli, and cabbage. It helps the body metabolize estrogen. Emma learned that hormonal contraceptives deplete the body of key nutrients such as B vitamins[10] — something she wished her doctor had told her.

- She made the switch to nasal breathing. While Emma was not a habitual mouth breather, she did always breathe through her mouth during exercise. She worked to ensure that she breathed only through her nose, even on a 100-km cycle. This left her feeling much calmer during exercise and throughout the rest of the day.
- She began practicing breath holds and long, slow breaths. Emma never considered herself a fast breather, but each month, around the same time she experienced PMS symptoms, she noticed that her breath felt shallow. She would struggle to take a full, deep inhalation, almost as though her body was not capable of getting the oxygen it required. By becoming aware of her breath, she felt better able to control it. She now uses breath holds to reset her system to get sufficient oxygen into her body.
- Emma began practicing meditation. She found that stopping for 15 to 20 minutes a day to "reset and reenter" had a profound effect on her PMS symptoms and on her daily life. Her PMS lows became much easier to deal with, and she felt better able to pull herself out of the "PMS hole" she found herself in on a monthly basis. Her concentration became sharper, and she began experiencing the best sleep she had ever had.

Emma had always been told that PMS is normal, that symptoms including fatigue, brain fog, bloating, and low moods are par for the course, and that she should "deal with it and take a painkiller." She was shocked to realize that nobody had ever explained why she experienced these symptoms, what was happening in her body to make her feel this way. Now she understands that her feelings of breathlessness are largely caused by the drop in $CO_2$ during the premenstrual phase of her cycle.

Emma's PMS has not completely disappeared, but every month her symptoms are less severe and more manageable. She has lost the extra two kilos she was carrying, she no longer has dramatic mood swings or brain fog, and her bloating is much less extreme. Her quality of life has improved because, in her words, she has much less of a battle to fight each month.

For women who suffer from PMS, the connection to hyperventilation is big news. It means that many symptoms previously believed to be hormonal and unavoidable are actually the result of a hormone-driven change in breathing patterns. That is something that can be addressed with breathing exercises and by moderating blood sensitivity to $CO_2$.

If you suffer from PMS, keep an eye on your breathing. If your BOLT score decreases, your breathing gets faster, or you experience air hunger, then practice breath holds, begin light, slow, and deep breathing, and work to restore full-time nasal breathing. That should help relieve your symptoms.

## HOW PREGNANCY AFFECTS BREATHING

It makes sense that breathing would change during pregnancy. After all, you are now breathing for two. Oxygen demand is higher due to a 15% increase in metabolic rate and a 20% increase in oxygen consumption.[11] The space within the abdominal cavity, where the diaphragm rises and falls, becomes incrementally smaller as pregnancy progresses. The increase in sex hormones in the system leads to a significantly higher incidence of hyperventilation,[12] Early on, there is a rise in minute ventilation of around 40% to 50%,[11] levels of blood $CO_2$ drop, and the ventilatory responses to hypoxia and hypercapnia increase[13].

The changes in pregnancy that lead to hyperventilation are believed to be caused by a heightened response to blood $CO_2$. There is a close relationship between blood sensitivity to $CO_2$ and the relative ratio of the hormones, progesterone, and estrogen. As well as maintaining pregnancy,[14] progesterone acts as a respiratory stimulant in men and women. Levels of the hormone increase around 100-fold during pregnancy.[15]

Sex hormones are instrumental in respiratory changes during pregnancy. Even back in 1979, researchers reported that the respiratory response to pregnancy was "largely mediated by the action of progesterone and, perhaps to a lesser extent, estrogens, at least in the first and second trimesters."[16] Estrogen, which increases around 80-fold during pregnancy, is known to improve the functioning of progesterone receptors.[13] The 1979 paper stated that breathlessness during pregnancy is likely to be caused by hormones, but at that time, the relationship between hormones, functional respiratory change, and the development of symptoms was not clearly defined.[16]

More recent work has demonstrated that hyperventilation at rest, even during the first trimester of pregnancy, is linked to an increase in ventilation with no change in respiratory rate.[17, 18] It is now understood that hyperventilation during pregnancy is caused by alterations to the blood acid-base balance, cerebral blood flow, metabolism, variations in sleep patterns, and changes in the central chemoreflex drive to breathe, triggered by the increased concentration of sex hormones.[12]

There are, of course, mechanical factors to consider too. For instance, as the size of the fetus and therefore the uterus increases, there is progressively less room for the breathing muscles. During the second half of the pregnancy, residual lung volume decreases by as much as 22% and respiratory resistance becomes greater. The diaphragm is displaced upward by about five centimeters, increasing its ability to generate tension as muscle fibers lengthen.[19] The diaphragm may have to work harder as load increases, but widening of the chest prevents further loss of lung volume.[20] The gradual extension of the abdominal muscles causes their fibers to lengthen by up to 115%, their thickness reduces, and their angle of function changes. This inhibits their ability to stabilize the pelvis—which may be a factor in back pain during pregnancy.[19].

Around 70% of healthy pregnant women report breathlessness during their daily activities. This often begins during the first trimester, suggesting that mechanical changes to the diaphragm and lungs are not to blame. It is more likely that breathlessness is caused either by hyperventilation associated with pregnancy or by a heightened perception of respiratory discomfort as the result of increased ventilation.

Not surprisingly, the incidence of sleep-disordered breathing increases among pregnant women. The physiological and anatomical changes intrinsic to gestation can unmask or exacerbate obstructive sleep apnea (OSA).[21] If this is left untreated, the limitations in upper airway flow can lead to serious consequences for both maternal and fetal health. While not the focus here, it should be noted that, generally in the realm of respiratory disorders, uncontrolled maternal asthma has been found to be associated with an increased risk of spontaneous abortion.[22]

Healthcare providers should screen expectant mothers for OSA to ensure the well-being of both mother and baby. This is especially important in pre-eclampsia, a primary cause of maternal and fetal illness and mortality, which sleep-disordered breathing has been proven to increase the risk and severity of. It is believed that the repetitive limitations to airflow that occur during sleep-disordered breathing are linked to surges in nocturnal blood pressure and poor health in both mother and baby—and may be just as damaging as full apneas.[21]

One 2016 paper about OSA during pregnancy describes sleep apnea as a modern epidemic.[23] It is now accepted that the condition is widespread in women, particularly during pregnancy. According to current evidence, sleep-disordered breathing is present in 50% of high-risk pregnancies and in 15% of otherwise healthy, obese pregnant women. It should be no surprise that pregnancy contributes to sleep disorders. By its nature, it causes anatomical, physiological, and hormonal changes, including narrowing of the upper respiratory tract, which can increase the risk of OSA or worsen existing apneas.[24]

During pregnancy, OSA contributes to a five-fold increase in maternal mortality due to complications including pulmonary embolism[23] (a blockage of an artery in the lungs). A 15-year study of maternal deaths in Michigan found a connection with OSA and sleep-disordered breathing and demonstrated that, even after the birth, OSA presents a risk for women.[25]

Maternal OSA has also been linked to poor fetal outcomes, fetal growth restriction,[23] low birth weight,[26] preterm delivery,[23] cesarean section, and preeclampsia.[27, 28] It has been connected to a low Apgar score in babies in the five minutes after delivery.[24] The Apgar score is a generalized measure of health that assesses appearance (skin color), pulse (heart rate), grimace response (reflexes), activity (muscle tone), and respiration (breathing rate and effort).[29] A 2012 study set out to determine whether poor pregnancy outcomes were related to OSA. It concluded that babies are at an increased risk of complications in the areas previously listed when the mother has sleep apnea. This can impact the health of the child long term.[24]

Children born significantly preterm commonly suffer from medical problems and growth restrictions in early childhood.[30] They frequently have lower weight, height, and head circumference than their classmates. The preterm children were much more likely than normal term children to have serious dental malocclusions, and deep bite and overjet were also prevalent.[30] According to pediatric dentist Dr. Kevin Boyd, restricted fetal growth can cause problems that will result in suboptimal airway health once the baby is born. In Chapter Eight, we discussed how dental problems and compromised airways in children can lead to childhood mouth breathing, and subsequent cognitive, developmental, and behavioral issues.

When fetal development is poor due to frequent drops in blood oxygen, as can be the case for mothers with OSA, the baby may have cognitive problems that progress into childhood and may not receive appropriate care. A 2020 review confirmed that children with restricted inter-uterine growth and small birth weight had significantly lower cognitive scores than those born at an average gestational age.[31] While these children had similar cognitive scores to those born preterm, they were unlikely to receive the follow-on care or to be included in the rehabilitation programs that are available to preterm babies.[31]

Another review explored the role of placenta health in chronic disease later in adulthood.[32] Much research has demonstrated how low birth weight contributes to the onset of certain diseases, including obesity, heart disease, stroke, and diabetes. Chronic hypoxia and elevated stress levels, both symptomatic of sleep apnea, cause changes to the organs of the unborn baby. The review cites a study of 187 men and 47 women that found that sudden cardiac death was linked to a thin placenta at birth. Fetal growth and lifelong health can be strongly influenced by the health of the placenta, which requires continual adequate oxygenation through healthy breathing during pregnancy.

## ANXIETY DURING PREGNANCY AND AFTER

Anxiety in new mothers is common. As a woman takes on a new role and new responsibilities, it could be considered an appropriate adaptive response.[33] However, some mothers suffer with severe, invalidating anxiety, depression, and other mood disorders in the period shortly before and after the birth of their child. Hormone fluctuations can play a part, as can psychological issues—perceived or real challenges and fear—which may increase in the case of an unexpected or unwanted pregnancy,[33] or when assisted reproductive technology has been used.[34]

It is now generally acknowledged that new mothers are vulnerable to postpartum depression, but the prevalence of anxiety disorders during pregnancy has not been as widely studied. Many women experience new or worsening anxiety symptoms in the months before and after birth: 21% of women have clinically significant anxiety during pregnancy, and 64% of these women continue to suffer with anxiety after giving birth.[33] Research suggests that prenatal anxiety is a major factor in susceptibility to postnatal depression. Untreated anxiety and depression, which often exist comorbidly, can have a serious impact on the mother and baby.[33] Anxiety during pregnancy can contribute to numerous problems, including preeclampsia, more time off work, nausea, increased visits to healthcare providers, spontaneous early labor and delivery, low birth weight, difficulty breastfeeding, and a more difficult birth with an increased likelihood of PTSD.

Pregnancy-related or postpartum anxiety can produce feelings of constant worry, fatigue, nervousness, insomnia, mood swings, poor focus or memory, hot flashes, nausea, and sleep disturbance. At its worst, postpartum anxiety inhibits the mother's ability to care for her child, causing considerable distress and resulting in a sickly infant or even infanticide.

There isn't much information about generalized anxiety in pregnant women and new mothers, although it is believed that anxiety is more prevalent in postpartum women than in the general population. In one study, between 10% and 50% of new mothers with anxiety also displayed symptoms of depression.[35] In another, 65% with generalized anxiety also reported depression, panic disorder, or agoraphobia. It is believed that generalized anxiety lasting more than six months may be more common in postnatal women[33] and that anxiety in new mothers is actually more common than depression.[35] It can be challenging to achieve a clear diagnosis of anxiety during pregnancy because it is normal for women to experience a certain level of worry at this time.[36] Also, there is no data about preexisting anxiety disorders in women before becoming pregnant, so it is impossible to ascertain to what extent anxiety is pregnancy related.

Generalized anxiety disorder during pregnancy can present as nervousness, fatigue, difficulty concentrating, persistent "worry" thoughts, muscle tension, and sleep disturbance. Due to the physiological changes of pregnancy, especially hormone-induced hyperventilation, pregnant women may be at greater risk for panic disorder. While there is research suggesting that pregnancy may provide some kind of protection against panic symptoms, the role of premenstrual hormone changes in panic disorder suggests that fluctuations in sex hormones make new mothers more vulnerable to anxiety and panic disorder.[36] One review has confirmed this increased susceptibility,[37] and some researchers hypothesize that this may be due to the sharp drop in progesterone after delivery.[37]

During pregnancy, progesterone levels are high. This supports the pregnancy, but it also causes hyperventilation and a reduction in blood $CO_2$. After the baby is born, progesterone drops and $CO_2$ rises, triggering panic symptoms. Too much blood $CO_2$ can cause panic attacks in patients who have a high sensitivity to blood $CO_2$, as the increase in air hunger triggers feelings of fear.[38] Conversely, panic symptoms can be triggered by hyperventilation when blood $CO_2$ drops to levels that are too low. The important thing to understand is that by improving functional breathing patterns, it is possible to normalize levels of blood $CO_2$ so that they are neither too high nor too low. It is also possible to reduce the body's sensitivity to $CO_2$ so that normal fluctuations do not cause panic-inducing air hunger.

Panic symptoms include breathlessness, hyperventilation, chest pain, a sense of choking or nausea, dizziness, and paresthesia (numbness and sensations like pins-and-needles). All of these are also symptoms of breathing pattern disorders.

The symptoms of panic attacks point to a correlation with poor oxygenation and sympathetic activation. Cognitive function abruptly declines, feelings of exhaustion occur, the patient becomes increasingly anxious to prevent further attacks, and quality of life suffers. In pregnant women and new mothers, the anxiety around future attacks can become severe enough to cause agoraphobia and social isolation.[33] There is also evidence that anxiety in the mother during pregnancy impacts on infant temperament, producing babies who are more "difficult," exacerbating maternal anxiety and stress.[34]

During and immediately after pregnancy, women are also more vulnerable to experiencing other mental disorders such as OCD and PTSD. Left untreated, these problems can have a significant impact on the physical and mental health of mother and child and other family members.[33] For the most successful results, researchers recommend an integrated treatment approach in which medicines are prescribed alongside psycho educational options, such as relaxation exercises and cognitive behavioral therapy. There is no research into the therapeutic benefit of breathing exercises for postpartum anxiety and depression, but a considerable body of research does clearly indicate the link between blood $CO_2$, sensitivity to $CO_2$, and these psychological disorders.

While a few studies discuss the hormonal implications of abortion and miscarriage, there is nothing in the literature to connect hormonal fluctuations in abortive pregnancy to respiratory health. In women who suffer very early pregnancy loss, the luteal phase is shorter for the next few cycles.[39] Early pregnancy loss is also associated with lower levels of luteal estrogen and progesterone. Heightened anxiety, depression, and insomnia are, not surprisingly, common after miscarriage. This is partly due to stress and to fluctuations in sex hormones. A breathing practice would help moderate hormone-induced hyperventilation during this difficult time,[40] regulating important factors that influence sleep and mood.

**Important: The breathing exercises in this book should not be practiced if you are in your first trimester of pregnancy.** Practice relaxation and work to gently restore nose breathing. In your second trimester, you may practice gentle relaxation, nasal breathing, and slow breathing. Throughout your pregnancy, it is very important to approach any exercises very gently. You should not practice any breath holds while pregnant.

## HORMONAL CONTRACEPTIVES AND THE BREATH

Progestogens and estrogens combined in oral contraceptive pills have been in widespread use since the 1960s. While much publicity has been given to the potential side effects in terms of cardiovascular health, little research has been done into the effects on breathing and the respiratory system.[41]

One 1979 study did find that women taking a progesterone-only oral contraceptive pill had a significantly greater minute ventilation than women ovulating normally, except when the control subjects were in the late luteal phase of their cycle.[16] This added weight to the idea that progesterone acts as a respiratory stimulant, a theory that has since been confirmed.

In terms of respiratory symptoms, a 1999 paper found no indication that hormonal contraceptives influenced asthma severity in women with mild asthma.[42] In a 2001 cross-sectional study of the general population in Copenhagen, no marked increase in asthma, asthma medication, wheezing, or coughing on exertion was found in women using oral contraceptives,[43] although some studies showed that asthma symptoms were slightly worsened by hormone replacement therapy (HRT) in postmenopausal women. In a 1995 study, researchers found that women who had previously taken oral contraceptives had a higher risk of developing asthma,[44] in contrast to a 2006 Australian study that reported a 7% decrease in adult-onset asthma for every year of oral contraceptive use.[45] A study of women in Northern Europe again found the opposite—that oral contraceptive users displayed a higher risk of developing asthma—but when examined alongside body mass index data, it was unclear whether the hormone pill or body weight was the primary factor in the asthma symptoms.[41] A 2015 paper reported that hormonal contraceptive use reduced asthma exacerbations in nonobese women,[46] while they increased the risk of asthma in obese women.[47]

An investigation of bronchial hyperactivity (BHR) showed less variability in symptoms over the course of the menstrual cycle in women using hormonal contraceptives, but the study did not describe how levels of BHR were affected by contraceptive use.[41] It makes sense that women whose asthma symptoms vary a lot through their menstrual cycle may experience more stability by using a hormonal contraceptive, but studies have returned contradictory results as to the relationship between overall asthma susceptibility and contraceptive use.

Clearly, observational research examining the connection between oral contraceptives and respiratory health often produces results that are difficult to analyze. Studies are subject to the problem of "confounding by indication." This is the scientific term for the difficulty in assessing a risk factor or treatment in relation to an outcome when there are "confounding" variables that could also be affecting the outcome. This is one reason why a study may draw inaccurate conclusions. For example, in studies into the side effects of a medication, patients who are prescribed the medication may be inherently different from people who do not take it—they are, after all, taking the drug for a reason. This very fact can distort the findings of research. For example, oral contraceptives are often used to treat polycystic ovary syndrome (PCOS). PCOS is linked with asthma, lower lung function, diabetes, and cardiovascular disease. Therefore, PCOS may be a significant factor confounding (complicating) the relationship between oral contraception and respiratory disorders. This, however, has not been considered in any of the studies described. The relationship is further complicated by the fact that hormone contraceptives can sometimes cause irregular menstruation.[41]

In general, the scientific literature on this topic is inconsistent and problematic. The makeup of oral contraceptives has changed over time—modern pills have a higher progesterone content and lower estrogen compared with those that were used some years ago. Each pill used in the early 1960s was roughly equivalent in terms of dosage to seven of today's pills.[48]

The 2012 review concludes that it is "likely and biologically plausible" that oral contraceptives affect the airways in diverse ways. While some studies indicate that asthma can be caused by contraceptives in some women, others demonstrate the opposite. It is important, therefore, for healthcare professionals to be aware of the possibility that hormonal contraceptives might affect respiratory health in different ways and to listen to their patients and assess them on an individual basis. The likelihood that these medications impact the airway is sufficient for researchers to advocate that respiratory symptoms and disorders be included in trials of new oral contraceptive pills.

I recently talked to Georgie, a healthy 25-year-old woman who is very fit with a high level of endurance. In the weeks before we spoke, Georgie had stopped taking her combined oral contraceptive pill and returned to her natural 28-day cycle. She tracks her cycle daily, logging her temperature via a fertility and ovulation app called "Natural Cycles." She also takes her BOLT score every day. Georgie's average BOLT score is around 30 or 31 seconds at rest, but during the midluteal/luteal phase of her cycle, there is a marked decrease of between 6 and 10 seconds. At the same time, she experiences increased anxiety, lower motivation and a lack of focus.

Since coming off the combined contraceptive pill, she has noticed the drop in her BOLT score is not so severe. Georgie told me:

> I know it usually takes around three months for the hormones to fully adjust back into their natural rhythm when you come off the pill, but for me an awareness of how my hormones fluctuate, especially in terms of respiratory function, is comforting. It improves my understanding about how to train in an athletic sense, and it helps me to know when I need to look after myself a little more.

Besides oral contraceptives, other methods of contraception are also in common use. Nonoral options include inter-uterine devices (IUDs) and implants, both of which release a synthetic progesterone hormone called levonorgestrel. There are also injectable medications. Most list depression and anxiety as side effects,[9] though no direct link has yet been made to breathing pattern disorders or respiratory health.

It is possible, though the link has not been investigated, that the recognized psychological side effects of hormonal contraceptives are linked to low levels of blood $CO_2$ triggered by the hormone changes, just as hyperventilation is a common factor in the luteal phase of the menstrual cycle. The low levels of blood $CO_2$ intrinsic to hyperventilation are associated with panic attacks, and panic symptoms lessen when levels of $CO_2$ are normalized. Breathing exercises that normalize blood biochemistry and decrease the ventilatory response to $CO_2$ should help alleviate cyclic depressive symptoms and create a positive feedback loop in which panic symptoms are better controlled.

In very rare cases, contraceptive devices have been known to negatively affect the health of the respiratory system in a directly physical manner. In one case, a young woman who was experiencing shortness of breath and severe chest pain attended the emergency department, where an X-ray revealed that her IUD had become displaced and was in her abdominal cavity. The device was removed, resolving her symptoms. IUDs should be regularly checked that they are still correctly positioned. A misplaced IUD should be considered by doctors where the cause of symptoms is not clear.[49] In another case, a single-rod subdermal contraceptive implant migrated into the lung of a 37-year-old woman.[50] Only those with the relevant training should ever undertake the insertion and removal of these implants.

## INFERTILITY AND BREATHING

In 2007, Austrian scientists examined changes in end-tidal $CO_2$ pressure during the menstrual cycle.[51] End-tidal $CO_2$ provides a measure of how much $CO_2$ is in the blood. Researchers examined 160 women with a history of regular menstrual cycles, measuring levels of blood $CO_2$ every day. The women's menstrual cycles were monitored using ultrasound and by recording levels of hormones, including estrogen and progesterone, in the blood and urine. The change in end-tidal $CO_2$ during the menstrual cycle was found to follow a regular pattern. They concluded that this could provide a promising method of natural family planning, and that it should be possible to identify the fertile phase of the menstrual cycle by measuring end-tidal $CO_2$.[51]

While $CO_2$ levels can help identify what's going on with the hormones, there are clear aspects of health that can cause complications for fertility. One such factor, described in a 2018 study, is psychological stress.[52] The connection between stress and infertility has been debated for years. Women who experience infertility report heightened feelings of depression and anxiety, and it is clear that infertility causes stress. What is less certain is whether stress can cause or contribute to infertility.

According to the 2018 review, recent research has documented the effectiveness of psychological interventions in reducing mental distress and significantly increasing rates of conception. The review concludes that therapeutic approaches to relieve stress may be the most effective way to achieve both goals for women struggling to conceive. Cognitive behavioral therapy (CBT) is suggested, but it is worth remembering that research has found slow, diaphragm breathing to be as effective as CBT in treating patients with panic attacks.[53] Slow, deep breathing works via different mechanisms, addressing the biochemical trigger for stress as well as the psychological factors. It would therefore make sense that breathing reeducation could be useful in supporting women with infertility-related stress. At the very least, it will certainly do no harm!

Citing stress as a factor, a 2015 study examined the influence of sleep on fertility. Stress certainly contributes to poor sleep, and the review set out to examine by which mechanisms sleep disorders might affect fertility. In the United States, infertility affects 15.5% of all women and 24.3% of women who have never had a child.[54] According to the review, many more women than men have insomnia. Menstrual transitions, pregnancy, and menopause all create a vulnerability to sleep continuity disturbance, and so women are more at risk for sleep problems throughout their lives. Traditionally, it was believed that mood swings, lifestyle changes, or hormonal fluctuations create a susceptibility to insomnia. However, the study suggests that the opposite may be true—a disturbance in sleep may influence fertility. If, for example, insomnia is caused by hyperarousal, the body is reacting to a real or perceived threat. In this instance, insomnia may be the evolutionary response to less-than-optimal circumstances for reproduction.

Sleep disorders and disturbances are increasingly recognized as pertinent to women's health and well-being, particularly in relation to the menstrual cycle, pregnancy, and menopause.[54] Little is currently known about how and to what extent fertility is affected by sleep quality and quantity, but sleep problems are frequently comorbid with infertility. The review concludes that, at the very least, treatment of sleep disorders would enhance the quality of life for women with fertility problems. At best, one or more sleep disorders represent "moderating factors for infertility or response to treatment." If this is indeed the case, treatment for sleep disorders may increase the chance of natural conception, improve the response to fertility treatment, and boost the potential for successful carriage to term.[54]

Again, as we discovered in Chapter Seven on sleep disorders, correct breathing plays a vital role in sleep quality. This is yet another therapeutic reason to address breathing in sleep disorders, whether it impacts fertility directly or indirectly.

A study reported in *Reuters Health* in 2018 further examined the link between infertility and sleep disorders,[55] suggesting that women who have trouble sleeping may be more than three times as likely to experience infertility and that women with insomnia are four times more likely to struggle to conceive. The study specifically examined women with sleep disorders other than OSA. Difficulty conceiving is often caused by a hormone imbalance called polycystic ovarian syndrome, though blocked fallopian tubes, anatomical problems with the uterus, sexually transmitted infections, smoking, diet, age, and excessive alcohol consumption can also play a role.

The 2018 study examined data from 16,718 women, all newly diagnosed with sleep disorders over a 10-year period, 2000 to 2010, alongside a control group of 33,436 women with no sleep problems. At the start of the study, the women ranged in age from 20 to 45. Results, before age and other health issues were taken into account, showed that women with sleep disorders were around 2.7 times more likely to experience infertility. With age and other medical conditions factored in, women with sleep problems were 3.7 times more likely to be infertile. Sleep disorders are frequently related to chronic health problems such as high cholesterol, hypertension, and lung disease. Women who sleep badly are also more susceptible to irregular menstrual cycles, depression, anxiety, and thyroid disorders.

While the study did not examine whether a direct causal link exists between sleep disorders and infertility, and researchers lacked data on certain things that impact fertility, the results indicated that poor sleep may be a factor for women struggling with infertility. CBT is the standard first-line approach for treating insomnia, but breathing exercises can be effective in addressing sleep disorders and the underlying stress that may be at their root. If you are trying for a baby, a gentle practice of slow breathing, sleep, and relaxation will boost your physical and mental resilience and health.

## MANAGING MENOPAUSE

At a certain point in every woman's life, menstruation will spontaneously and permanently cease, and menopause will begin. While this is a natural event and one that all women experience, there is little scientific literature examining this characteristic change in sex hormone levels, and most women don't really know what to expect. This is not really surprising in light of the gender imbalance present in scientific studies, but it is an issue that is currently receiving growing attention. In medical terms, it is not even entirely clear when menopause begins—the "menopause state" is confirmed after 12 consecutive months without a period[41]. This happens at a median age of 51 years, although an extensive 2009 study reported an increase toward 54 years.[56]

Before menopause, many women experience a phase called perimenopause. This is the body sending up flags of the coming hormonal changes. Levels of estrogen rise before the production of sex hormones ceases, and you might experience hot flashes, night sweats, sleep disturbances, vaginal dryness, irregular periods, mood swings, recurrent depression, and short-term memory loss.[41] Perimenopause begins, on average, at the age of 46 and lasts for about five years.[41]

One thing that is known is that while menopause is a natural progression, smoking significantly impacts the age at which it occurs. Women who smoke enter menopause about a year and a half earlier than those who don't.[41] This already points to an obvious link between menopause and overall well-being and more specifically, respiratory health.

Early menopause is a known risk factor for various illnesses, including cardiovascular diseases and osteoporosis. Early menopause is also directly linked to mortality in general[57]. There are correlations between natural menopause and lung health, but studies have largely failed to factor in other things during a woman's life that are known to affect the function of the lungs.[57]

As women live longer, they will spend more years in postmenopause, and scientists recognize that this makes it essential to understand how hormonal shifts during this period affect the health of the lungs.[57] Fortunately, the fact that progesterone levels drop after menopause means that there is a large study population available in which reduced hormone levels can be examined, and scientists are beginning to explore these connections in more detail.

A 2009 paper found that not only were estrogen and progesterone levels significantly lower in postmenopausal women, the pressure of blood $CO_2$ at rest was much higher too[58]. This is because the central chemoreflex drive to breathe is lessened after the menopause. This change is related to the decrease in sex hormone concentrations and complex blood acid-base interactions. This finding has important implications in understanding why sleep-disordered breathing becomes more common after menopause. It is also useful in determining the effects of HRT on ventilatory control and on blood pH, at rest and during exercise, in both healthy women and those who are unwell.[58]

The authors of a 2020 study published strong evidence of a connection between early menopause and reduced lung function. This was the first long running study to confirm a relationship between pulmonary health and early natural menopause. Using data about lung function collected when participants were 7 and 53 years old, researchers found that women whose menopause occurred before they were 45 had poorer lung function than those who experienced menopause aged 45 or later. This is the first study to take into account factors earlier in the lives of the women, such as childhood asthma, socioeconomic status, and parental smoking.[59]

By identifying that this relationship exists, scientists have made it possible to assess women with a higher potential risk of lung problems or those women who might be likely to develop lung disease when menstruation ends. Early menopause triggers a susceptibility to respiratory disease and a vulnerability to environmental factors such as air pollution that has not previously been recognized. It is unclear whether changing hormone levels directly accelerate the decline in lung function in some women, but a clear link between estrogen fluctuations and pulmonary health exists.

Women whose respiratory function is poor before menopause may be at an even greater risk, especially if they are subject to other factors, for example, regular exposure to toxins at home or at work. Women who have an existing lung condition, such as COPD, and experience early menopause may subsequently suffer a more serious and progressive version of the lung disease.[59] The study recommends that the impact of menopause on asthma be reevaluated. It also suggests that immune dysfunction connected with the main estrogen of menopause may be significant in a chronic condition called bronchiectasis, a disorder of the airways that mainly affects postmenopausal women.

A high proportion of the women in this study who experienced early menopause had also had early menarche. It is believed that these women may be generally at higher risk for lung dysfunction or disease. Interestingly, women in this same group were more likely to smoke and to use hormonal therapies. Women in the study cohort who were still menstruating had the lowest rate of respiratory symptoms and diseases.

While this study represents a step forward in research on the topic, more work is needed to understand the mechanisms of menopause and lung function. However, it is important that early menopause is understood to be a risk factor in respiratory health.

## IMPACT OF HORMONE REPLACEMENT THERAPIES ON THE BREATH

As menopause occurs, many women choose to take a HRT for either shorter or longer periods. There has been some uncertainty about the safety of these medications, largely because of reports from the Women's Health Initiative study, which condemned the therapy as unsafe due to links with increased risk of coronary heart disease and breast cancer.[60] The uptake of HRT declined as a result of this publicity. It was subsequently shown that the risk of breast cancer was low and only relevant for women with a very long exposure to a combined HRT regimen, and that for some, estrogen may actually reduce susceptibility. More recently, these findings were again contradicted in research published in the *British Journal of Cancer*, which reported that women taking combined HRT are nearly three times more likely to develop breast cancer than nonusers, with risk increasing with longer HRT use. The "Breast Cancer Now Generations Study" provided a comprehensive update about HRT use, suggesting that many previous investigations were not so thorough and may have "underestimated the increased risk of breast cancer by up to 60%.[61] Importantly, the heightened risk level appears to return to normal once HRT use ends.[61] There is not thought to be increased risk for coronary disease.[60]

Overall, the link between menopause and lung health is still not well understood. Despite the fact there has been a certain amount of research focus on HRT, the underlying condition of menopause itself has barely been studied. What literature there is on HRT and respiratory health returns confusing results.

Research into asthma and other respiratory symptoms tends to indicate an increased risk for women who take HRT, especially nonsmokers and women with a lower BMI. However, studies of lung function suggest a beneficial or at least a neutral connection with HRT.[41] As we discovered earlier, studies often contradict each other for various reasons. There may be differences in BMI between study populations, clinical practice around HRT use isn't always the same, the type and duration of HRT differs, and there are variations in study design and even in the assessment of menopause. There are also complex problems around distinguishing the effects of HRT from symptoms of menopause itself. Fundamentally, as studies have explained, more knowledge of biological mechanisms is needed before it is possible to return truly accurate results.

In 2017, *Science Daily* reported the results of new research, presented at the European Respiratory Society International Congress, which demonstrated that oral HRT can slow the decline in lung function in middle-aged women.[62] The study followed 3,713 women for two decades between the early 1990s and 2010 and found that those who took HRT for two years or longer did better on lung function tests than women who had never taken HRT. Lung function is at its best during the midtwenties. From then on, it decreases incrementally. One thing that accelerates lung decline is menopause—which raises the question, could HRT at least partly counteract it?

The women's lung health was tested at the start of the survey and again 20 years later. The measurement used was *forced vital capacity* (FVC), which assesses the volume of air that can be exhaled from the lungs after taking the deepest possible breath. Women who used HRT lost, on average, 46 milliliters less lung volume over the 20-year period than those who had never taken it. To put this finding into context, 46 milliliters is approximately the amount of lung volume that would be lost by a woman who smoked a pack of cigarettes every day for three years. While researchers do not believe this is likely to be clinically significant for healthy women, for women who have airway disorders, the decline in lung function could lead to increased breathlessness and fatigue, decreased ability to work, and poorer quality of life.[62]

While the study does not advocate either for or against HRT, the findings do demonstrate the importance of female sex hormones for the maintenance of healthy lungs in middle-aged women. This research provides another piece in the puzzle in understanding the relationship between menopause and lung health. The fact remains that women and their doctors need to be better informed about the health changes that happen after menopause. Women with existing respiratory conditions such as asthma should be closely observed during the menopausal transition, and advice about medication should be more personalized and take changing hormonal levels into account.

## OSTEOPOROSIS AND BREATHING PATTERN DISORDERS

Osteoporosis is a condition prevalent in postmenopausal women that might, at first, appear to have no connection with breathing.[63] It is a disease of low bone mineral density or excessive bone loss and is a common cause of bone fractures in older women. Osteoporosis affects 200 million women worldwide, with nearly one in two women over the age of 50 likely to suffer an osteoporosis-related fracture. In women over 45, the condition accounts for more days of hospitalization than diabetes, heart attack, or breast cancer.[64]

It can cause repeated fractures of the vertebrae attached to the ribs, which may lead to an excessive curve in the spine called thoracic kyphosis. Each time one of these thoracic vertebrae is broken, lung capacity shrinks, with a reduction in forced vital capacity of 9%. While research has examined the link between osteoporosis and respiration in terms of this impact on mechanical function, very little work has been done to measure lung health in women with osteoporosis but no diagnosis of chronic respiratory disease.

The fact that women with osteoporosis commonly complain about breathlessness prompted a 2018 study.[63] Researchers theorized that the fragility of the rib cage typical of bone loss and osteoporosis negatively impacts respiratory function by inhibiting the body's responses to normal breathing stimuli, and thus affecting the blood acid-base balance. In simple terms, the fragility of the ribs causes instinctive changes to breathing patterns, designed to protect weakened bones.

To test this theory, scientists assessed lung function, arterial blood gas levels, central respiratory drive, and breathing patterns of women with bone fragility who had no respiratory illness, kidney disease, or anemia, and who were not taking any medication known to alter blood pH. The women's results were compared with a control group of women who did not have bone fragility.

The results showed for the first time that women with osteoporosis or bone loss who had never smoked displayed disturbances in blood gas exchange and changes in breathing patterns compared to age-matched healthy women. The differences were not the result of anatomical changes or other conditions such as cardiorespiratory disease. This is the first study to look at gas exchange and breathing patterns where participants were selected to minimize confounding factors, such as respiratory disease, smoking, medications, and anatomical considerations.

Lung volumes at rest and during exercise were similar in all the women, but the differences in breathing patterns and gas exchange values between women with or without bone fragility were significant, even though all the values fell within normal reference ranges. Differences included changes in the ventilatory response to $CO_2$, lower levels of arterial $CO_2$ and oxygen, a higher arterial to alveolar oxygen gradient suggesting defective diffusion of oxygen from the blood to the lungs, and higher pH levels in the blood.

Interestingly, bone loss has been linked to depressive symptoms. Post-menopausal women are at increased risk of depression at the same time of life they are vulnerable to bone loss. While several studies have found a relationship between bone loss and depression, none have identified the reason for the connection[64]. Osteoporosis and bone loss are often undiagnosed until a woman suffers a fracture. However, a 2018 review found that depressive symptoms are indicative of bone loss, may help identify women with these conditions, and should trigger further investigation of bone health.[64]

According to a 2019 paper, the biochemical and physiological effects of psychological stress are recognized as contributing factors in osteoporosis.[65] Researchers looked at evidence pointing to stress-associated mental health disorders as risk factors for osteoporosis. They suggested that therapies to address psychological health could have benefits for bone-loss patients. Research into this topic is limited, but the studies that do exist indicate that a personalized, multifaceted approach may improve patient outcomes, particularly in those who are at a higher risk of developing osteoporosis.

A further link exists between osteoporosis and anxiety.[66] A 2018 study of 192 women found that those with high levels of anxiety were more prone to osteoporosis-related fracture. Anxiety levels were connected to age, depressive symptoms, years since menopause, and age at menopause. Scientists concluded that anxiety levels in postmenopausal women were associated with, and predictive of, reduced bone mineral density in the lumbar spine and hips.

While it is interesting to explore the connections between osteoporosis and breathing, there is currently no research to indicate a direct link between menopausal depression and anxiety, physical symptoms of bone mineral loss, and breathing pattern disorders. However, it is the case that addressing poor breathing can significantly improve quality of life by reducing susceptibility to a huge range of mental and physical conditions.

## SLOW, DEEP BREATHING AND MENOPAUSE SYMPTOMS

It has been proven that slow, deep breathing can reduce certain hormonal symptoms of menopause. A 2012 study explored the potential of parasympathetic activation via slow, deep, diaphragmatic breathing to reduce the frequency and severity of hot flashes. Paced breathing can reduce the stress response, relaxing the body and mind.[67]

For the study, scientists designed a nine-week, three-arm clinical trial in which participants used an audio CD to practice guided paced breathing exercises. One group practiced at 6 breaths a minute once a day for 15 minutes. A second group practiced the same exercise twice a day. The third group practiced 14 breaths a minute for 10 minutes each day (normal breathing). Nearly 80% of the women who completed the study found the exercises easy to do and to fit into their daily routine. All of the participants across the three groups reported reductions in hot flashes. Women who practiced paced breathing twice a day saw the biggest improvement (52%). Those who practiced 6 breaths a minute once a day saw a 42% improvement and those practicing normal breathing experienced a 46% improvement. The researchers concluded that paced breathing provides a workable intervention that can be easily applied, and a larger study is needed to fully assess the impact of the breathing exercises on hot flash reduction.

The ebook, *Recognizing and Treating Breathing Disorders*, cites earlier studies that demonstrate women who are unable or "unwilling" to take HRT have successfully used breathing retraining to reduce hot flashes.[68, 69]

This research is backed up by an email I received from a client who wrote that she had noticed significant benefits after implementing the breathing techniques. She said, "I have noticed a 90 to 100% decrease in night sweats when I go to bed with my mouth taped, and this is after only one week." This points to better regulation of the autonomic nervous system and corresponds with research that connects nocturnal sweating with sleep apnea.[70] According to the 2013 paper, incidence of night sweats is three times higher in people with untreated sleep apnea than it is in the general population. By using MyoTape to ensure nasal breathing during sleep, night sweats, apnea, and the associated insomnia may all be alleviated.

## WHAT'S NEXT FOR FEMALE RESPIRATORY HEALTH?

The scientific literature exploring the role of female sex hormones in respiratory health is complicated and incomplete[41]. Women differ significantly in hormonal profiles over the course of their lives, and assessment of hormonal status is still a problem in that menopause cannot be confirmed until 12 months after it actually occurs. Even then, it is often difficult to determine because of the use of hormonal medications.

It is important that research begins to investigate hormonal influences on respiratory health in sufficiently large studies. Future work needs to take into account real life factors, such as smoking, which has an antiestrogen effect. For instance, establishing a clear connection between asthma and HRT is likely to be heavily influenced by understanding the role of smoking.

There is enough evidence to be sure that sex hormones do influence respiratory health and disease throughout the course of a woman's life. However, the understanding of this impact is limited.

Some research covers asthma and lung function, but hardly any investigates COPD. It seems fairly clear that women who reach puberty early and have irregular periods also suffer with more asthma and poor lower lung function. Asthma and respiratory symptoms are known to fluctuate during the menstrual cycle, and this suggests the possibility of therapeutic interventions.

Changes in respiratory health around menopause are likely but very understudied and difficult to measure due to HRT use. Better understanding of these areas has great potential to improve treatment and outcomes for women with asthma and COPD. The 2012 review of the literature on respiratory health in women from menarche to menopause concludes firmly with this statement, "The era for investigating respiratory health in 2,000 men and 29 women has passed."[41]

# CHAPTER FOURTEEN
## SUGAR, SUGAR

---

## WHAT IS DIABETES?

Diabetes is a long-term disease that affects the way the body metabolizes blood sugar or glucose, an important source of energy. Glucose comes from the food we eat, especially foods rich in carbohydrates. During digestion, those carbohydrates are broken down into simple sugars that enter the bloodstream via the intestines.[1] When this happens, beta cells in the pancreas secrete insulin, which is a hormone.[2] Hormones are chemical messengers produced by the body and released into the blood to trigger specific responses. Insulin's job is to enable the cells to absorb blood sugar to release energy. The relationship between insulin and glucose is similar to that of carbon dioxide ($CO_2$) and oxygen. Just as $CO_2$ is needed to release oxygen from the blood, insulin is necessary to unlock the energy in blood glucose.

In a healthy system, insulin helps regulate blood sugar, making sure there is never too much (*hyperglycemia*) or too little (*hypoglycemia*) glucose in the blood for the body's vital systems to function.[3, 4] In a diabetic body, this process is compromised, either because the pancreas produces insufficient or no insulin (type 1) or because the body is unable to use insulin properly (type 2). When this happens, glucose can't be absorbed by the cells, and levels of blood sugar become chronically high.

## TYPE 1 DIABETES

Type 1 diabetes is an autoimmune disorder that results in excessive sugar in the bloodstream. People with this type of diabetes are not able to produce their own insulin due to an immune system malfunction that destroys the insulin-producing beta cells of the pancreas. Instead, they have to inject insulin every day to keep blood sugar under control.

This type of diabetes tends to occur during childhood or early adulthood. Its cause has not yet been determined, but scientists believe it begins with a genetic predisposition and is initially set off by an immune system activated by, for example, a viral infection, environmental triggers, or a genetic condition.[5] The immune system attacks the beta cells in the pancreas, producing a single insulin-destroying antibody.

According to TrialNet, an international network of researchers working to understand type 1 diabetes, if you have a relative with type 1 diabetes, you have a 1 in 20 chance of developing the disease, compared to a risk factor of 1 in 300 for the general population.[2, 6] In children under the age of five years, incidence is increasing. In the United States, figures suggest that 1 child in every 400 to 600 is affected, and 15% to 20% of new diagnoses are in children under five.[7] Because type 2 diabetes is also to some extent hereditary, people often confuse the two conditions, but it is important not to lump the two types of diabetes together.

## TYPE 2 DIABETES

This is the more common type of diabetes, affecting around 90% to 95% of adult diabetics. Type 2 diabetes manifests as difficulty using and producing insulin, otherwise known as insulin resistance. Blood sugar levels become too high because the body can't respond normally to insulin. This causes the system to compensate by producing ever-increasing amounts of the hormone. Over time, the pancreas becomes exhausted by its efforts to meet the demand for insulin. It becomes unable to produce sufficient insulin, and blood sugar levels rise even higher.[3, 4]

Whenever imbalances exist, the body's systems will try to restore homeostasis. If any aspect of those systems is faulty, long-term adaptations occur that can drain the body's resources, impacting overall health. One example of the body's attempt to restore homeostasis, of course, is the biochemical response to habitual overbreathing.

According to key statistics from Diabetes UK, contributing factors in type 2 diabetes include obesity, age, genetic predisposition,[8] socioeconomic status, and ethnicity,[9] In part, this is because people from deprived backgrounds are more likely to experience physical inactivity, a poor diet, and tobacco use.[10]

The onset of type 2 diabetes can be difficult to identify, as it progresses more slowly and without the acute metabolic disturbances seen in type 1 diabetes.[11] As many as half of all type 2 diabetics may be undiagnosed.[11]

## WHY DIABETES LEAVES YOU BREATHLESS

Abnormal respiratory function is a feature of both types of diabetes.[12] A 2017 study describes the negative impact type 2 diabetes has on lung health.[13] Researchers explain that insulin resistance, chronic low-grade inflammation, and damage to the veins and autonomic nervous system all contribute to the lung deterioration associated with type 2 diabetes, causing physical changes that include changes to the tissues.[13]

Diabetes is recognized as a risk factor for sleep-disordered breathing, sleep apnea, and daytime sleepiness.[13] Researchers recommend that patients with type 2 diabetes should be considered at risk of pulmonary dysfunction.[13] The paper notes that in previous studies, declines in lung function could be detected up to three years before type 2 diabetes was diagnosed.[13] In another paper, which examined lung health in Native Americans with diabetes, impaired pulmonary function was observed before diabetes occurred. What's more, the risk of diabetes increased by 2% for every 1% decrease in forced ventilatory capacity,[14] a measure of lung volume.

Also, both types of diabetes can cause a type of nerve damage called neuropathy. Neuropathy can affect the *phrenic nerve*, an important nerve responsible for motor control of the diaphragm.[15] This is one factor that may lead to respiratory symptoms, respiratory failure, and even death in diabetics.

When the body is not able to process blood sugar properly, complications occur on a "microvascular" and "macrovascular" level—both in the small and large blood vessels. The blood vessels essentially become "clogged" with excess glucose. On a microvascular level, this affects the tiny blood vessels in the skin and eyes and can lead to problems that include blindness,[16] damage to the retinas and nerves, and kidney failure.[16] On a macrovascular level, it affects the feet,[17] impacts organs including the heart and brain, and can lead to heart attack and stroke.[12] The first obvious sign of these problems may be excessive breathlessness.

According to the National Kidney Foundation, around 30% of type 1 diabetics and 10% to 40% of type 2 diabetics will eventually suffer from kidney failure.[18] One outward symptom of kidney failure is breathlessness. Acute breathlessness can be caused by a serious condition called diabetic ketoacidosis or metabolic acidosis, which involves disruptions to the blood acid-base balance that adversely affects the respiratory system.[19] Metabolic acidosis can lead to respiratory failure and contribute to the development and progression of disease. Much like respiratory acidosis, this type of acidosis commonly causes hyperventilation, a fast breathing rate, and a decrease in blood $CO_2$ that evolves into overbreathing with an increased tidal volume.[19] Left untreated, it can be fatal.[19]

Dysfunctional breathing is prevalent in type 2 diabetes. One study found that patients with type 2 diabetes had significantly lower end-tidal $CO_2$ and a much higher respiratory rate than a control group of healthy people. Scientists concluded that lung function was impaired in the diabetic patients and that they would benefit from a program to improve it.[20]

Earlier research, which investigated lung function in patients with type 1 diabetes, identified the lung as a "target organ" for diabetes.[21] Another paper examined 45 patients with type 2 diabetes and found a "strong and inverse relationship" between the duration of the diabetes and diminished lung volumes, concluding that poor blood sugar control was directly related to decreases in the volume of the lungs[22]. Several other studies have also associated diabetes with reduced lung function and respiratory muscle weakness.[23–26]

Gas exchange in the lungs occurs in the alveoli, where a thin membrane separates capillary blood from the air. Any damage to this membrane will negatively affect the lung's ability to absorb oxygen into the blood and release $CO_2$. Scientists have suggested that changes in lung function, especially reduced gas exchange, may occur in patients with diabetes as a result of damage to the alveoli.[27]

A study of yogic techniques, including breathing exercises and relaxation, found that the exercises led to better lung function in type 2 diabetic patients, improving forced expiratory volume and forced vital capacity.[28] Researchers suggested that the increase in lung function was due to practices designed to improve respiratory muscle stamina and lung expansion and to conscious breathwork, which relaxed the respiratory process, supporting better lung elasticity and function.[28] Like previous research in healthy patients and people with a range of conditions, yoga was found to be helpful in diabetes, reducing obesity, improving oxygenation, opening the airways, and increasing recruitment of the alveoli.[28]

Diabetics should find breathing exercises helpful. Light, slow, deep, breathing reduces stress, which we know is instrumental in the onset and progression of disease. Lower sensitivity to $CO_2$ helps maintain homeostatic balance in the blood acid base, and nasal breathing from the diaphragm supports healthy lung volumes and respiratory muscle function.

In addition, functional breathing harnesses $CO_2$, an important vasodilator. Poor vasodilation is a major issue in diabetes and can compromise circulation in the legs, leading to painful ulcers.[29] One 2015 study reported that $CO_2$ therapy was beneficial in treating foot ulcers in diabetic patients by increasing blood flow to the affected area.[30] In that experiment, synthetic $CO_2$ was dissolved in water and applied directly to the feet to improve tissue oxygenation, just as the Romans and ancient Greeks used to do, bathing in waters rich in carbonic acid to cure a variety of illnesses.

## NICK'S STORY

Nick Heath is an Oxygen Advantage instructor. He is also a type 1 diabetic. Nick was just 11 years old when he was diagnosed. For 14 years, he received "standard care" for his condition, but the results were mediocre at best. At the age of 25, he began to eat better and exercise regularly. His blood sugar improved, and at the time, he thought it probable that he had achieved the best control he was ever likely to have over his diabetes. Despite this improvement, over the next few years, he still felt that something was amiss. Nick was doing everything he could from a nutritional and exercise perspective, but he was still unable to maintain consistent energy levels, and he often felt drained.

When he was 30 years old, Nick found the *Oxygen Advantage*. After his first night using a lip tape to ensure nasal breathing during sleep, he woke up noticeably refreshed and full of vitality. He emailed his wife at work to say that either he was crazy or taping was the best thing ever. Inspired by his newfound energy, which seemed more stable and long-lasting than any previous change, he also began applying the slow breathing and breath-hold techniques from the Oxygen Advantage. After a few months, he noticed his blood sugars were improving considerably and he needed 10% to 20% less insulin.

Nick's college major was meteorology, qualifying with a PhD. This background as a research scientist made him eager to learn how the breathing exercises were having such a dramatic impact on his diabetes. He spent several years exploring the impact of correct breathing techniques on diabetes and chronic disease and found evidence to explain the positive effects of slow breathing and breath-hold exercises on his blood sugars.

Slow breathing has been shown to improve the function of the autonomic nervous system by reducing activation of its stress-driving sympathetic branch[31]. It reduces oxidative stress[32]—an imbalance of antioxidants and free radicals that contributes to the aging process and can lead to cell and tissue damage[33]. Lack of oxygen in fat cells has been directly linked to the development of insulin resistance in mice.[34] Slow breathing also lowers blood glucose[35] and increases oxygenation of the tissues.[31, 36] This enhanced uptake of oxygen into the blood and cells could be crucial in understanding why slow breathing is so helpful for diabetics.

Studies have shown that the root cause of autonomic dysfunction in diabetes might be tissue hypoxia[37]—a condition in which part of the body is deprived of adequate oxygen. Slow breathing practice supports optimum gas exchange and better oxygenation, helping the body restore autonomic balance. This, in turn, reduces stress[38] and anxiety,[39] helping control fluctuations in blood glucose. As part of the fight-or-flight stress response, the body releases stored glucose from the liver into the blood. If insulin function is poor, that extra blood sugar cannot reach the cells and sugar concentrations in the blood rise.[40] Research has also shown that slow breathing can increase insulin sensitivity,[41] particularly in type 2 diabetics. This means that insulin is more able to do its job and the body can metabolize blood sugar better.

Nick also discovered the power of taping his mouth at night to reduce sleep-disordered breathing. (This technique is described in detail in Chapter Seven.) An intimate two-way link between type 2 diabetes and sleep apnea has been established.[42] One 2010 pilot study reported that 40% of its 37 long-term type 1 diabetic subjects had OSA.[43] While Nick didn't believe he had sleep apnea, when he taped his mouth to ensure nasal breathing at night, he experienced much deeper, more restorative sleep. This resulted in better morning blood sugars. As anyone living with type 1 diabetes will know, managing the condition is a full-time job. The increased energy Nick felt as a result of taping meant he felt better able to control his diabetes throughout the day.

Another reason for Nick's improved quality of sleep could be that better breathing helped balance his autonomic nervous system, improving autonomic function. Diabetics tend to have lower parasympathetic tone at night, which may result in a disrupted circadian rhythm.[44] Slow breathing is known to increase parasympathetic activity. (We examined this in the context of the vagus nerve in Chapter Four.) By nasal breathing during sleep, a practice that results in slower breathing and stimulates the vagus nerve, it is likely that Nick improved his circadian rhythms.

Nick also began a breath-hold practice. As a surfer, he primarily used the exercises to improve his confidence in the water. However, his research led him to understand that breath holds, or *intermittent hypoxia*, were a key component of his increased diabetes control too. The positive results Nick experienced can be explained by three factors:

1. Hypoxia lowers blood sugar, independent of insulin sensitivity.[45]
2. Hypoxia strengthens the innate function of the immune system.[46]
3. Hypoxia increases insulin sensitivity.[47]

**Important:** It is never advisable to practice breath holds while in the water. If you take part in any water sports, you should only practice these breathing exercises on dry land so you can enjoy the benefits when in the water.

Of the three techniques, slow breathing, taping, and breathholding, Nick found that taping at night had the greatest impact. He wakes every morning energized, with good blood sugars, ready for a great day. Since beginning with a breathing practice, he has seen a marked improvement in his quality of life and in his diabetes. His average blood sugar measurements are the best they have ever been.

## DIABETES CONTROL AND THE BREATH

Functional breathing is a keystone habit that forms the foundation of good health,[48] and diabetes is no exception. Studies have explored the potential of deep breathing and controlled intermittent hypoxia (IH) as a holistic intervention to relieve symptoms associated with both type 1[49, 50] and type 2 diabetes.[47, 51, 52] Trials have focused on the possible applications for improving blood sugar, biological functioning, energy, stress, and well-being. Controlled IH is a periodic dropping of blood oxygen saturation with adequate recovery between sets. Because it is controlled, it differs from the unhealthy oxygen decrease seen in sleep apnea. IH can be achieved with breath holds or by using breathing equipment and altitude tents.

Research into breathing techniques would be immensely valuable for medics, certified breathing instructors, and other holistic practitioners who are interested in using the principles of IH breath training to improve the health of their diabetic patients. Studies indicate that integrating periodic breath holds (IH breathing training) into diabetic care plans is an excellent step toward improving quality of life.

**Important: If you have diabetes, it is vital that you monitor your blood sugar levels regularly during practice of any kind of breathing exercises. Breath holding can cause blood sugar levels to drop too quickly.**

To monitor blood sugar levels, consider investing in a continuous glucose monitoring (CGM) device—a readily available gadget that allows you to check your blood sugar levels in a noninvasive way. They are not cheap, but, as the range of products on the market expands, they are becoming more accessible. If you have type 1 diabetes, it's likely you already own a CGM, but they are equally valuable for any type 2 diabetic interested in making lifestyle choices that will improve their condition.

As Nick also discovered, good quality sleep is an essential part of diabetes management. Many aspects of sleep-disordered breathing can be addressed simply by making the switch to nasal breathing during sleep. Healthy breathing while asleep has many positive effects on the body's systems that are beneficial for many conditions, including diabetes. This is worth paying attention to since sleep deprivation is associated with insulin resistance, and poor sleep quality, sleep apnea, and insomnia have all been shown to increase the risk of type 2 diabetes.[53]

## DIABETES AND RESPIRATORY DISEASE

Type 1 and type 2 diabetics have a higher risk for four major respiratory diseases.[54, 55] A research paper published in *Diabetes Research and Clinical*

*Practice* analyzed the link between type 1 and type 2 diabetes and four common respiratory diseases: chronic obstructive pulmonary disease (COPD), chronic bronchitis, emphysema, and asthma.[54, 55] The study looked at data from 53,146 adults, all aged 20 years or more. Of the participants, 781 had type 1 diabetes, 4,277 had type 2 diabetes and 48,088 were nondiabetic. Respiratory diseases were present in 26% of type 1 diabetics, 21% of type 2 diabetics, and 13% of nondiabetics. A number of different examinations also showed that type 1 diabetics were 62% more likely to suffer a respiratory disorder than nondiabetics, while type 2 diabetics were 26% more vulnerable. The most common disease was asthma, and type 1 diabetics were found to be 51% more at risk of asthma than nondiabetics. In type 2 diabetes, the increased likelihood of asthma was 38%.[54, 55]

Impaired immune function is a common feature of diabetes. In type 2 diabetes, researchers have identified oxidative stress as one possible pathway by which innate immunity is disrupted.[56] In type 1 diabetes, the immune response is, by nature of the condition, dysregulated. One theory points to systemic inflammation as a link between diabetes and lung dysfunction.[12] Exaggerated inflammatory responses in the lung may be the result of an impaired ability to regulate inflammatory mechanisms.[12] (The connection between inflammatory responses and breathing was explored in depth in the chapter on the vegas nerve, Chapter Four.)

Equally, even before type 2 diabetes is diagnosed, the lung may be the primary location for the activation of inflammatory processes. This might explain why lung function is already worse before the onset of diabetes. A 2012 study describes lower lung volumes in type 2 diabetics with inadequate glycemic control than in those whose blood sugars were well-regulated. Patients with poor blood glucose control also had much higher blood levels of inflammatory markers, indicating that inflammation is involved in the decrease in lung function and fibrosis in type 2 diabetics.[12] The paper suggests that both systemic inflammation, which involves chronic activation of the immune system[57], and inflammation in the lungs[58] may contribute to the "complex interplay between respiratory and metabolic dysfunction."[12]

In type 1 diabetics, abnormal growth during childhood (stunting)[59] may affect the proper growth and development of organs including the lungs. While the duration of diabetes has an inverse relationship with lung function in type 2 diabetics, there isn't strong evidence to support the same connection in type 1 diabetes.[60] However, a 2011 study did find a significant difference in the incidence of restrictive breathing disturbances depending on whether or not "extreme stunting" was present.

Another study states that children with type 1 diabetes have increased airway resistance and that they are more likely to have abnormal lung function later in life, with long-term problems, including decreased lung volume, less ability to diffuse $CO_2$, and poor diabetes control. Researchers concluded that progressive abnormalities in lung function might adversely interfere with the effectiveness of intrabronchial insulin treatment.[61]

In a 2020 Swedish cohort study of more than one and a quarter million children, of whom 9.5% had asthma and 0.3% had type 1 diabetes, scientists found that children with asthma were more likely to develop type 1 diabetes, but the reverse was not the case. Asthma was associated with a small but significant increased risk of being diagnosed with type 1 diabetes compared with non-asthmatic children.[62] In an article for *MedPage Today*, physician Michael Yafi suggested that, "It may seem plausible that some factors, like early exposure to viruses, would play a role in the development of these two diseases."[63]

Yet another paper looked at changes in the thickness of the lung cell basement membrane in patients with pulmonary diseases. The study examined participants with diabetes, asthma, bacterial pneumonia, pulmonary tuberculosis, idiopathic pulmonary fibrosis, sarcoidosis, and even lung cancer and found that the basement membrane of cells *was only thicker in diabetes and asthma*. What this means is that diabetes and asthma have physiological similarities,[64] and that explains why the Oxygen Advantage breathing techniques used successfully for asthma may also be effective for diabetics. With this understanding and given that respiratory illnesses are so prevalent in people with diabetes, it seems essential to include breathing exercises into diabetes treatment along with other forms of wellness maintenance such as nutrition and exercise.

## THE IMPORTANCE OF EXERCISE

It's no secret that people who are physically active are healthier. Exercise boosts the immune system, supports cardiovascular health, and is important for weight control and self-esteem. Exercising your muscles more often and pushing them to work harder improves their ability to use insulin and absorb glucose.[65] When the muscles are better able to metabolize glucose, the insulin-producing cells don't have to work so hard. However, exercising with diabetes can be challenging, and it is important to consult with your healthcare professional to receive appropriate guidance on diet and medication before changing your exercise regime.

You may find that you get more out of your exercise time and enjoy it more if you incorporate a mixture of resistance training and a variety of aerobic exercises such as cycling, swimming, and jogging. You will also notice gradual improvements in your health if you simply reduce periods of inactivity throughout the day and evening.[4]

When it comes to sedentary lifestyle choices, too much time spent watching TV can be particularly damaging. Research indicates that every two hours spent watching TV instead of doing something more active increases the chance of developing diabetes by 20%, raises the risk of heart disease by 15%, and makes it 13% more likely that you'll die early.[65] TV watching is unhealthy, not just in its inactive nature. While it's true that there are links between time spent on the couch and weight gain or obesity—something all diabetics must avoid—it is also the case that it's easy to slip into unhealthy dietary habits when watching television.[65]

The good news is that it is possible to see benefits with relatively small lifestyle changes. While there are obviously increased advantages in terms of cardiovascular health if you can work your way up to longer, more intense periods of exercise, the risk of developing type 2 diabetes can be reduced by 30% simply by walking briskly for half an hour every day.[65]

Another benefit of exercise is that it helps rid the body of excess fat. That much is relatively obvious. But if you have never thought about where that weight goes, you may be surprised to learn that it is not burned off as heat or energy. A 2014 study published in the *British Medical Journal* found that fat primarily leaves the body via the lungs, as $CO_2$.[66] In fact, 84% of the atoms in every fat molecule is exhaled as $CO_2$, with the rest ending up as water, which is eliminated in urine, sweat, and other bodily fluids.[67] According to the paper, replacing one hour of rest with an exercise, such as jogging, which increases the metabolic rate by seven times removes an extra 39 grams of carbon from the body. While the researchers point out that this is easily countered by overeating, they state that since weight loss requires the unlocking of carbon from fat cells, the maxim, "eat less, move more" remains a good starting point.[66]

## A HEALTHY HEART VERSUS A DIABETIC HEART

Lower levels of oxygen in the blood of diabetics are common, while reflex responses to insufficient oxygen are blunted. These abnormalities can lead to serious cardiovascular/renal complications.[65]

The heart function of people with type 2 diabetes becomes abnormal. Instead of working optimally, the metabolic systems of the heart change, becoming less able to process blood sugar. In this state, the body oxidizes (a chemical reaction involving oxygen) more fatty acids such as oils, cholesterols, fats, and steroids. The word *metabolism* refers to the entire spectrum of biochemical processes that take place within the body. This particular change in metabolic function results in greater oxygen consumption by the heart muscle tissue, independent of contraction.[68]

## BREATH HOLDS, HYPOXIA, AND DIABETES

Type 1 diabetics generally suffer from low-grade chronic hypoxia, which may be the root cause of many diabetic complications.[51] An interesting 2013 study looked at the effects of a single bout of IH on cardiorespiratory control in 15 patients with type 1 diabetes.[51] The research, which was the first of its kind, examined the benefits of breathing hypoxic air using a facemask. Just one session with the mask produced beneficial changes in aerobic efficiency and ventilatory responses to hypoxia (too little blood oxygen) and hypercapnia (too much blood $CO_2$).[51] Wearing a mask is not the same as practicing breath holds, but the same effect of reducing oxygen can be achieved with either method.

The researchers explain that, while it might seem counterproductive for diabetics to practice IH training, when used correctly, the technique helps the body to adapt to hypoxia. The study notes that more research is needed in regard to prolonged exposure to IH of more than two weeks. However, the improvement seen in breathing efficiency does indicate that IH training may be beneficial in the treatment and maintenance of type 1 diabetes, particularly as negative side effects are minimal.[48]

## STIMULATING BLOOD SUGAR TRANSPORT IN MUSCLE

IH has been found to "significantly" stimulate "glucose transport in muscle" in both lean and obese patients.[45, 48] Research dating back 25 years shows that IH was already established as being beneficial. In 1995, scientists from the University of East Carolina's Department of Biochemistry set up an experiment to see whether hypoxia-driven glucose transportation (absorption of blood sugar into the muscle cells) was still possible in insulin-resistant muscle. The results showed that when IH was used alongside insulin, there was a substantial increase in muscle glucose transportation.[45, 48] Insulin used together with the practice of hypoxia reduced a diabetic's blood glucose more than either insulin or hypoxia on its own.

Scientists found that muscle contraction and insulin stimulate the transport of blood sugar to the muscle cells through separate pathways, and that breath holds work on the muscle contraction pathway.[45, 48] This is exciting news because it indicates that the pathway for blood sugar transport is still present in diabetics, including those with insulin resistance (type 2 diabetics). The presence of this pathway explains how diabetics can potentially lower their blood sugar by using breath-hold exercises under the guidance of a professional certified breathing instructor.[45, 48]

## OXYGENATING THE BRAIN

When the body is at rest, the brain consumes around 20% of the body's total oxygen supply. It should follow that during IH, the system would compensate to ensure an adequate oxygen supply to the brain. As $CO_2$ is a major driver of cerebral blood flow, it might make sense that reducing blood $CO_2$ would result in less blood flowing to the brain, but previous research has returned conflicting results.

In 2017, a new study examined how the two blood gases react by analyzing whether decreases in oxygen would increase blood flow to the brain or would be offset by reduced $CO_2$.[48, 69] The outcome of the trial indicated that IH raises oxygen extraction in the brain, and that even when levels of blood $CO_2$ are low, blood continues to flow to the brain. The overall results showed an increase in brain blood flow and that these increases were substantially stronger at the fifth rather than at the first bout of hypoxia, implying a cumulative effect.

Notably, although the participants reduced their $CO_2$ by a relative amount, their brain blood flow still rose considerably. This indicates that the IH-induced brain blood flow is more significant than the reduced circulation brought about by low blood $CO_2$.[48, 69] Results showed a substantial increase in oxygen extraction in the brain after the first bout of IH, which continued throughout the remainder of the procedure. Conversely, the extraction of oxygen in the muscles fell, implying that during hypoxia, the brain's need for oxygen is prioritized over that of the muscles.[48, 69]

The research authors noted that normal levels of oxygen in the tissues and blood, together with exposure to IH, cause dilation of the blood vessels in the brain and improve blood flow to the brain. While the oxygenation of muscles decreased during repeated IH, oxygen extraction in the brain increased. This, in combination with improved blood flow, helped maintain oxygen-dependent brain metabolism during acute, moderately intense IH. The study concluded that normal IH causes compensatory responses in both the heart and the blood vessels in the brain, which could have potential applications for training and optimizing brain blood flow.[69]

Research from the University of Rochester demonstrated that major increases in brain blood flow take place at a certain level of oxygen uptake.[70] Since both breath holds and high levels of $CO_2$ cause the blood vessels in the brain to dilate, it seems possible that, by employing high $CO_2$ breath holds, brain blood flow would increase even more:

> This research supports practicing breath holds before a workout, competition, or presentation, as increased brain blood flow helps focus & prepare the mind.[48]

For the purposes of this book, it is important to distinguish IH from breath holding. IH involves a controlled reduction in blood oxygen saturation to between 82% and 95%. This may be done between 3 and 15 times per day.[71-73] Most of the studies with IH use expensive equipment, which will be out of reach for many people.

With breath holding after an exhalation, blood oxygen saturation can be lowered to between 80 and 88% within a few days of practice. Of course, breath holding is not the same as IH. However, the point is, exposing the body to short, controlled doses of hypoxia may be beneficial.

Be aware that breath holding can generate a feeling of moderate to strong air hunger, which can be stressful. If you choose to practice breath holding, do so gently. Do not expose your body to high stress.

It can also be helpful to use a good quality pulse oximeter to monitor your blood oxygen saturation as it drops. If you have cardiovascular issues, are pregnant, or have other serious medical conditions, please do not practice breath holding.

## EMPTYING THE STOMACH

Both type 1 and type 2 diabetics are susceptible to a disruption of normal stomach contractions, which can cut off the digestive process. "Gastric emptying of solids is delayed in 30% to 50% of patients with diabetes."[74] This is the result of effects the disease has on the nervous system. Diabetes can negatively impact the vagus nerve, compromising the stomach and other muscles of the digestive tract.[75] As a result, food cannot pass through the digestive system as rapidly as it should. However, research indicates that hypoxia with oxygen levels of 10% and 6% causes an increase in gastric vagal nerve activity in just a few seconds.[76] It is possible to activate and therefore treat the vagus nerve by practicing slow breathing at six breaths per minute with a technique called heart rate variability biofeedback (HRVB).[77] (There is more detailed information about HRVB in Chapter Four.)

## SLOW BREATHING TO LOWER BLOOD SUGAR

The functioning of the two branches of the autonomic nervous system (ANS) is relevant in diabetes too. The sympathetic branch of the ANS raises blood sugar through direct nerve stimulation of the liver and indirectly through the release of the hormone adrenaline. The liver is controlled by both the sympathetic nervous system (SNS) and parasympathetic nervous system (PNS). When the SNS is triggered, the hormone adrenaline causes the liver to convert stored glycogen into blood sugar. Adrenaline increases insulin resistance.[48, 78] Simultaneously, the SNS suppresses the release of insulin from the pancreas. The pancreas is also controlled by nerves from both the SNS and PNS.[48, 78]

The important point here is that when the SNS is activated, stimulating the stress response, the pancreas can no longer release insulin. Conversely, when the PNS is stimulated, insulin production increases.[48] Slow breathing helps activate the PNS, which is "beneficial, especially for type 2 diabetics who still produce insulin."[48]

Research shows that the body of the diabetic tends to be in a chronic fight-or-flight state. When the SNS is overactive, we automatically breathe faster than usual and are more reactive to stress. The good news is that, by breathing slowly and lightly, it is possible to offset this imbalance. In this way, we can use the breath to consciously move into a parasympathetic mode.

Adding to the benefits of slow breathing, controlled intermittent breath holds also activate the SNS, strengthening the nervous system and making the body more resilient to stress.[48] Sympathetic activation is part of a healthy ANS, as long as it doesn't become chronic, getting out of balance with the parasympathetic branch.

## THE BENEFITS OF SLOW BREATHING FOR DIABETICS

In 2017, one of the most highly regarded scientific journals, *Nature*, shone a spotlight on the benefits of slow breathing for diabetics.[31] The publication cites research-backed findings that a reduced rate of respiration boosts the ANS, enhances arterial function, and increases blood oxygen saturation in type 1 diabetics: "Oxygen-induced impairment in arterial function is corrected by slow breathing in patients with type 1 diabetes."[31] The improved balance in autonomic function that comes from stimulating the PNS and suppressing sympathetic responses provides an antioxidant effect. The report suggests that slow breathing could represent a simple beneficial intervention in diabetes.[48] There is practical evidence that just two minutes of slow breathing can greatly enhance general health in diabetics.

Study participants were able to increase their arterial function. The arteries are important as part of the cardiovascular system. They are elastic blood vessels that carry blood away from the heart. Participants were also able to improve their blood oxygen saturation and key autonomic markers, measures of various processes regulated by the ANS, such as breath rate and blood pressure.[48]

## BREATH HOLDING AND BLOOD PRESSURE CONTROL

Type 1 diabetics show poor baroreflex sensitivity, which is compounded during periods of low blood sugar. As discussed previously, the baroreflex is a homeostatic mechanism that maintains blood pressure at near constant levels by controlling various functions such as heart rate. Greater baroreflex sensitivity implies a more responsive, flexible, healthy system, while low baroreflex sensitivity is an index of poor health and can indicate issues including cardiovascular disorders. Baroreflex sensitivity is also one of the key markers of the ANS.[79] Slow breathing has been found to improve the parasympathetic activity of the baroreflex in both diabetics and healthy subjects.

In a review of arterial function in type 1 diabetics, researchers found that slowing the respiratory rate to six breaths per minute increased the baroreflex sensitivity of type 1 diabetics to the extent that measurements were similar to those of the nondiabetic control group.[31] An even more interesting aspect of this study is the hypothesis that tissue hypoxia contributes significantly to diabetic autonomic disorders. By breathing slowly and allowing $CO_2$ to accumulate in the blood, it is possible to alleviate tissue hypoxia. This discovery could have major implications for the long-term complications associated with diabetes.

## DIAPHRAGMATIC BREATHING TO FILL A THERAPEUTIC NEED

2019 research from Pakistan explored using diaphragm breathing exercises for diabetics in developing countries where the cost of medications such as insulin can be a barrier to treatment. Scientists stated that breathing exercises are "very useful" and, if practiced regularly, can minimize hyperglycemia and prevent major complications associated with type 2 diabetes.[80]

The study sought to determine the effects of diaphragmatic breathing exercises on blood sugar levels and HbA1c (a reading of average blood glucose levels over two or three months) in 64 diabetic women. While studies from countries, including China, Japan, India, and Russia, where yoga is a common practice, have found significant improvements in blood sugar levels, diaphragmatic breathing exercises are not common in Pakistan. However, in this context, breathing exercises provide an accessible approach to diabetes control because patients can practice at home without the expense of medication and without any harmful side effects. Cost is an important consideration for diabetic patients in developing countries like Pakistan.

The study cites 2012 research into the therapeutic effects of diaphragmatic breathing on oxidative stress in type 2 diabetics. This earlier paper concluded that, while breathing exercises alone may not produce significant results, breathing could be successfully incorporated as an add-on therapy to standard care to improve blood sugar and HbA1c.[32]

I was first directed to research on this topic by my friend and colleague Dr. Jonathan Herron, from Dungannon in Northern Ireland. He has several diabetic family members and has lost one relative to diabetic complications. His masters thesis in biomedical science focused on novel therapies to treat diabetes. In his extensive work with diabetic patients, he has noticed a direct correlation between higher blood sugars and chronic hyperventilation, which suggests that correction through reduced breathing techniques would have a positive effect on HbA1C, lessening the need for drug therapy.

In fact, the Pakistani study did find that diaphragmatic breathing exercises were beneficial, especially when combined with other techniques like walking, meditation, and guided imagery, especially when the breathing is practiced regularly. It was noted that results in this study were negatively affected by the fact that participants didn't always practice the exercises. It recommended that medical practitioners working with diabetics should motivate their patients to adopt a routine practice of breathing exercises at home, stating, "Quality of life of type 2 diabetic patients can be improved significantly if patients' compliance with these exercises is assured." The study concluded that it would be valuable to investigate further effects of the breathing exercises with a larger sample of participants.

# CHAPTER FIFTEEN

# SEIZURE CONTROL AND THE BREATH

---

## WHAT IS EPILEPSY?

Epilepsy is a chronic neurological disease involving the brain.[1] It affects around 50 million people of all ages worldwide,[2] making it one of the most common neurological conditions. The disorder makes the sufferer susceptible to recurrent seizures that negatively impact health and quality of life. The risk of early death is three times higher in epileptics than the general population. In many parts of the world, suffers also experience discrimination and stigma.[3]

However, according to the World Health Organization, as many as 70% of people with epilepsy could live seizure-free if properly diagnosed and treated.[3] The condition is usually treated with anticonvulsants, but the effectiveness of those medications varies depending on the type of seizure condition.[4, 5]

Seizures can be caused by anything that interrupts necessary connections between nerve cells in the brain. Common nonepileptic triggers include low or high blood sugar, high fever, alcohol or drug withdrawal, and a brain concussion.[3] When a person has two or more seizures that are not provoked by any of these factors, he or she is considered to have epilepsy. Epilepsy has many possible causes—tumors, strokes, brain damage from injury or illness, an imbalance of neurotransmitters (the nerve-signaling chemicals), or a combination of these—but in many cases, there is no discernible basis for the disease.[6]

Epileptic seizures caused by identifiable factors, including brain tumors and lesions, are classified as symptomatic. Seizures where the cause is unknown are called idiopathic.[7] In this chapter, we focus on idiopathic seizures.

The brain controls and regulates all the voluntary and involuntary responses in the body. It is made up of nerve cells (neurons) that communicate with each other through electrical activity. When part of the brain receives a burst of abnormal electrical signals that temporarily interrupt normal brain function, a seizure occurs.[6]

In a healthy, normal system, all the electrical signals that travel between nerve cells are related to necessary processes such as memory, logic, decision-making, the deliberate or involuntary movement of muscles, and the functioning of the senses. For these signals to successfully transmit from one nerve cell to another, the strength of the electrical signal needs to be high enough—just as a mobile phone requires enough signal strength to make a call or an electrical socket must have the correct voltage to power your appliances.

The nerve cells also need to have a high enough "excitability" threshold so that this strong signal won't overpower them. In mammals, this threshold is normally around 50 microvolts[8, 9] (one microvolt is equivalent to around one millionth of a volt). When the seizure threshold is normal, electrical signals can pass between nerve cells in a functional way. It is important that no vital information is lost when signals are transmitted and that any irrelevant signals are repressed so that they don't interfere with the brain's usual processes. If the neuronal excitability threshold is too low for any reason, accidental signals can be amplified, causing the functioning of the central and peripheral nervous systems to be disrupted or suppressed.

This disruption is comparable to the changes in blood biochemistry that occur during abnormal breathing patterns.[10] In fact, this comparison draws a further parallel with epilepsy in that the levels of carbon dioxide ($CO_2$) and oxygen found in relation to chronic hyperventilation also tie in with susceptibility to seizures. Studies have reported a connection between epilepsy and the breath and even drawn conclusions that breathing exercises can help reduce the frequency and severity of seizures.[11]

Seizures can alter respiratory parameters, including the perception of respiration and fullness of breath.[12] During a seizure, respiratory rate, breathing pattern, and breathing quality may change. The patient may experience breathlessness, coughing, and secretion of mucus, and it is believed that neurogenic pulmonary edema (acute onset of pulmonary edema following a significant central nervous system insult)[13] may contribute to sudden unexplained death in epilepsy patients. Apnea (involuntary breath holding) and cyanosis (a blue tinge to the skin) are "normal" during several types of seizure, and hyperventilation is common in mesial epilepsy,[14] a form that is often hard to treat.[15] Coughing, shortness of breath, and choking can all occur when a seizure interferes with breathing and the rhythm of the heart.

Over time, these issues can lead to increased risk of cardiovascular disease and stroke.[16]

Observation of breathing after a seizure can even help healthcare practitioners identify the type of seizure. For example, respiration after a generalized tonic-clonic seizure tends to be regular, loud, and deep with prolonged inhalation and exhalation. After general nonepileptic seizures, breathing is faster with short in and out breaths.[17]

## JENNY'S STORY: SEIZURE CONTROL AND GREATER CONFIDENCE

Jenny was 13 years old when she began having epilepsy. At first, she had only small complex partial seizures and was able to manage her symptoms. However, by the time she finished college, postictal psychosis had become a problem. Postictal psychosis is an episode of psychosis that commonly occurs after a cluster of seizures. For Jenny, this would continue for three or four days after a seizure, with symptoms including paranoia, insomnia, and hearing voices. Her daytime seizures could be triggered by something as simple as tiredness or even by just catching her reflection in a mirror. Sometimes her panic attacks were so severe she ended up in hospital. She was advised that neurosurgery would help, and she went ahead with the procedure.

Jenny's epilepsy had improved after surgery, and five years after the surgery, Jenny was able to take a full-time job for the first time. The position gave her the option to work from home, which was helpful when she had epilepsy symptoms. While neurosurgery meant her daytime seizures stopped altogether, nocturnal seizures became a greater issue. The aftereffects of these were less severe, but the day after a seizure she still experienced a throbbing headache, memory impairment, and an unpleasant coppery taste in her mouth. Even though she no longer suffered from daytime seizures, she would sometimes feel an aura, as if a seizure were imminent. This could be extremely frightening and trigger severe panic attacks. The resulting chronic anxiety caused her to lose self-confidence.

Things changed for Jenny after she read online that light nasal breathing to address hyperventilation and regulate oxygen intake could help stem the onset of a panic attack. After getting my book *Anxiety Free: Stop Worrying and Quieten Your Mind*, she made the switch to full-time nasal breathing. She saw the connection between her anxiety, overbreathing through her mouth during sleep, and poor sleep quality. She realized that her habit of breath holding during sleep followed by overbreathing (sleep apnea) was causing her daytime sleepiness, poor concentration, forgetfulness, dry mouth, and headaches.

Once Jenny began to breathe lightly through the nose during the day, her next nocturnal seizure was much less severe. She got out of bed without noticing the metallic taste in her mouth that normally followed a seizure. Now, if she feels herself beginning to panic, she is able to avert the panic attack by keeping her mouth closed. Her nocturnal seizures are so much better that she sometimes has to look at the sleep app on her phone to see whether she has had a seizure. Jenny still takes an anticonvulsant, but by addressing her breathing habits, she has been able to gain more control over her condition. If the daytime aura comes on, she focuses on her breathing until the feeling passes. Her seizures have now completely stopped.

## THE BIOCHEMICAL LINK

The neuronal excitability threshold—the level of tolerance the nerve cells have for the strength of the signals passing between them—is highly sensitive to and dependent on the concentration of $CO_2$ in nerve tissues. Hyperventilation, and the resulting low $CO_2$ pressure in the brain, causes nerve cells to fire in a spontaneous and asynchronous way. This means that when levels of $CO_2$ and oxygen in the blood, muscles, and cells are disrupted due to poor breathing patterns, weak or inappropriate electrical signals may be strengthened and relayed through some areas of the brain, interfering with the normal signals and causing the seizure threshold to drop.[18]

According to the author and breathing afficionado, Dr. Artour Rakhimov, between 70% and 100% of epileptics can lower their neuron excitability threshold and induce seizures by deliberate hyperventilation.[19] Evidence demonstrates that hyperventilation can cause seizures,[20] but research has not so far identified the exact $CO_2$ level that can trigger seizures in people with epilepsy. This makes sense because many factors influence the transmission of electrical signals in the brain. While the concentration of arterial $CO_2$ is key, metabolic rate, which is affected by things like body position, posture, and exercise, also plays a role. So does the availability of calcium and magnesium ions in tissues, as well as the levels of amino acids, neurotransmitters, and other substances. Hypocapnia (low blood $CO_2$) provides the necessary condition for a reduced seizure threshold and the onset of seizures, but it is not the only factor leading to epileptic symptoms. Nonetheless, numerous studies have shown that hyperventilation reliably triggers seizures in epileptics (and patients suffering from explainable seizures), indicating that the threshold of nerve cell excitability is closely related to or controlled by respiration, with some lesser contribution from other states of homeostatic imbalance, such as sleep deprivation, stress, low blood sugar, infection, fever, alcohol intake, and overheating.[21]

The first research paper to explore the beneficial effect of $CO_2$ in epilepsy was published in the 1928 *Journal of Clinical Investigations*.[22] Scientists reported that inhaling air rich in $CO_2$ reduced the severity and duration of seizures due to the effect of the gas on nerve and muscle cells. A 1956 study returned the same results.[23] In 1999, another research paper explored the effects of hyperventilation on the brain's sensory responses and concluded that

> Increased neuronal excitability caused by hyperventilation-induced hypocapnia leads to spontaneous and/or asynchronous firing of cortical neurons.[24]

In simple terms. this means that the low levels of blood $CO_2$ that occur as a result of hyperventilation create abnormal activity in the nerve cells of the brain.

The conclusions of a 2005 paper are even more comprehensive, stating that, as well as altering respiration and vascular tone, abnormal $CO_2$ levels affect blood pH, consciousness, and seizure threshold.[25] Outside of the brainstem, the mechanisms by which $CO_2$ levels influence the function of neurons are unknown, but research suggests that $CO_2$-induced changes in nerve cell function are pH-dependent. The authors conclude that their findings demonstrate a mechanism for the bidirectional effects of $CO_2$ on neuronal excitability in the forebrain.

Sometimes, seizures may be triggered, worsened, and prolonged by low blood sugar levels. These are called "hypoglycemic" seizures.[26] It is known that chronic overbreathing results in poor blood sugar control, exacerbating the symptoms of hypoglycemia.[27].

Because one of the roles of $CO_2$ is as a vasodilator, hypocapnia (low $CO_2$) can lead to vasoconstriction, or narrowing of the blood vessels, which in turn can cause the carotid arteries to go into spasm, another key trigger for seizures. The carotid arteries are blood vessels that carry oxygen-rich blood to the brain, neck, and face.

At the same time, overbreathing from the upper chest reduces oxygenation of the organs, including the brain. This can lead to respiratory alkalosis, in which the blood pH is too high. This compounds the abnormal electrical activity, further lowering the seizure threshold.[9] A 2006 study from researchers in Finland reported that the suppression of alkalosis with 5% ambient $CO_2$ "abolished" seizures in juvenile rats within 20 seconds.[28]

This link with $CO_2$ forms the basis for the exchange breathing method (EBM) protocol, an emergency seizure-recovery method in which the first-aider administers an outward breath into the subject's nose during seizure. In a 2019 study, EBM was administered 28 times during different seizures in one subject. The least number of breaths given to stop a seizure was 1, and the most 10. Typically, 3 breaths were needed. In this case, this breathing method stopped the seizures at least three times faster than diazepam, without the postseizure side effects, such as drowsiness and bad moods. Researchers concluded that, since this simple technique can be used any time, it can be easily incorporated into existing treatment protocols, even applying it as soon as a seizure begins.[29]

## CHRONIC HYPERVENTILATION AS A SEIZURE TRIGGER

As we've already discussed, hyperventilation is a respiratory behavior where an irregular increase in the speed and depth of the breath results in abnormal exchange of gases in the lungs and low blood $CO_2$ levels.[30] Clinical and research evidence demonstrates a strong link between this habitual overbreathing and epilepsy. In early studies investigating the relationship between hyperventilation and seizures, scientists described the objective and subjective experiences accompanying low blood $CO_2$, commenting that, "there are few drugs the effects of which upon the neuromuscular system are so rapid and so striking as the effect of voluntary hyperpnea"[31] (deliberately increased rate and depth of breathing)[32]. It was found that seizure sufferers have an unusually high sensitivity to changes within a fairly narrow range of blood $CO_2$ concentrations.

According to Robert Fried's book *Breathe Well, Be Well*,[33] hyperventilation is a major cause of fits in epilepsy. The author refers to numerous studies dating back to the 1930s that have made the connection between overbreathing and seizures. In 1954, scientists stated that, "In persons who are predisposed to epileptic fits, simply overbreathing, often results in an attack."[34] A research paper from 1975, *Hyperventilation: The Tip and the Iceberg*, explained how low blood $CO_2$ causes constriction of the blood vessels, leading to a reduction in the amount of oxygen reaching the brain.[35] These effects are immediate, which is why hypocapnia can quickly result in feelings of faintness, dizziness, and visual disturbance. The paper also states that grand mal seizures may be triggered by hyperventilation.

Although research has clearly identified the role of $CO_2$ in cerebral circulation, many studies still conclude that the cause of seizures is neurological. The rationale behind this idea is that $CO_2$-driven changes to the blood acid-base balance create an unstable environment for the nerve cells of the brain. Further studies have suggested that anxiety can act as a seizure trigger because it leads to hyperventilation, lowering blood $CO_2$ levels.[36] Patients were prone to hyperventilating when they felt anxious, and while they did not display any obvious signs of overbreathing, they experienced a 50% drop in $CO_2$ and an increase in both EEG and clinical seizure activity. Separate research into cerebral blood flow and metabolism acknowledges the role of $CO_2$ as a vasodilator. A 2008 study examining sexual dysfunction in men with epilepsy points out that sex can itself prove problematic because of hyperventilation,[37] which is commonly associated with orgasm, can trigger seizures. In *Freedom from Asthma*, Alexander Stalmatski argues that epileptics, like asthmatics and people with a variety of other related conditions, always hyperventilate, suggesting that, "With reconditioning of their breathing patterns . . . the establishment of proper levels of $CO_2$, it is possible to prevent seizures without drugs."[38]

In clinical settings, hyperventilation is used to activate seizures for monitoring. I asked a friend who is a brain doctor about the connection between epilepsy and hyperventilation. My friend explained that hyperventilation is used

> especially by the child neurologists as a bedside tool to diagnose absence seizures (petit mal seizures) in children. Hyperventilation

causes blood to be alkaline by driving out $CO_2$. . . . This low blood pH causes constriction of the blood vessels, hence low oxygenation triggers the seizures. Even though children are more sensitive, in adults with chronic hyperventilation due to anxiety attacks, for example, the brain can suffer the metabolic and oxygenation changes.

I am increasingly surprised that breathing retraining to reverse hyperventilation is not widely considered in the treatment of seizures. Especially, since it is also widely recognized that common seizure triggers including alcohol, low blood sugar, and stress produce an increase in breathing volume that may deplete blood $CO_2$ to the seizure threshold.

According to an exhaustive 1990 review by Robert Fried and Mary Claire Fox, research has proven that the dramatic effect of inhaled $CO_2$ on EEG activity can be replicated by limiting the rate of respiration.[30] While, at the time of publication, no evidence existed to indicate that $CO_2$ could be controlled by self-regulation, the researchers believed that there would be broad clinical application for such a technique, commenting that "physiological equilibrium" could be restored by increasing oxygenation of the cells and tissues or by enhancing blood flow and metabolism. As Fried and Fox explain, studies have demonstrated that the cause of seizures is metabolic and vascular, and that the connection between hyperventilation and seizures is so strong as to indicate that one causes the other.

Alongside the Fried/Fox review, a significant body of research demonstrates a connection between hyperventilation and epilepsy symptoms. In 1981, a study compared the effect of 15 minutes of moderate exercise against 3 minutes of hyperventilation in 43 young patients with epilepsy.[39] Results were measured in terms of EEG discharges—abnormalities in EEG readings consisting of repetitive sharp waves or spikes. The epileptic subjects were compared to a control group of 20 young people who had either no organic brain injury or in whom brain injury had not caused epilepsy. Researchers found that the number of EEG discharges decreased in nearly all participants during exercise but increased during hyperventilation. The paper concluded that moderate exercise inhibits seizure activity, while hyperventilation exacerbates it.[39]

A 1984 study found that the concentration of blood $CO_2$ had a direct impact on the duration of seizures.[40] The researchers induced hypocapnia by hyperventilation to the point where concentration of $CO_2$ in the alveoli was only 2%. The duration of seizures increased significantly compared with the normal $CO_2$ level of 5%, even though oxygen concentration remained constant at 92%. While different levels of oxygen did not produce any notable changes to seizure duration, seizures became progressively longer as the amount of $CO_2$ in the alveoli decreased. This finding was confirmed in a 2008 paper, which reported that moderate hyperventilation caused a significant increase in EEG seizure duration compared to normal ventilation.[41] In 1993, scientists examined 19 patients with complex-partial seizures, reporting that hyperventilation triggered a "marked activation" of the epileptic focus—the area of the brain from which the seizure originates.[42]

There have been attempts to determine whether the degree of hypocapnia correlates with an increased frequency of petit mal or absence seizures and if there is a critical concentration of $CO_2$ at which these seizures are reliably induced.[43] In a 1996 study, scientists monitored 12 children who had newly diagnosed absence epilepsy. EEG readings and percentage of $CO_2$ in expired air were recorded during quiet respiration and hyperventilation. These readings were taken while the children breathed four different gas mixtures:

1. Room air
2. 100% oxygen
3. Room air with 4% $CO_2$
4. A gas containing 4% $CO_2$ and 96% oxygen

When the children were breathing quietly, a reduction in EEG spikes was seen when the breathing gas contained extra $CO_2$ (3 and 4), but a higher concentration of oxygen in inspired air (2) caused no changes. Seizures were triggered in eight of the children with each trial of hyperventilation, but the level of $CO_2$ that induced seizures was found to differ among the children. The study concluded that it would be helpful to discover whether sensitivity to blood $CO_2$ could help predict the likely response to antiepileptic drugs, and that more research was needed into the possible use of $CO_2$ for the remission of seizures.

A study from 2001 examined patients who suffered nonepileptic seizures, 41% having coexisting epilepsy and found the most frequent features of nonepileptic seizures included fear, anxiety, and hyperventilation.[44] Another paper found that typical absence (brief, generalized) seizures are "easily precipitated by hyperventilation" in approximately 90% of untreated patients. Similarly, a study of children who had epilepsy with myoclonic absences concluded that the seizures were easily provoked by hyperventilation.[45] This finding was repeated in a 2009 study, which observed myoclonic absence seizures in three patients which were triggered by hyperventilation.[45] Researchers concluded that "hyperventilation is most effective in activation of generalized absence seizures during routine EEG studies."[46] Research from 2011 repeated the finding that hyperventilation is an effective way to activate epileptic seizures in patients with epilepsy.[47] In a study of children aged between 3 and 11 years, hyperventilation induced seizures in all patients.[48] It's worth noting that around 10% of seizures in children with epilepsy are absence seizures, otherwise called petit mal seizures.[49] These seizures have a significant impact on quality of life.[50]

$CO_2$ has long been recognized for its anticonvulsant properties.[51] In 2007, the science news website *Science 2.0* reported research that presented $CO_2$ as a "new—and completely free—way to prevent fever-related epileptic seizures" in small children.[52] Scientists believed that $CO_2$-enriched air could be used to stop seizures. The research showed that fever-related seizures, which are common in children under the age of five, could be safely suppressed within 20 seconds simply by adding 5% $CO_2$ to inhaled air. Experimental research indicates that these childhood seizures may increase the risk of epilepsy developing later in life.

The study suggested that $CO_2$ therapy could also be effective in stopping other types of epileptic seizure.[52] This theory was tested in 2011 research when scientists set out to discover whether inhaling 5% $CO_2$ would stop seizures in epilepsy patients.[53] A pilot study of seven people demonstrated a "rapid termination of electrographic seizures" even though the 5% $CO_2$ was applied after the seizure had begun. The researchers concluded that inhaled $CO_2$ could be used for acute treatment of epileptic seizures.[53]

A follow-on review of this study stated that the research demonstrated the "feasibility" of hypercapnia as a clinical treatment.[51] While more work is needed to ensure safety and efficacy—for instance, it is important that hypercapnia does not progress to acidosis during a prolonged seizure—the review suggests that this is a worthwhile avenue, concluding, "Carbon dioxide inhalation could prove to be an easy and inexpensive intervention for acute seizures in the hospital, and possibly in the home as well."

A further study from 2014 sought to discover whether inhaling 5% $CO_2$ could suppress hyperventilation-induced absence seizures and irregular electrical discharges in the brain known as "spike and wave discharges."[54] Researchers concluded that treatment with $CO_2$ may help treat these seizures. A 2019 clinical review reiterated earlier findings, stating that the "spike and wave" neuronal discharge typical of absence seizures is triggered by voluntary hyperventilation in more than 90% of patients with absence epilepsy. The paper describes the use of hyperventilation to quickly diagnose patients with absence epilepsy as "commonplace." While scientists are still unclear whether a single mechanism exists to prompt absence seizures, the review suggests that the changes in blood pH (alkalosis) brought on by hyperventilation may contribute.[55]

In the 2014 study, 12 participants who had hyperventilation-induced absence seizures were examined while breathing either room air, 5% $CO_2$, or 100% oxygen. Compared to hyperventilation in normal room air, the 5% $CO_2$ decreased the frequency and duration of seizures after hyperventilation and reduced the number of "spike and wave" discharges. This pilot study added yet more clear evidence that hypercapnia could provide a way to treat hyperventilation-related seizures.[54]

## COMORBID HEALTH PROBLEMS IN EPILEPSY

The *Cold Spring Harbor Perspectives in Medicine* published a paper in 2015 that suggested that epilepsy encompasses more than spontaneous recurrent seizures and should be classified as a "spectrum disorder."[7] For many epileptics and their families, what causes the greatest impact are the many conditions that exist alongside the primary symptoms. Comorbid conditions can include psychiatric and behavioral disorders like anxiety, depression, attention-deficit hyperactivity disorder (ADHD), learning disabilities, intellectual disability, and autism.

Traditionally these comorbidities were thought to be secondary to uncontrolled seizures and adverse reactions to medication. However, they are now acknowledged as integral to epilepsy. In some cases, the comorbid conditions predate the seizures and can be attributed to an underlying disorder of neuronal networks.[56] A 2007 study states that even a single seizure can cause modifications to receptor expression and distribution, altering neurodevelopment—the growth of neurological pathways in the brain that influence things like intellectual functioning, reading ability, memory, focus, and social skills—leading to cognitive and behavioral changes.[57]

The most common psychiatric comorbidity in epilepsy is depression. This is interesting because depression is linked with dysfunction in the hippocampus and limbic structures of the brain, areas of the brain that are both frequently involved in epileptic circuits. The connection between depression and epilepsy is bidirectional. People with epilepsy are more likely to develop depression, and those epileptics with depression more commonly suffer refractory seizures, seizures that are uncontrolled or difficult to treat.[58]

It can be difficult to achieve a clinical diagnosis of anxiety in patients with epilepsy, but the unpredictable nature of the disease and the fear of seizures often leads to some level of anxiety. Approximately 30% of adults with epilepsy have depression and 10% have bipolar disorder.[58] Both these disorders are related to increased risk of suicide. The same is true in children, but symptoms are harder to identify here. Research has demonstrated that children with newly diagnosed epilepsy are around three times more likely to also have a mood disorder.

Physical health problems also affect many people with epilepsy. The *Centers for Disease Control and Prevention National Health Interview Survey* found that adults with epilepsy were more likely to also have cardiovascular and respiratory disorders, inflammation, obesity, diabetes, and other conditions, including arthritis, pain in the upper or lower spine, and severe headaches.[59] Epileptics also have a higher incidence of sexual dysfunction,[37] early mortality, and sudden unexplained death.[60]

Another concern for people with epilepsy is the impact of seizure medication on bone health. Epileptics are more prone to fractures due to decreased bone mineral density.[61] The antiseizure medications carbamazepine, phenytoin, and phenobarbital cause a decrease in bone mineral density by triggering release of the CYP450 enzyme, but non-enzyme-inducing AEDs are also linked to altered bone health.[61] We looked at the link between bone mineral loss and breathing pattern disorders in Chapter Thirteen.

In all cases, whether comorbidities are psychological or physiological, understanding the relationship between epilepsy and its associated conditions can have a significant positive impact on quality of life for people living with the disease. Indeed, scientists consider this to be a priority for future research. More to the point, many of the problems that exist alongside epilepsy, including anxiety disorders, diabetes, heart problems, and respiratory conditions, can also be contributed by breathing pattern disorders such as chronic hyperventilation.

## EPILEPSY AND BLOOD FLOW TO THE BRAIN

Cerebral blood flow is known to change during seizures, specifically in the epileptogenic zone, the area of the cortex that initiates the seizure.[62] Blood flow to the brain decreases between seizures and increases during them. Immediately after a seizure ends, cerebral blood flow becomes very low, and it remains low for several minutes. Unfortunately, these changes in blood flow prevent proper oxygenation of the brain. A 2017 study reported that the most severe long-term result of repetitive epileptic seizures was neuronal degeneration.[63] Researchers state that while the primary cause of this is overstimulation of the neurons, new findings indicate that hypoxia, or lack of oxygen caused by abnormal blood flow, "may be to blame for as much as half the neuronal death caused by the condition."

Research has found that cerebral blood flow can be improved with breathing exercises. Again, $CO_2$ plays a key role. One 2011 study tested the potential for simple breathing exercises to increase cerebral oxygenation and/or blood flow.[64] Scientists examined 18 participants aged between 19 and 39 years and recorded levels of end-tidal $CO_2$ and brain oxygenation. Subjects were asked to complete paced breathing exercises that included breath holds on both inhalation and exhalation. The exercise involved walking slowly for three steps while inhaling, holding the breath for three steps, exhaling for three steps, holding the breath for three steps and so on.

The researchers found that the main parameter influencing cerebral circulation is the level of $CO_2$ in the blood, and that an increase in $CO_2$ concentration of around 70% may as much as double blood flow.[65] When more blood flows to the brain, the brain receives more nutrients and oxygen, and this may have a significant influence on its physiology. People trained in breathing exercises can increase their levels of blood $CO_2$ by learning to control tidal volume[64] (the amount of air that moves in and out of the lungs with each inhalation and exhalation). This means that it is possible to improve cerebral blood flow simply by moderating the breathing.[66]

A second study, also from 2011, explored cerebral oxygenation in people who were experienced in yogic breathing techniques.[67] Six participants, who were each able to breathe at an extremely slow rate, performed an identical periodic breathing exercise with a respiratory rate of two breaths per minute. In all six subjects, the results showed a periodic change in cerebral blood flow and oxygenation. This result was repeated in a 2016 paper by the same research team.[68]

Given that much of the neuronal damage caused by epilepsy is caused by lack of oxygen to the brain, it is promising to realize that breathing exercises can so simply improve cerebral blood flow and therefore brain oxygenation.

## SLEEP MATTERS IN EPILEPSY

Epilepsy and sleep-disordered breathing (SDB) are both relatively common conditions.[69] However, they occur comorbidly more frequently than expected, leading to considerations that a connection exists between the two. It is understood that epilepsy can aggravate obstructive sleep apnea (OSA) because it causes an increase in light sleep. Epileptic medications can also produce side effects (such as weight gain) that increase the likelihood of SDB, and epileptic seizures can trigger central apneas.

It is also the case that SDB can impair epilepsy control due to repetitive hypoxia and disrupted sleep. While this area lacks research, some evidence suggests that, if SDB can be treated, seizure control will improve, as will quality of life and general health and well-being.

According to a 2018 article in *Epilepsy Foundation*, "there has never been a prospective, multi-center trial to evaluate the effect of OSA treatment on seizures in people living with epilepsy."[70] More research is needed, particularly in the field of pediatrics. Healthcare professionals who may not be aware of the connection between sleep disorders and epilepsy need to be educated. However, there is some limited research into the relationship between the two disorders. A 2008 paper exploring sleep-study abnormalities in epileptic children describes the relationship between SDB and epilepsy as "complicated and reciprocal."[71] Researchers have looked in detail at the link between epilepsy and sleep, and whether one affects the other, but little has been done to understand the mutual interaction of epilepsy and sleep disorders, particularly in children. The 2008 paper examined questionnaire-based survey responses from 486 patients with partial seizures and 492 age- and gender-matched controls. It found that sleep disturbances affected 39% of adults with epilepsy, compared to 18% of the control group.[71]

A 2019 Australian study published in *Neurology* found that 26.5% of participants had moderate to severe SDB, as defined by an apnea-hypopnea (AHI) index of "greater than 15."[72, 73] (We looked at the AHI in Chapter Seven.) This study found that daytime sleepiness was an accurate indicator of sleep disorders in epileptics, but that age and body-mass index also contributed to the condition.

The small amount of research into this topic means that much evidence is conflicting, both in terms of prevalence and diagnostic criteria. A 2019 study states that OSA is twice as common in people with epilepsy than in the general population, and as in other OSA cases, its incidence increases with age.[74] According to this review, subjective self-reporting of daytime sleepiness is particularly unhelpful as a diagnostic tool for OSA in epileptics, because a diverse range of comorbidities can cause tiredness in epilepsy.

The prevalence of sleep disorders in epileptic children is under-recognized.[71] Children with epilepsy often experience changes in the way they sleep—how quickly they fall asleep, their total sleep time, sleep architecture, and spontaneous arousals—and they are more likely to suffer from broken sleep and daytime drowsiness.[71]

Many things can cause sleep disruption in children with epilepsy, including the epilepsy itself and antiepileptic medications. These children present with conditions including SDB, OSA, and limb movements during sleep. The poor quality of sleep that results has a negative impact on seizure control that may logically be related to hyperventilation caused by mouth breathing during sleep. Sleep deprivation can trigger seizures, and frequent seizures cause broken sleep, creating a vicious cycle. Even when seizures occur during wakefulness, they can have a negative impact on sleep.[71] Antiepileptic drugs can cause marked weight gain in children. Aside from a general feeling of tiredness and poor health, this increases the likelihood of SDB as excess fat on the abdomen and tongue restricts the movement of the diaphragm and narrows the airways.[75]

According to a 2019 paper, several small retrospective studies have found that positive airway pressure treatments such as CPAP can produce a significant reduction in seizures for people who have comorbid epilepsy and OSA[74].

A 2018 article in *Epilepsy Foundation* reported that patients treated with positive airway pressure had a 63% chance of a reduction in seizures of up to 50%.[70] This was compared with a 14% chance for those who were untreated.

Apnea, hypercapnia (too much blood $CO_2$), and oxygen desaturation (when blood oxygen levels drop below normal) can all occur during and immediately after a seizure, especially with generalized tonic-clonic seizures.[74] The respiratory disturbances that occur during apnea suggest activation of the central autonomic network, an intricate system of structures in the brain that performs a key role in the working of the autonomic nervous system.[76] This may contribute to sudden unexpected death in epilepsy (SUDEP), the leading cause of epilepsy-related death in patients with drug-resistant epilepsy. People who die from SUDEP generally have a history of nocturnal seizures and centrally mediated post-seizure cardiorespiratory dysfunction.[77] They often die during sleep, and while sleeping prone (face down), but it is unknown whether OSA contributes to sudden death.[76]

A 2018 study explored the relationship between SUDEP and SDB in 30 participants and reported that cardiorespiratory dysfunction was more common in patients at high risk of SUDEP, while SDB was found in 88% of sleep-study results.[77]

While epilepsy and SDB often coexist, one of the difficulties faced by medical practitioners when identifying abnormal events that are related to sleep disorders rather than epilepsy is the fact that signs of nocturnal seizures can overlap with symptoms of SDB.[77] A 2014 paper describes the case of a three-year-old child who demonstrated EEG activity during seizure that could also be associated with a particular form of OSA. The child's seizures were characterized by increased respiratory rate, paradoxical breathing, and oxygen desaturation.[78] In this case, cardiorespiratory sleep study results initially led to a misdiagnosis of severe OSA.

Excessive daytime sleepiness and sleep disorders are known to be common in adults with epilepsy, and one 2006 study found that children with epilepsy also reported worse daytime sleepiness than a control group. In this study, researchers concluded that further research using screening questionnaires and formal sleep studies is needed to accurately assess the prevalence of sleep disorders in children with epilepsy.[79]

A 2008 study evaluated abnormal results in 40 epileptic children who had each been referred for a sleep study because of various problems with sleep.[71]

Snoring was observed in 83% of patients, and SDB including obstructive hyperventilation, sleep apnea, and upper-airway resistance syndrome was found in 42.5% of the children. Children who had poor seizure control also experienced poor quality sleep, a higher arousal index, and a higher percentage of REM sleep states compared to those who were either seizure-free or had good seizure-control.

Those children who had both epilepsy and OSA generally had a much greater body mass index and longer sleep latency—the amount of time it takes to get to sleep. Significantly, they also demonstrated more severe oxygen desaturation than children who had sleep apnea uncomplicated by epilepsy.[71] A considerable number of the children with epilepsy who were referred for polysomnography presented with SDB, including OSA. This study concluded that treatment of OSA by removing the tonsils and adenoids may lead to an improvement in sleep disturbances, which might in turn result in better seizure control and quality of life. The researchers suggested that physicians should routinely screen for snoring and other signs of OSA when examining children with epilepsy.[71] However, there is an argument that as with SDB in nonepileptic children, developing the airways and training in full-time nasal breathing should be considered before resorting to surgery.

Research into the link between SDB and epilepsy is still very limited. It is unclear whether epilepsy causes OSA or whether OSA exists comorbidly alongside epilepsy. But the evidence linking seizure frequency and duration to chronic hyperventilation, coupled with the research confirming that mouth breathing during sleep is a common in both OSA and chronic hyperventilation, would indicate that improving or eradicating SDB may help with seizure control.

## THE VAGUS NERVE CONNECTION TO EPILEPSY

Electronic stimulation of the vagus nerve using implanted devices has been used in the treatment of epilepsy and depression for several decades.[80] More recently, noninvasive devices have been developed. As we discovered in Chapter Four, vagal stimulation can also be achieved naturally by practicing a breathing rate of six breaths per minute.

The vagus nerve innervates a wide range of organs, but its function can be most easily assessed in relation to the rhythm of the heart. Heart rate variability (HRV) is indicative of vagal tone. As we know, low vagal tone correlates with lower parasympathetic activity and is linked to a wide range of mental and physical conditions and early mortality.[80]

People with epilepsy, particularly those whose seizure control is poor, have lower vagal tone, leading researchers in a 2017 study to theorize that natural stimulation of the vagus nerve might improve seizure control.[80] Interestingly, the most common self-reported seizure trigger for people with epilepsy is stress, a fact that points to an autonomic imbalance.[81] The paper discusses three natural methods for increasing HRV and parasympathetic tone—stress reduction, nutrition, and exercise—but does not mention the relationship between slow diaphragmatic breathing and vagal tone. None of the three suggestions mentioned in the study were found to reduce seizures. But the researchers do report that patients have been known to experience increased vagal tone and a subsequent reduction in seizures by listening to music by Mozart.[80] Equally, as already discussed, slow breathing has been found to reduce the onset and duration of seizures. This may have some relation to activation of the parasympathetic nervous system as well as counteracting the biochemical effects of hyperventilation. The study concludes that much more work is needed to examine the impact of the various methods for optimizing HRV on seizure occurrence.

Vagus nerve stimulation is widely used to treat patients over the age of 12 years who have refractory epilepsy.[82] A retrospective study published in 2007 examined the data to find out whether the procedure had any adverse implications for younger children. Scientists reviewed statistics for 26 children, aged between 3 and 17 years, who had been treated with vagus nerve stimulation implants between 1998 and 2004. The children predominantly suffered with symptomatic-generalized epilepsy. Seventy-seven percent presented with moderate to severe intellectual disability, and 65 had more than 30 seizures every month. The duration of treatment in the studied children ranged from one month to eight years.

After treatment, frequency of seizures reduced more than 50% in 54% of the children. Two became seizure-free, 23% experienced seizure reduction of less than 50%, and four developed the ability to end seizures using the implant. OSA was found in four of the children after placement of the implant.[82] The study concluded that vagus nerve stimulation is an effective treatment for children with refractory epilepsy but that an overnight sleep study should be used to identify patients with preexisting OSA before the device is implanted.[82]

A small study of adults also made the connection between vagus nerve stimulation and SDB in epileptic patients.[83] The 2020 paper followed three cases representative of SDB brought on by vagal activity in refractory epilepsy. Of the three participants, two had sleep apnea and the third a condition called stridor, which presents as a high-pitched wheezing. This paper drew the same conclusion, as the 2007 study involving children, that given the high incidence of OSA in people with refractory epilepsy, patients should be screened for SDB before being treated with a vagus nerve stimulation implant. However, researchers also suggest that SDB is a rare complication of vagus nerve stimulation and, where sleep apnea occurs, it must be investigated alongside data regarding the firing of the nerve stimulator.

A more recent study looked at the outcome of vagus nerve stimulation treatment in terms of HRV and electrocardiogram (ECG) readings in patients with drug-resistant epilepsy.[84] Participants were 32 patients who had received vagus nerve stimulation implants at the same hospital, and 32 healthy age- and gender-matched controls. Researchers found that those people who failed to respond to vagus nerve stimulation—defined as having less than a 50% seizure reduction one year after treatment—had significantly lower preoperative vagal tone than those who responded well to the treatment. In simple terms, patients whose parasympathetic tone was worse received less benefit from the treatment. This would indicate that it is possible to predict the level of seizure reduction after treatment.[84] It would also suggest that patients who are able to improve their vagal tone, something it is possible to do using breathing exercises, would gain more benefit from the vagus nerve stimulation implant in terms of relief from epilepsy symptoms.

A 2018 study evaluated the effects of vagus nerve stimulation on HRV in 20 epileptic children.[85] Researchers also investigated whether antiepileptic drugs had any negative impact on HRV. Prior to treatment with vagus nerve stimulation, all of the children showed increased heart rates, less variability in heart rate, and more extreme frequency readings (whether low or high) than children in a control group. "Remarkable" improvement was seen after six months of treatment, but this did not continue incrementally, and no further changes were seen after 12 months. HRV was still markedly lower than in healthy children. Base levels of HRV were also found to be further reduced in patients who had lived with epilepsy for longer and those in whom epileptic focus was localized—where partial seizures arise from one part of the brain, such as the temporal lobe.

When a child has epilepsy, the autonomic nervous system is heavily balanced toward the sympathetic branch. Although vagus nerve stimulation seems to offer substantial benefits in the short term, increasing vagal tone and redressing the balance with the parasympathetic nervous system, HRV remained lower than in healthy children, even after long-term treatment. The researchers concluded that, while factors including epilepsy duration, age, epileptic focus, medication, and seizure frequency may all lead to reduced HRV, epilepsy itself may contribute to impaired autonomic regulation of the cardiovascular system.[85]

It is worth noting that a vagus nerve stimulation implant, while it activates the parasympathetic branch of the ANS, does not address the biochemical influence of $CO_2$ or the effects of dysfunctional breathing. The study does not record whether children were examined for signs of chronic hyperventilation, which plays a key role in seizure onset, frequency, and duration. Unlike the implant, the breathing exercises in this book can be used to naturally stimulate the vagus nerve while simultaneously rebalancing blood gases and addressing underlying breathing pattern disorders.

## EPILEPSY AND MIGRAINE: IS THERE A LINK?

In the 1999 book *Breathe Well, Be Well*, Robert Fried explains that, in general, medical practitioners are largely unaware of the role hyperventilation plays in many common disorders.[33] Fried lists conditions, including hypertension, migraine, chronic muscle fatigue, idiopathic epilepsy, stress, headaches, panic attacks, and depression. Even though medical education teaches the physiological disturbances that hyperventilation causes, there is still a long way to go before the connection is fully understood or integrated into treatments.

We know that healthy or unhealthy breathing has a profound effect on the heart and that it can increase or decrease the diameter of the blood vessels depending on how much $CO_2$ is in the blood.[33] Blood vessels constrict when levels of $CO_2$ are low, and this contributes to idiopathic seizures and migraine. It also plays a role in Raynaud's syndrome, a condition in which spasms in the arteries cause reduced blood flow to the fingers and toes.

In this book, we have already examined menstrual migraine in women, and its relationship to cyclical hormone-induced hyperventilation. But are migraines and epilepsy also related? Fried acknowledges that it may be unexpected to read about migraines and epilepsy in the same chapter of his book but states that it is "still a matter of conjecture that migraine and epilepsy are entirely different entities." He makes the case that epilepsy is as much an arterial blood vessel problem affected by breathing as migraine is and that the distinction between the two conditions can be ascribed to whether the affected arteries are inside or outside of the skull.[33]

According to an article in *Neurology Advisor*, "patients with migraine are more likely to have epilepsy, and patients with epilepsy are more likely to experience migraine." The article states that patients with seizure disorders are twice as likely to suffer with migraines, a fact that can often lead to misdiagnosis.[86] It is certainly the case that both migraine and epilepsy can be relieved by breathing training and nutritional management.[33] Indeed, as far back as 1907, the neurological researcher Sir William R. Gowers described similarities between migraine and seizure disorders[33] in his book *The Border-land of Epilepsy*. In particular, he identified hyperventilation as a contributing factor.[87]

One 2019 study describes comorbidities that frequently occur alongside vestibular migraine[88]—migraine in which disruptions to balance, such as vertigo, are present. Many of the study participants reported feelings of anxiety, depression, and insomnia following the onset of vestibular symptoms. Changes in function affecting the senses, pain perception, and muscle strength were diagnosed, and some of the patients experienced phobic disorders, including claustrophobia and agoraphobia prior to symptoms occurring. In 42.7% of participants, abnormal eye movements were observed. This ocular disturbance is called nystagmus, and it causes the eyes to make uncontrolled, repetitive movements that can affect balance and coordination and impair vision. In the study, nystagmus was induced by hyperventilation in 22.5% of the patients.[88]

Connecting the eyes with breathing is not without precedent. In his 1942 book *The Art of Seeing*, Aldous Huxley wrote, "There is a regular correlation between attentive looking and quite unnecessary, indeed positively harmful, interference with breathing."[89] He went on to explain that any improvement in the quality of circulation is immediately reflected in better vision. Huxley, who had problems with his eyesight for his whole life, tells how he saved himself from blindness when doctors had failed to help. He connects quality of sight with better circulation and correct breathing. Since the entire body suffers when we fail to breathe correctly, it makes sense that the eyes would also be affected.[90] In fact, in extreme cases, breathing-related visual loss can be caused by retinal hemorrhage, for instance, in patients with asthma who experience a sudden rise in intra-abdominal or intra-thoracic pressure due to exacerbations.[91]

Ultimately, Fried asks the primary question, "Why do some people get seizures when others do not?" He maintains that epilepsy is not the result of disease of the nervous system and that seizures are, like migraines, due to arterial blood vessel spasms rather than a "massive discharge of neurons in the brain." He suggests that the electrical discharge seen in seizures is the result of the seizure, not its cause.[33] He confirms from his own research that hyperventilation precedes seizure and describes a method for biofeedback-assisted breathing reeducation to reduce the frequency and severity of seizures in patients who do not respond to anticonvulsant drugs.[30]

## SEIZING CONTROL OF SEIZURES WITH BREATH RETRAINING

The many links between $CO_2$ and epilepsy—the influence of $CO_2$ on the electrical activity in the brain, the abnormal fluctuation in $CO_2$ levels that precedes grand mal seizures, and the abnormal levels of blood $CO_2$ in patients with petit mal and grand mal seizures—indicate that the gas plays a signifi-cant role in triggering epileptic seizures[30]. While research into the potentially therapeutic effects of breathing exercises is limited, some papers do explore slow diaphragmatic and nasal breathing.

A 1990 study looked at the impact of diaphragm breathing training on seizure frequency.[30] Subjects were taught diaphragm breathing techniques by an instructor who worked with each person, instructing him or her on the correct movements of the chest and abdomen. Where necessary, the tutor used practical methods including a book positioned on the abdomen to help the subject achieve the correct movement. During the breath training, participants were asked to practice a specific respiratory pattern that resulted in an end-tidal $CO_2$ reading of 5%. The breathing rate used to produce this pattern was around 12 to 14 breaths per minute, approximately the same as normal respiration.

The study focused on two factors, chronic hyperventilation and seizure activity. The researchers reported that, in every case, patients presenting with idiopathic epilepsy also demonstrated moderate or severe chronic hyperventilation. The control group contained several participants who had moderate to severe hyperventilation but did not experience seizures.[30]

The results of this study produced considerable evidence to support the theory that end-tidal $CO_2$ biofeedback is "essential in the therapeutic correction of abnormal respiration." Scientists reported that it was not enough to adjust the rate of respiration.[30] Both statements are consistent with the exercises in this book. The BOLT score provides a simple way to get biofeedback about $CO_2$ sensitivity, while the exercises teach reduced breathing volume as well as a slower respiratory rate.

In previous pilot studies, the same researchers discovered that patients only became aware of their need to breathe from the diaphragm once they could see the difference in end-tidal $CO_2$ compared with chest breathing.[92, 93] The "knowledge of results" presented by end-tidal $CO_2$ biofeedback is believed to play a vital role in the lasting benefits of breath training. In a similar way, the BOLT score can be used as a measure of progress when practicing breathing exercises.

In the 1990 study, the breath training procedure caused significant improvements to habitual breathing patterns.[30] In particular, participants showed notable reductions in respiratory rate, which researchers explained was due to the moderating effect of diaphragmatic breathing. EEG readings were also interesting, normalizing, as a result of the breath training, in participants with epilepsy. It was believed that the changes in EEG could be due to greater blood flow and metabolism in the brain. Improved cerebral circulation would be an expected result of reducing respiratory alkalosis, which negatively affects oxygen delivery to the brain. Conversely, a combination of low $CO_2$ and the ensuing alkalosis would be likely to further inhibit oxygenation of the brain.

Abnormal EEG readings in people with moderate to severe chronic hyperventilation are consistent with the practice of using voluntary hyperventilation to induce epileptic seizures in EEG examinations. Remember, EEG readings record the electrical signals in the brain, so they will pick up any spike and wave discharges or misfiring messages. Atypical readings are also common in migraine and are associated with hypoxia (lack of blood oxygen) and the narrowing of the blood vessels in the brain.

In the 1990 study, respiration training to correct overbreathing led to a significant reduction in seizure activity in patients resistant to anticonvulsant medications.[30] The number of participants was too small to accurately conclude which variables predicted the reduction in seizures, and none of the patients was seizure-free after the seven-month trial, but those who experienced grand mal seizures had none during the training period. In all participants, the frequency and severity of seizures, as well as the type of seizure, was considerably modified by the breath training. The researchers suggest that the stress-reducing effects of diaphragm breathing were also a key factor in reducing seizures.

The study findings indicate that at least some forms of epilepsy go hand-in-hand with a considerable imbalance of the autonomic nervous system.[30] Whatever causes chronic hyperventilation, the result is a narrowing of the blood vessels in the brain, leading to poor brain blood flow and metabolism, and predisposing susceptible people to seizures. Disrupting the blood acid-base balance inhibits oxygen delivery to the brain and interrupts the reflexive relationship between the heart and the lungs. Diaphragm breathing exercises to correct hyperventilation can reduce seizures by raising the seizure threshold.

One suggestion made in several earlier studies is that the link between overbreathing and seizure activity may actually be airflow stimulating the nasal mucosa.[94] Research has reported that when air is blown into the nasal cavity, it triggers epileptic areas of the brain.[95] Also, in some types of epilepsy, nasal hyperventilation has been found more likely than oral hyperventilation to induce epileptic EEG activity.

On a day-to-day basis, we spontaneously alternate our breathing from one nostril to the other. Certain yogic breathing practices explore this, focusing the breath in one nostril at a time, a technique that scientists call unilateral nostril breathing. Interestingly, studies have found that unilateral nostril breathing has a greater impact on the same-side brain hemisphere.[94, 95] Right nostril breathing produces abnormalities in the right side of the brain, and left nostril breathing affects the left side of the brain. It is unclear what causes this phenomenon, but researchers suggest that a reflex involving stimulation of the olfactory nerve by nasal airflow is involved.[94, 96]

These ideas are expanded in 2016 research. Based on the same ancient yoga breathing technique of single nostril breathing, new evidence suggests that altering nasal airflow between the nostrils can influence brain activity.[97] Researchers observed that when nasal breathing was through only one nostril, cognitive function improved. This method has also been shown to trigger seizure activity in epileptic patients. The paper hypothesizes that rather than vasoconstriction being solely responsible for seizure onset, seizure activity may be related to the way the air stimulates the nasal mucosa.[97] Scientists have found that, in some types of epilepsy, nasal hyperventilation was more likely than oral hyperventilation to stimulate epileptic EEG activity in the brain and that this effect was inhibited by applying local anesthetic to the nasal mucosa.

Although the mechanism, extent, and significance of these findings remain unclear, evidence from studies of epileptics and arousal during sleep indicates that a nasal airflow stimulus has some sort of activating effect on the brain. This underlines the importance of reduced nasal breathing exercises, in which the amount of air breathed is lessened. It is possible to switch to nasal breathing and still hyperventilate if other aspects of poor breathing patterns are not addressed.

In 1984, an article published in the journal *Psychosomatic Medicine* described the use of breathing exercises to self-regulate $CO_2$ and control seizures.[92] The study followed 18 participants between the ages of 10 and 42 years, 11 of whom were male and 7 female. All those who took part suffered moderate to severe chronic hyperventilation and idiopathic, medication-resistant seizures. The subjects were given diaphragmatic breathing training with end-tidal $CO_2$ biofeedback. This was very effective, producing a rapid correction of breathing patterns. The patients' breathing even became comparable to that of people in an asymptomatic control group. Ten of the participants remained in the study for at least seven months. Following the treatment, EEG power spectrum readings had normalized in eight people, as had cardiorespiratory synchronicity. These people experienced a significant reduction in the frequency and severity of their seizures.

In 1993, doctors from the Boston Neurobehavioral Institute (Harvard Medical School) applied the same principle to the treatment of two children with severe developmental problems. Parents, caretakers, and teachers were taught to modify the children's breathing to eliminate hyperventilation in order to prevent seizures. The technique was successful in both cases.[98]

It is widely recognized that poor health is associated with lower parasympathetic tone.[99] This is certainly the case in people with epilepsy. Those people who have intractable—hard to control—seizures have lower vagal tone than those whose epilepsy is controlled. A 2010 study links the fact that slow breathing exercises are known to increase parasympathetic tone in healthy people with the theory that slow breathing exercises in people with epilepsy might cause a similar increase in parasympathetic tone and reduce seizure frequency. Slow breathing improves conditions including hypertension, asthma, anxiety, and post-traumatic stress disorder, and it affects cortical activity and seizure thresholds through the chemoreceptors, baroreceptors, and pulmonary stretch receptors. The researchers suggest that slow breathing might also reduce seizure activity by lessening anxiety.

Few epileptics are aware of the link between seizures and breathing, but various studies demonstrate that breath retraining can successfully reduce the severity and frequency of epileptic seizures, just as hyperventilation can be (and is) used to induce seizures for EEG studies. While many factors contribute to epilepsy, and research on the therapeutic application of breath retraining is still limited, hyperventilation is known to play a significant role as a seizure trigger. Therefore, breathing exercises to correct hyperventilation and normalize the imbalance of blood $CO_2$ are likely to prove helpful for people with epilepsy. Epilepsy is not caused by poor breathing, but it is certainly exacerbated by it. While there is not enough research to conclusively demonstrate that breathing reeducation will be effective for everyone who suffers with epileptic seizures, the benefits of healthy breathing patterns, for general well-being and for reducing the feelings of anxiety and panic that can happen as the result of living with an unpredictable condition, will doubtless help build a better quality of life. To my understanding, while not all forms of epilepsy are breathing-related, it simply doesn't make sense for children and adults affected by epilepsy that chronic hyperventilation and breathing pattern disorders are not addressed in treatment.

## NICKY'S STORY: OVERBREATHING AND OVERREACHING

I am including Nicky's story for several reasons. She shared her journey and research because her own life has changed so much for the better. More important, her story also illustrates what happens when we try too hard, go at a new idea all guns a-blazing, and try to apply perfectionism to a breathing practice. Overall, Nicky's experience is one of courage and persistence, and it provides invaluable insight.

Nicky wouldn't have described herself as anxious. After all, she never had panic attacks. She liked to be in control of her life and was organized, efficient, and had good attention to detail. She wasn't aware that anything was wrong with her breathing, but she would frequently lose her train of thought in conversation, and her focus was poor. Her heart often raced, and she sometimes had palpitations, which her doctor assured her was normal. But she was irritable, hypersensitive to noise, and had ongoing digestive issues. She knew this was related to a low level of intermittent anxiety, but she couldn't pinpoint why, as her life was not particularly stressful. If she drank coffee, it would often bring on feelings of anxiety, and alcohol, which she drank only rarely, would cause disturbed sleep. She was exercising for at least an hour most days, but this seemed to make her more tired rather than fit and energized. She recovered slowly and had sore, aching muscles most of the time.

Nicky did everything at a hundred miles an hour, driven by a never-ending to-do list. If something went wrong, her reaction was emotional, angry, or tearful. She had strong physiological reactions to many of her thoughts, regularly had nightmares, and was beginning to have night sweats.

She noticed that her breathing was irregular and that she frequently sighed and yawned. Sometimes she would find herself breathing gently, become frightened, and try to breathe more deeply to correct it. After all, she had learnt in yoga that deep breathing is good for you. When she couldn't sleep, she used deep breathing to relax.

Nicky also had nocturnal epilepsy, irregular grand mal seizures, only ever between 1 and 5 a.m., and intermittent partial complex seizures during the day. Before a grand mal seizure, she would experience extreme hyperventilation. Her husband would try to wake her, hoping to stop the ensuing seizure, but neither of them knew if this was actually helpful. After a grand mal seizure, she would sleep for two days, and during the following weeks, she would have hundreds of very intense partial complex seizures, like aftershocks with diminishing frequency. Her concentration and memory were badly affected. She could get lost driving around her own small town.

A brain scan found no physical cause for Nicky's seizures. She felt like a zombie due to the side effects of her medication, and she was told that she was at risk of going into "status." This is where seizure after seizure occurs until the heart fails. Her neurologist said that her seizures had to be fully controlled, and she was prescribed Lamotrigine. On it, she had no more seizures, but she still had regular episodes of nighttime hyperventilation.

Then in 2016, Nicky took part in a breathing course. She had decided to attend the instructor training, alongside the group course, to try to fix her husband's chronic snoring. At the start of the course, her BOLT score was just 8 seconds, and she breathed at 20 breaths per minute during rest. Her breathing was irregular, audible, and 50% through the mouth. Her blood $CO_2$ levels were between 26 mmHg and 32 mmHg, while a reading of between 35 mmHg and 40 mmHg is considered normal.

As the week of training progressed, she experienced a high level of stress. She was frustrated that none of her healthcare providers had identified the link between her breathing dysfunction and many of her health problems. She had, for example, suffered severe postnatal depression with both of her children, after births that were out of control and full of fear and pain. The course also triggered an incredibly strong cleansing reaction and a mounting concern over her seizure threshold.

The breathing course had opened Nicky's eyes to the fact that her breathing was incredibly unhealthy. But it also became apparent that she should have learned much more slowly how to breathe functionally. She should not have been in a group course at all, given the extent of her hyperventilation and epilepsy, combined with her perfectionist tendencies. Instead, her training should have begun with awareness, then suppressing sighs, then full time nasal breathing, and moved slowly on to posture and diaphragm breathing. Only once her BOLT score was about 20 seconds should she have begun practicing with air hunger.

After the course, it took Nicky two distressing weeks to be able to breathe without trying to control every breath. She had resolved to stop breathing in the old way immediately but couldn't work out how to breathe functionally.

She tried to implement everything she had learned at once. As a result, she found herself on the edge of a panic attack most of the time. She experienced the following problems:

- She started using her diaphragm properly and it ached constantly, making it impossible to switch her focus away from her breathing.
- She changed her posture overnight and again experienced pain. Sitting was uncomfortable, and she preferred to stand.
- She stopped sighing and tried to breathe through her nose at all times. She tried to retrain her breathing while speaking and began to lose weight because she didn't like the effect eating had on her breathing.
- She tried to do the breathing exercises as taught but the reduced breathing destabilized her respiration.
- She experimented with her breathing, counted her breaths, and tried all sorts of things to no avail. By lying down and reducing her breathing she could get her breathing rate down to four or five breaths per minute, which felt good. When she stopped the practice, her breathing became rapid again. She wondered whether going from one state to the other was dangerous.

By now, she had become very concerned about her seizure threshold. Her husband had to go away for a night, and she was terrified to go to sleep without him there to wake her if her breathing changed. During the day, she was so focused trying to work out how to breathe that she could barely do anything else.

Her breathing instructor advised her to ease up, stop taking her pulse, stop practicing breath holds and counting her breaths, and just breathe softly and gently through the nose, one step at a time. She finally had a breakthrough when, one morning, in desperation and with a panic attack imminent, she began to read the chapter *Nine Healthy Breathing Habits in Five Days*, from Tess Graham's book *Relief from Snoring and Sleep Apnea*.[100] The instructions in the book enabled Nicky to finally let go of control and start to breathe easily again.

Four months later, the improvements in Nicky's health were extraordinary. She lost six kilos as her metabolism stabilized, and she didn't need to drink so much water. The hyperexcitability and asynchronous firing of brain neurons that, at times, caused her to be overreactive, emotional, fragile, hostile, irrational, anxious, and fast, which she thought were part of her personality, vanished. Raising her $CO_2$ levels led to a much calmer outlook. Her memory and cognitive function improved. She taped her mouth every night, and her sleep quality became so good that she needed less sleep, no longer needing to go to the toilet during the night or experiencing nightmares. Exercise no longer left her feeling exhausted or achy, and her capacity for exercise increased.

However, her BOLT score was still only 16 seconds, and her lack of progress was frustrating. She wanted to achieve the level of super health that she knew was available with a BOLT score over 40. To teach, she also needed to improve her BOLT score. She had the time, energy, motivation, and commitment to do the work, but her breathing instructor's advice was just to relax and not focus on her BOLT score.

At this point, her breathwork consisted of daily yoga or a walk, during which she reduced her breathing, and one or two meditation sessions where she lay on her back and practiced reduced breathing. She was still unable to do the reduced breathing exercise as it was taught to her. Two or three times a week, she had bad breathing days when her head and sinuses would feel constricted, and she would be less able to focus.

She developed tension in her neck and shoulders. Her instructor suggested that she try the Himalayan rock salt drink (a quarter teaspoon of rock salt in warm water three times a day) and see what happened. This had been suggested in the course, but she had overlooked it. She took the drink twice that day and has been taking it ever since. The tension problem resolved immediately, and it has not returned.

In September 2016, without consulting her doctor or specialist, Nicky started to come off Lamotrigine at a rate of 25 mg every few weeks. This process took five months. She felt safe reducing the dose as she considered the recurrence of some complex partial seizures to be a warning system that would let her know the epilepsy was still there. She also felt that as long as her mouth was taped at night, she wasn't likely to hyperventilate enough to bring on a grand mal seizure.

From her research, she understood that her BOLT score should be around 35 before epilepsy would be controlled, but she decided to go ahead and reduce the drug anyway. Everything was fine until she got down to

25 mg per day (down from six pills per day to one), and then her nervous system reacted. Her nervous excitation and feelings of irritability returned, and she struggled to get any work done. Her capacity for exercise reduced again. She lost confidence in the future and in her breathing practice, and she was nervous about having come off her medication with a BOLT score of only 16.

Nicky realized that with such a low BOLT score, her breathing was still too unstable for her epilepsy to be under good control. She needed to make some progress, and it seemed that by practicing strong breath holds she might achieve this, but her breathing coach had told her not to practice breath holds at all. She had also been warned that the intense detoxification caused by strong breath holds could induce exacerbations of disease, which in her case meant grand mal seizures.

She was confused and frustrated. However, she persisted in seeking help and working to understand her breathing. She also consulted physical therapists and began to release long-standing physical tensions and imbalances.

Fast-forward to 2019, and Nicky noticed that, despite all the changes she had made, speaking still left her feeling exhausted. She experienced tension in her abdomen when she spoke for long periods, and she found herself cancelling social engagements due to a sense that she didn't have enough breath to go out and talk for the evening. She also had a phobia of public speaking.

Nicky's ambition was still to become a breathing educator, but she wasn't sure how this would work. She consulted speech therapist Hadas Golan, who identified the problem: Nicky was speaking for too long without taking a breath, exhaling too much air, bringing it below the resting expiratory level, leading her to gasp and overinflate her lungs on the inhalation. This habit creates a lot of tension in the secondary breathing muscles and abdominals. While Nicky still hyperventilates when she talks, she now uses practice of reduced breathing, after teaching, to recover.

Nicky also began taking a selection of supplements. In the book *Normal Breathing*,[101] author Doctor Artour Rakhimov identifies that levels of calcium, magnesium, potassium, and sodium tend to run low in overbreathers, and Nicky began adding these minerals to her diet.

Now, Nicky's end-tidal $CO_2$ reading is between 38 mmHg and 40 mmHg at rest. Her BOLT score is around 20 seconds. She has not had either type of seizure since she took the first breathing retraining course. In fact, she believes the breathing practice probably saved her life. She is planning to train as an instructor in New Zealand and works to raise awareness of breathwork. One of her goals is for breathing dysfunction to be screened for in general practice, and she is taking steps to promote this.

## ADVICE TO FELLOW PERFECTIONISTS AND OVERBREATHERS

1. Before training as a breathing instructor, it is important to do a course yourself to ensure that your own breathing health is sufficient.
2. A client can be quite sick while appearing to be normal and high functioning. A detailed health questionnaire is an important part of any breathing assessment.
3. For anyone with a serious health condition, breathing retraining cannot be undertaken in a five-day course. Ongoing, long-term support is likely to be necessary.
4. People with epilepsy must learn very gently and slowly. Weekly sessions are enough.
5. If you have anxiety or control tendencies, the work should be taken very slowly, especially if you also have a serious health condition.
6. Long breath holds must not be practiced by anyone with epilepsy.
7. Chronic hyperventilators may not be able to relax the breathing muscles. When muscles are underoxygenated, they become "jumpy." This may also affect the diaphragm.
8. The body compensates for anemia by increasing breathing. This is an appropriate physiological response, and iron levels should be restored before attempting breathing retraining. If you have a history of anemia, you should check your iron levels regularly.
9. Overbreathers tend to run low in macronutrients.
10. If you have had a dysfunctional breathing pattern for a long time, there are likely to be biomechanical issues. It may benefit you to seek help from a physical therapist.
11. Even though breathing is something we all do, it is easy to misunderstand instructions. If there is anything that feels wrong or seems

to cause physical or mental stress, stop the practice, and seek specialist advice, especially if you have a serious health condition.

12. Never come off your medication without consulting your doctor.

13. Never underestimate the power of this work and the changes in the mind and body that can result from a few simple breathing exercises.

# CHAPTER SIXTEEN
# JOIN THE BREATHING REVOLUTION

---

U ntil recently, knowledge of the power and application of optimal breathing has been limited to elite sports, advanced yoga practitioners, research scientists, and other high-level professionals. In the last few years, we have witnessed the beginning of a breathing revolution. Since I started my own journey with the breath, my aim has been to bring these resources to as many people as possible. I believe the exercises and understandings in this book can truly change lives for the better. Just as it is human nature to leave things undone until they become necessary, it has perhaps taken a global respiratory pandemic to underline that we can't take anything, not even our breath, for granted.

I am grateful this topic is now getting the attention it deserves. The negative effects of oral breathing have been debated in dentistry since 1910, especially the issue of whether mouth breathing affects craniofacial development in children. All the while, millions of children and adults have continued to suffer the health impacts of poor breathing while an industry argues about whether the problem exists.

I feel sorry for the dentists, orthodontists, and medical doctors who tried to highlight the importance of nasal and functional breathing patterns, only to be ridiculed by their peers. I know Professor John Mew and his son Dr. Mike Mew from the United Kingdom well. I have visited their clinic and observed them working with patients. Both have done their best to highlight the importance of nasal breathing and received bad press within the industry. Doctors William Hang, Kevin Boyd, James Bronson, Tamara Gray, Carlos O'Connor, and James Bartley, along with Joy Moeller, Licia Paskay, Barbara Greene, Samantha Weaver Moeller, and Marc Moeller, to name but a few, have also worked tirelessly in their quest to help children and adults.

I have often wondered why an industry populated with highly intelligent people armed with dental and medical degrees has failed to realize the importance of nasal and functional breathing. Breathing retraining is safe, simple, and economically viable. It applies to major fields of dentistry, respiration, sleep, mental, and physical health.

This same question was raised during a recent panel discussion held by the Academy of Applied Myofunctional Sciences (AAMS). The answers presented by each of the panelists suggested a lack of cooperation between dentistry and medicine, lack of scientific research, and similar arguments. These are all valid points. However, I wasn't so guarded in my comments. My belief is that the real reason breathing does not receive attention from the medical and dental industries is that its therapeutic applications do not promise significant profit. One thing is certain: if there were a promise of lucrative return—the kind of money generated by big pharma and sleep medicine—there would be interest. For breathing to be properly integrated into medicine, it seems necessary for there to be either the promise of profit or the avoidance of the kind of loss that might be encountered when patients raise a lawsuit on realizing they were not offered the best treatment.

I am not claiming that breathing is a cure-all. It is not a magic bullet. My intention is not for people to replace traditional treatments with breathing exercises expecting a miracle. However, there is a role for functional breathing alongside medicine.

I can't help but think back to 1994 when I had an operation to fix my nose so that I could breathe better through it. The surgeon performed a successful procedure, but nobody told me I needed to stop my habitual mouth breathing. I continued to experience sleep-disordered breathing for four years until I discovered the importance of nasal breathing in 1998.

Three decades later, my four-year-old daughter had surgery to remove her tonsils and adenoids. After the operation, there was no follow-up or advice to suggest we should help her learn to breathe through her nose. It is never sufficient to treat the nasal obstruction. It is crucial for the long-term outcome to change the behavior of breathing. This fact is regularly overlooked.

To realize the potential application of breathing exercises, it is necessary to practice. You can read this whole book and understand the importance of light, slow, and deep nasal breathing, but your efforts will be wasted unless you apply the exercises to your health.

To begin with, set aside some time each day to devote to breathing practice. It will be the best investment in your health and well-being. Wake up 20 minutes earlier in the morning, sit down on a chair or the floor, cross-legged or in the lotus position, close your eyes, and draw your attention to your breathing. Gently soften and slow down your breath for 15 minutes to generate a tolerable air hunger.

As you go about your day, take some attention out of your mind and direct it to your breath. Slow down your breathing with lateral expansion and contraction of the lower ribs. Go for a walk or head to the gym and apply light, slow, and deep breathing while you exercise. Remember the mantra *LSD, Light, Slow, and Deep.*

This book contains breathing exercises for everyone. Some stress the body, others relax it, up-regulating and down-regulating your nervous system.

Most important, when you think of functional breathing, remember it is not limited to the studio, to your practice, or to your workout. Functional breathing patterns are relevant during rest, sleep, and physical exercise, for life. On a day-to-day basis, it is likely that much of your attention is directed outward. Modern life is full of distractions. Emails, text messages, social media alerts, work, and family all fight for your attention—to the point that you surrender your attention outward. It is increasingly rare for us to bring our attention inward.

For me, this mindfulness of the breath has been life changing. The ability to shift my attention from my mind to my breath, to create space between thoughts, has given me a new outlook and focused my abilities beyond what I would have thought possible. You can trust that time given to breathing practice will never go to waste. Functional breathing is a game changer for health and performance.

As you begin your practice, be patient. Progress does not always travel in a straight line. We all have ups and downs over the years, and you will have some bumps along the road. Persevere and make a continued effort to bring good breathing into your way of life, and you will reap the rewards.

To assist you, our mobile apps, which are available free of charge, contain guided exercises and instruction. We have two apps available: ButeykoClinic is for children, teenagers, and adults and focuses mainly on health. OxygenAdvantage is designed to help adults with health and sports performance.

I close by wishing you the very best in your application of functional breathing patterns.

# CHAPTER SEVENTEEN

# IS NASAL BREATHING YOUR FIRST LINE OF DEFENSE AGAINST CORONAVIRUS?

---

Throughout this book we have examined the importance of nasal breathing. In the case of respiratory infections, research indicates that where facemasks fail, the nose may provide a natural filter for dangerous pathogens. We know that the nose filters, warms and humidifies air on its way into the body, where mouth breathing does not. But as we discussed in Chapters Three and Ten, it may also help protect you from a high viral load and the severe form of COVID-19. Let's look at the research in more detail.

COVID-19 is a new disease. Little direct research is currently available about its development, although knowledge is growing every day. However, studies that have been published on similar illnesses may be significant. One key paper from 2005, shortly after the outbreak of SARS (severe acute respiratory syndrome coronavirus) reported that nitric oxide inhibits the replication cycle of the virus. Although the total number of deaths relating to COVID-19 has far exceeded those recorded during the 2002–2003 SARS epidemic, the current mortality rate is still much lower than that of SARS, which killed 9.6% of those infected.[1]

Many people have asked why coronavirus is considered to be so much more serious than the annual outbreak of influenza. In simple terms, COVID-19 behaves very differently from flu and is much less well understood. It has a very high viral load, and where flu results in a crippled immune system, this new virus attacks a very specific type of cell called a type 2 pneumocyte.[2, 3]

Type 2 pneumocytes are responsible for the production and secretion of a molecule called surfactant, which reduces the surface tension of fluid in the lungs and contributes to the elastic properties of the alveoli. It facilitates oxygen transport to the blood and prevents lung collapse and edema. Now imagine this function is compromised and it is easy why coronavirus can be deadly for even a young, healthy person, and why it can cause damage to organs including the heart.

In laboratory tests using Vero E6 cells, the authors of the 2005 study found that nitric oxide has an antiviral effect, specifically inhibiting the replication of the virus during early stages of infection. Their research showed that NO inhibits viral protein and RNA synthesis—essential stages of viral reproduction in SARS.[4]

Nitric oxide (NO) is produced in the paranasal sinuses. This means that by breathing through the nose, we harness various properties of NO including its pathogen-killing power. NO is understood to be a vasodilator—it plays a role in the dilation of the blood vessels in the lungs so that oxygen can be properly absorbed from the air. But according to a 1999 paper by scientists Lundberg and Weitzberg[5], another biological function of nitric oxide is the effect it has on the growth of various pathogens, including viruses. What this tells us is that nitric oxide in the nasal airways could represent an important first line of defense against infection. The existence of nitric oxide in exhaled air was first discovered in 1991.[5] Later studies clearly demonstrated that almost all of this NO originates in the upper airways, with only minor input from the lower respiratory tract and lungs.

Nitric oxide (NO) has also been proven to be important for its role in surfactant production.[6, 7] It controls production of surfactants by the alveolar cells and preserves surfactant function.

A paper published in 2009 by the scientists responsible for the research into the SARS virus, states that: "NO is involved in local host defense in the upper airways."[8] The research, which also used isolated laboratory cells, suggests that while it is unclear whether NO acts directly on microorganisms or if it works in combination with other components to produce its toxic impact, it may help keep the sinuses sterile. Interestingly, the study found that NO inhibits the replication of SARS in two distinct ways.[8]

Research from 1999 and 2000 found NO has "opposing effects" in viral infections, including flu and pneumonia, and it inhibits the replication of a variety of viruses. And research into the human rhinovirus (HRV), the primary cause of the common cold, concluded that humans actually produce more nitric oxide in response to HRV infection, theorizing that the gas plays a key role in viral clearance.

Without the regular inhalation and exhalation through the nostrils, nitric oxide in the nasal airways goes unused. Therefore, the simplest way to naturally increase NO is by nostril breathing. However, as we discovered in Chapter Three, evidence suggests that humming is effective in emptying the paranasal sinuses of accumulated NO, leading to far greater production of the gas.[9]

Much of the worry around coronavirus stems from uncertainty. However, what is certain is that large amounts of nitric oxide are constantly being released in the airways during nasal breathing, and that this gas has been found to have important antiviral functions that defend against the replication of flu-like illnesses. The mechanism of COVID-19 is still unknown, and it would be cavalier to state that nasal breathing will kill the virus. However, it has been consistently proven that nasal breathing leads to better overall health, and it makes logical sense, given that the primary defense to airborne viruses is in the nose and not the mouth, that breathing through the nose can support the body's natural resistance to infection.

## HOW DOES THE VIRUS SPREAD?

Just like other respiratory infections, the virus travels from person to person in droplets of bodily fluid such as mucus or saliva. When an infected person sneezes or coughs, the virus disperses into the air and onto surrounding surfaces. Droplets from coughs and sneezes can travel several feet and stay suspended in the air for up to 10 minutes, increasing the likelihood of infection for anyone who comes into direct contact with a sick person or touches a contaminated surface.

The biggest issue here is that because COVID-19 is a brand new virus in humans, no one has any immunity to it, and this increases both the fear factor and the potential for infection. However, Bruce Ayleward, assistant director general of the WHO explains that: "Panic and hysteria are not appropriate." "This is a disease that is in the cases and their close contacts," he says. "It's not a hidden enemy lurking behind bushes. Get organized, get educated, and get working."[10]

## PREVENTIVE MEASURES

Much of the advice around coronavirus focuses on hygiene practices such as frequent and thorough handwashing, self-isolating and catching sneezes in the crook of the elbow. The use of face masks has become synonymous with outbreaks of this type, and masks are now an accepted defense against spreading Covid-19. The Center for Disease Control (CDC) recommends that people wear masks in public settings, at events and gatherings, and anywhere they will be around other people. When you wear a mask, you protect others as well as yourself, but masks are not without controversy.

Toward the end of April 2020, social media users began sharing images online, claiming that continuous use of a mask forces the wearer to breathe in excess carbon dioxide ($CO_2$) from exhaled air, causing hypercapnia. Hypercapnia is the buildup of $CO_2$ in the bloodstream, and it's common in conditions such as COPD. It can lead to dizziness, fatigue, headaches, breathlessness, drowsiness, and disorientation. More severe symptoms include loss of consciousness, seizures, and coma.

While it can be dangerous to breathe in high levels of $CO_2$, the claim is inaccurate. It's true that medical masks have been found to cause headaches in healthcare workers who wear them for a long time, but there is no evidence that these masks are dangerous.

According to Reuters, a representative from the CDC explains: "The $CO_2$ will slowly build up in the mask over time. However, the level of $CO_2$ likely to build up in the mask is mostly tolerable to people exposed to it. You might get a headache but you most likely [would] not suffer the symptoms observed at much higher levels of $CO_2$. The mask can become uncomfortable for a variety of reasons, including a sensitivity to $CO_2$ and the person will be motivated to remove the mask. It is unlikely that wearing a mask will cause hypercapnia."

## SUMMARY:

- The mechanism of COVID-19 remains unknown and it is not confirmed whether breathing through the nose can inhibit this virus.
- However, it is logical to breathe only through the nose given that the primary defense to airborne viruses is in the nose and not the mouth, that breathing through the nose can support the body's natural resistance to infection.
- Breathe through your nose, especially in public places—on public transport, while exercising at the gym, and so on.

- While in public places, slow down your breathing and deliberately reduce the volume of air taken into your lungs.
- Be aware of your breath-hold time during rest. During a head cold, lower respiratory tract infection or respiratory symptoms, breath-hold time during rest is reduced. To test, exhale through nose, hold breath and time how long it takes for you to experience first definite desire to breathe. If it is less than 10 seconds, respiration is not optimal.
- You will find a suggested exercise protocol for COVID-19 recovery in Chapter Two.

# RESOURCES

---

MyoTape mouth tape for sleep can be ordered from MyoTape.com

Nasal dilators can be purchased from NasalDilator.com

The SportsMask can be found at SportsMask.com

A list of Oxygen Advantage® registered breathing instructors can be found at OxygenAdvantage.com/instructors

Downloadable app for sports performance: OxygenAdvantage

Downloadable app with exercises for children and adults: ButeykoClinic

Free children's breathing exercises can be found on YouTube by searching *Patrick McKeown, children*

## HRV MONITORS SUGGESTED BY DR. JAY WILES:

- Lief Therapeutics wearable ECG
- Oura Ring
- WHOOP Strap
- BioStrap
- HeartMath Inner Balance™ or emWave2®
- Polar H10 Chest Strap with the Elite HRV app

To find a myofunctional therapy specialist in your area, visit AomtInfo.org

# BONUS CHAPTERS

---

Available at **https://oxygenadvantage.com/thebreathingcure**

Chapter Eighteen: **Phenotypes of Obstructive Sleep Apnea**

Chapter Nineteen: **The Breath and the Singing Voice**

Chapter Twenty: **Adult Breathing Classification (ABC)**
Chapter Twenty-One: **The Subtle Art of Yoga Breathing**

# REFERENCES

———————————

Available at **https://oxygenadvantage.com/thebreathingcure**

# ACKNOWLEDGMENTS

When I changed career paths to teach breathing in 2002, it certainly raised a few eyebrows. It caused angst with some family members and drew a good hearty laugh from others.

Roll on 18 years, and my work continues, thanks to the help and support of many people. I've learned two things that could be considered guiding principles. First, follow your intuition. It might be the best thing you ever do. Second, with passion and effort, we are likely to attract the right people at the right time!

This book wouldn't exist without those "right people." I'm grateful to the initial "whoosh up" from the Irish media. Thanks to the *Galway Advertiser* and Mary O'Connor for the very first article on the Buteyko method for asthma. Written in April of 2002, it sourced my first three clients. And to the journalists who tested the technique for their asthma and wrote stories on it. Kevin Murphy from the *Irish Independent* and Sylvia Thompson from the *Irish Times*. Both took a dedicated interest in the Buteyko method, writing many articles over the years.

This book would not have been possible without the help of Johanna McWeeney, a tremendous writer, editor, and researcher who was able to convert medical jargon into reader-friendly tones.

Many thanks to Laird Hamilton for writing the foreword and to the team at XPT; Pj Nestler, Gabby Reece, and Jennifer Meredith.

To the breathing instructors Yasin Seiwasser, Robin Rothenberg, Nick Heath, Dr. Jonathan Herron, Lisa Seaman, Georgi Rose Lawlor, Dr. Jay Wiles, Kathleen Dixon, Alessandro Romagnoli, Leonardo Pelagotti, Dr. Paul Sly, Tim Anderson, and Magnus Appelberg. Thank you for sharing your experience with the breath. Soprano Claire Wild, thank you for checking the singing appendix.

To James Nestor, whose book *Breath* represents the greatest contribution to breathing in 20 years. It is one of the best books on breathing I have read.

The real-life examples in this book add the human touch. Some of the stories you will read are from clients I have worked with. Others are from readers who have written to me. Regardless, the personal element is very important. Knowing that these exercises have helped people makes the work worthwhile. It provides me with the motivation to keep driving forward.

To Dr. Joseph Mercola for reaching out to his 2 million members on Mercola.com, to inform them of the importance of nose breathing and functional breathing patterns. To Joy, Marc, and Samantha Moeller for their tireless dedication in advancing research into breathing and myofunctional therapy.

To the dentists and orthodontists Dr. John Mew and Mike Mew, Dr. William Hang, Dr. Kevin Boyd, Dr. Marinela Banica, Dr. James Bronson, Dr. Douglas Knight, Dr. Lynn and Dr. Ed Lipskis, Dr. Yue Weng Cheu, Dr. Louisa Lee, Dr. Frank Seaman, Dr. James Metz, Dr. Derek Mahony, and Dr. Tony O' Connor. Thank you for highlighting an issue vital to the development of our children. No doubt we often feel we are swimming against the tide. The time is now ripe for calm waters.

To Keith Pfeffer and Mary Glenn of Humanix Books for bringing *The Breathing Cure* to tens of thousands of people across the globe.

The invited podcasts by Brian Rose, Dr. Rangan Chatterjee, Brian Johnson, Ben Greenfield, XPT Performance, Dave Asprey, Darin Olien, Ben Pakulski, Robin Rothenberg, and Pat Divily. Thank you.

Currently, we are united with 290 Oxygen Advantage instructors and 400 Buteyko instructors from 50 countries. I never imagined the day where we would have such a reach to bring functional breathing to so many people.

Thank you, Ana Mahe, for doing such a great job in managing Oxygen Advantage and Buteyko Clinic International. To our team—to my wife, Sinead, and to Ana, Tina, Mladen, Vesna, Lucas, Matias, Johanna, Daniel, and Ronan—thanks so much. To Bex Burgess for her help over the years with illustrations and diagrams, some of which you will see in the book. And as always, Jana Antonova for website design.

Finally, to you, the reader. Thanks for parting with your hard-earned cash and trusting in the book. I hope it has been of use and will continue to be helpful to you for many years.

*Patrick McKeown, Galway, Ireland*

# Allergy-Proof Your Life

## Natural Remedies for Allergies That Work!

Inside *Allergy-Proof Your Life*:

- ✓ **What You Should Never, Ever Eat if You Suffer From Allergies**
- ✓ **Dangers and Limitations of Common Allergy Medications**
- ✓ **Top Foods & Nutrients to Help You Fight Allergies**
- ✓ The Gut-Allergy Connection Your Doctor Won't Tell You About
- ✓ And Much More ...

### Allergy-Proof Your Life

NATURAL REMEDIES FOR ALLERGIES THAT WORK!

- ✓ Asthma
- ✓ Nutritional deficiencies
- ✓ Seasonal allergies
- ✓ Itching & Hives
- ✓ Rashes & Eczema
- ✓ Congestion
- ✓ Inflammation
- ✓ Sinusitis
- ✓ Leaky or inflamed gut
- ✓ Rhinitis

Inside: Delicious Recipes for Allergy Relief

Michelle Schoffro Cook, PhD, DNM, ROHP
Award-Winning and Bestselling Natural Health Author

## FREE OFFER

## Claim Your FREE OFFER Now!

Claim your **FREE** copy of *Allergy-Proof Your Life* — a **$24.99 value** — today with this special offer. Just cover $4.95 for shipping & handling.

Plus, you will receive a bonus **FREE** report — *Over-the-Counter Health Hazards* — from one of America's foremost holistic physicians, David Brownstein, M.D.

We'll also send you a 3-month risk-free trial subscription to *Dr. David Brownstein's Natural Way to Health* which provides you with the most recent insights on emerging natural treatments along with the best of safe conventional medical care.

"*Allergy-Proof Your Life* is a great resource for all allergy sufferers. It helps you discover the underlying causes of your allergies, so you can heal them once and for all."
— *Dr. Brownstein, M.D.*

## Get Your FREE Copy of *Allergy-Proof* TODAY!
# Newsmax.com/Breathe

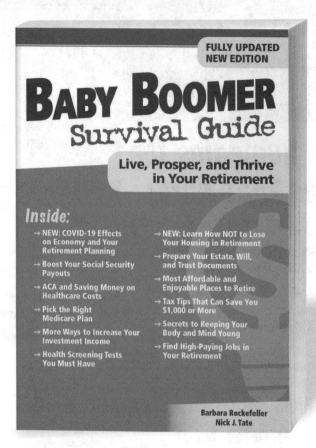

## This 351-page guide will show you how to:
- Get up to $103,200 MORE in Social Security payments
- Retire overseas on $1,250 a month or less
- Create your perfect retirement plan
- Boost your income in retirement
- Save THOUSANDS on Medicare and drug costs
- Know the best age for you to start collecting Social Security
- And much, much more!

# To get your FREE copy of the *Baby Boomer Survival Guide* go to:

# Boom511.com/Breathe

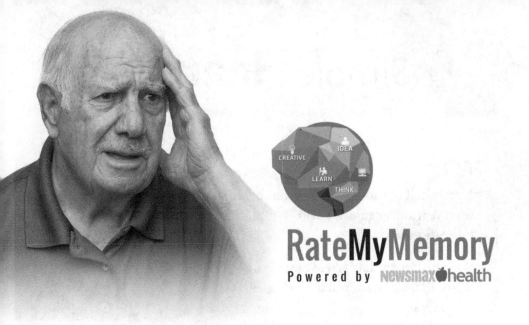

# Normal Forgetfulness?
# Something More Serious?

You forget things — names of people, where you parked your car, the place you put an important document, and so much more. Some experts tell you to dismiss these episodes.

"Not so fast," say the editors of Newsmax Health, and publishers of *The Mind Health Report.*

The experts at Newsmax Health say that most age-related memory issues are normal but sometimes can be a warning sign of future cognitive decline.

Now Newsmax Health has created the online **RateMyMemory Test** — allowing you to easily assess your memory strength in just a matter of minutes.

It's time to begin your journey of making sure your brain stays healthy and young! **It takes just 2 minutes!**

# Test Your Memory Today:
# MemoryRate.com/Breathe

# Simple **Heart Test**

Powered by Newsmaxhealth.com

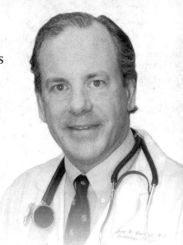

## FACT:

▸ Nearly half of those who die from heart attacks each year never showed prior symptoms of heart disease.

▸ If you suffer cardiac arrest outside of a hospital, you have just a 7% chance of survival.

## Don't be caught off guard. Know your risk now.

### TAKE THE TEST NOW ...

Renowned cardiologist **Dr. Chauncey Crandall** has partnered with **Newsmaxhealth.com** to create a simple, easy-to-complete, online test that will help you understand your heart attack risk factors. Dr. Crandall is the author of the #1 best-seller *The Simple Heart Cure: The 90-Day Program to Stop and Reverse Heart Disease*.

**Take Dr. Crandall's Simple Heart Test** — it takes just 2 minutes or less to complete — it could save your life!

## Discover your risk now.

- **Where you score on our unique heart disease risk scale**
- Which of your lifestyle habits really protect your heart
- **The true role your height and weight play in heart attack risk**
- Little-known conditions that impact heart health
- **Plus much more!**

## SimpleHeartTest.com/Breathe